ANTICANCER

PROPERTIES OF FRUITS AND VEGETABLES

A Scientific Review

ANTICANCER
PROPERTIES OF FRUITS AND VEGETABLES

A Scientific Review

Ajaikumar B Kunnumakkara
Indian Institute of Technology Guwahati, Assam, India

World Scientific

NEW JERSEY • LONDON • SINGAPORE • BEIJING • SHANGHAI • HONG KONG • TAIPEI • CHENNAI

Published by

World Scientific Publishing Co. Pte. Ltd.

5 Toh Tuck Link, Singapore 596224

USA office: 27 Warren Street, Suite 401-402, Hackensack, NJ 07601

UK office: 57 Shelton Street, Covent Garden, London WC2H 9HE

Library of Congress Cataloging-in-Publication Data

Anticancer properties of fruits and vegetables : a scientific review / [edited] by Ajaikumar B. Kunnumakkara.

p. ; cm.

Includes bibliographical references and index.

ISBN 978-9814508889 (hardcover : alk. paper)

I. Kunnumakkara, Ajaikumar B., editor.

[DNLM: 1. Neoplasms--prevention & control. 2. Anticarcinogenic Agents. 3. Chemoprevention. 4. Fruit. 5. Phytochemicals. 6. Vegetables. QZ 200]

RC268

616.99'405--dc23

2014016544

British Library Cataloguing-in-Publication Data

A catalogue record for this book is available from the British Library.

Typeset by Stallion Press

Email: enquiries@stallionpress.com

Printed in Singapore

Contents

Contributors

Ahmed S. Ibrahim
Department of Biochemistry
Faculty of Pharmacy
Mansoura University
Mansoura-35516, Egypt

Ajaikumar B. Kunnumakkara
Department of Biotechnology
Indian Institute of Technology Guwahati
Assam-781039, India

Amitava Khan
Department of Physiology
University of Calcutta
West Bengal-700009, India

Anirban Pradhan
Department of Physiology
University of Calcutta
West Bengal-700009, India

Apurba Mukherjee
Department of Environmental Carcinogenesis & Toxicology
Chittranjan National Cancer Institute
Kolkata, West Bengal-700 026, India

Atulya Mathew
Department of Pharmaceutical Biotechnology
Manipal College of Pharmaceutical Sciences
Manipal University
Manipal, Karnataka-576 104, India

Chandrasekharan Guruvayoorappan
Department of Biotechnology,
Karunya University,
Tamil Nadu,
India-641114.

Debdutta Ganguli
Department of Physiology,
University of Calcutta,
West Bengal-700009,
India.

Diaaeldin M. Elimam
Department of Pharmacognosy,
Faculty of Pharmacy,
Mansoura University,
Mansoura- 35516,
Egypt.

Dipesh Kr Das
Department of Physiology,
University of Calcutta,
West Bengal-700009,
India.

Farid A. Badria
Department of Pharmacognosy,
Faculty of Pharmacy,
Mansoura University,
Mansoura-35516,
Egypt.

Ganesan Padmavathi
Department of Biotechnology,
Indian Institute of Technology Guwahati,
Assam-781039,
India.

Gautam Sethi
Department of Pharmacology,
Yong Loo Lin School of Medicine,
National University of Singapore,
Singapore 117597.
And,
Cancer Science Institute of Singapore,
National University of Singapore,
Singapore 117599.

Indu Ramachandran
Cancer Research Program,
Division of Cancer Research,
Rajiv Gandhi Centre for Biotechnology,
Thiruvananthapuram,
Kerala-695014,
India.

Javadi Monisha
Department of Biotechnology,
Indian Institute of Technology Guwahati,
Assam-781039,
India.

Jaydip Biswas
Department of Environmental Carcinogenesis & Toxicology,
Chittranjan National Cancer Institute,
Kolkata,
West Bengal-700 026,
India.

Jayesh Antony
Cancer Research Program,
Division of Cancer Research,
Rajiv Gandhi Centre for Biotechnology,
Thiruvananthapuram,
Kerala-695014,
India.

Jesil Mathew Aranjani
Department of Pharmaceutical Biotechnology,
Manipal College of Pharmaceutical Sciences,
Manipal University,
Manipal
Karnataka-576 104,
India.

Jose Padikkala
Amala Cancer Research Center,
Amala Nagar,
Kerala-680 555,
India.

Krishnendu Manna
Department of Physiology,
University of Calcutta,
West Bengal-700009,
India.

Kunal Sikder
Department of Physiology,
University of Calcutta,
West Bengal-700009,
India.

Kunnathur Murugesan Sakthivel
Department of Biotechnology,
Indian Institute of Technology Guwahati,
Assam-781039,
India.

Madhumita Roy
Department of Environmental Carcinogenesis & Toxicology,
Chittranjan National Cancer Institute,
Kolkata,
West Bengal- 700 026,
India.

Mahuya Sinha
Department of Physiology,
University of Calcutta,
West Bengal-700009,
India.

Manoj K. Pandey
Department of Pharmacology,
Penn State College of Medicine,
Pennsylvania,
USA.

Minakshi Saikia
Cancer Research Program,
Division of Cancer Research,
Rajiv Gandhi Centre for Biotechnology,
Thiruvananthapuram,
Kerala- 695014,
India.

Naman Katre
Department of Biotechnology,
Indian Institute of Technology Guwahati,
Assam- 781039,
India.

Nilanjan Das
Department of Physiology,
University of Calcutta,
West Bengal-700009,
India.

Rakhi Sharma Dey
Department of Food and Nutrition,
Rastraguru Surendranath College,
Barrackpore,
Kolkata,
West Bengal- 700120,
India.

Ruby John Anto
Cancer Research Program,
Division of Cancer Research,
Rajiv Gandhi Centre for Biotechnology,
Thiruvananthapuram,
Kerala-695014,
India.

Sakshi Sikka
Department of Pharmacology,
Yong Loo Lin School of Medicine,
National University of Singapore,
Singapore 117597.

Sanjit Dey
Department of Physiology,
University of Calcutta,
West Bengal-700009,
India.

Sankar Jagadeeshan
Cancer Research Program,
Rajiv Gandhi Centre for Biotechnology,
Poojapura,
Thiruvananthapuram,
Kerala-695014
India.
&
Department of Genetics,
University of Madras,
Chennai,
Tamil Nadu-600 113
India.

Shantu G. Amin
Department of Pharmacology,
Penn State College of Medicine,
Pennsylvania,
USA.

Sushobhan Biswas
Department of Physiology,
University of Calcutta,
West Bengal-700009,
India.

Sutapa Mukherjee
Department of Environmental Carcinogenesis & Toxicology,
Chittranjan National Cancer Institute,
Kolkata,
West Bengal-700 026,
India.

Swaraj Bandhu Kesh
Department of Physiology,
University of Calcutta,
West Bengal-700009,
India.

S. Asha Nair
Cancer Research Program,
Rajiv Gandhi Centre for Biotechnology,
Poojapura,
Thiruvananthapuram,
Kerala-695014
India.

Ujjal Das
Department of Physiology,
University of Calcutta,
West Bengal-700009,
India.

Vaishali Bakliwal
Department of Biotechnology,
Indian Institute of Technology Guwahati,
Assam-781039,
India.

Preface

YES, CANCER CAN BE PREVENTED!

One of the most critical issues affecting planetary health and individual wellbeing is whether cancer can be prevented. While there are many monographs, articles and books praising the cancer-preventive properties of certain natural food stuffs, this book is unique. In the pages that follow, highly respected scientists provide clinically proven information as to which plant-based foods can prevent this insidious disease on a cancer-by-cancer basis.

Cancer is "an equal opportunity" disease because it affects men, women and children in every nation and culture. It has been estimated that approximately 12.7 million people are diagnosed with cancer every year, causing more than 7.6 million deaths, annually. If current trends continue, over the next ten years, approximately 127 million people will be diagnosed with cancer and it will cause death to 76 million. Moreover, the cost of cancer treatment is increasing exponentially, and in some instances, skyrocketing.

Clearly, there is an urgent need to avert the human and economic costs of this potentially lethal disease. The Ancients were well aware of the healing properties of certain foods. Hippocrates of Cos (460-370 B.C), the father of western medicine, said "*Let food be thy medicine and medicine be thy food*". Thousands of years later, cancer research scientists have shown the correctness of Hippocrates' dictum. It is now well established that the prevention of approximately 85% of cancers can be attributed to a healthy lifestyle, a key component of which, is a diet rich in plant-based substances.

Numerous lines of evidence show that increased intake of fruits and vegetables can reduce cancer risk because these foods contain a multitude of antioxidant chemicals. Antioxidants scavenge reactive oxygen species that are extremely harmful to biological molecules such as DNA, proteins etc. In other words, the antioxidants in these foods prevent or repair DNA damage or mutations, which are the main causes of cancer. Additional lines of evidence suggest that fruits and vegetables contain compounds that can stop activation of signaling pathways and over expression of proteins that are responsible for cancer cell survival, proliferation and their spread to other parts of the body. Because of their cancer preventive potential, the United States National Institutes of Health recommends a food regimen consisting of twelve servings of fruits and vegetables a day.

Although there is a dawning awareness that good nutrition is fundamental to good health; it is only recently that the general public has become aware of the role fruits and vegetables can play in cancer prevention. And, the vast majority of the general public has no knowledge of the impact that *certain* fruits and vegetables can have on preventing *specific* types of cancers. Moreover, to date, there is no comprehensive scientific article or other writing that shows the health benefits of fruits and vegetables on a cancer-by-cancer basis.

Thus, the goal of this monograph is to fill the void in cancer prevention literature. All of the authors are well known cancer scientists in the area of natural product research. A painstaking effort has been made to compile the most comprehensive and the best information available about the cancer preventive properties of plant-based foods and their active ingredients, as well as, how these ingredients work to prevent this debilitating and potentially deadly disease.

On a personal note, I would like to thank all of the contributors to this work for their efforts; without them this book would not have been possible. It is our hope that it will serve as a guide to anyone seeking excellent health, and that it will become an essential reference for scientists and students pursuing a course in health, nutrition and medicine. Finally, we hope that you, the reader, will find these pages sufficiently helpful and informative that they will inspire you to spread the word about the critical importance of fruits and vegetables in leading a cancer-free life.

Ajaikumar B Kunnumakkara, Ph.D.

1

Cancer Preventive and Therapeutic Properties of Fruits and Vegetables: An Overview

*Chandrasekharan Guruvayoorappan, Kunnathur Murugesan Sakthivel, Ganesan Padmavathi, Vaishali Bakliwal, Javadi Monisha and Ajaikumar B. Kunnumakkara**

INTRODUCTION

Cancer is one of the leading causes of death worldwide, accounting for one in every eight deaths — more than HIV/AIDS, tuberculosis, and malaria. According to GLOBOCAN (2008), approximately 12.7 million people are diagnosed with cancer every year, causing approximately 7.6 million deaths.[1] During the past several decades, numerous epidemiological and experimental studies have resulted in significant progress in understanding the molecular mechanisms of cancer development. These studies also suggest that lifestyle plays a critical role in the development of this disease. For instance, obese and diabetic patients have a greater susceptibility to cancer than lean and non-diabetic individuals. Moreover, it has been well established that a diet rich in saturated fats and red meats and low in fresh fruits, vegetables, and whole grains has been shown to increase the risk of cancer. According to the United States National Institutes of Health, "12 servings of fruits and vegetables a day" can prevent common diseases including cancer.

*Corresponding author: Ajaikumar B. Kunnumakkara, Ph.D., Assistant Professor, Department of Biotechnology, Indian Institute of Technology Guwahati, Assam, India.

This clearly shows the importance of fruits and vegetables in the prevention of this disease. In this chapter, we will discuss the common fruits and vegetables that are known to have anticancer properties. However, we will first place the subject in context, discussing the history, classification and development of cancer and its different treatment modalities.

Cancer

Cancer has been known since human societies first recorded their activities, but the formal study of cancer (i.e., oncology) was first documented in the seventeenth century. Cancer can be defined as a disease of uncontrolled division of abnormal cells. Cancer not only affects human and higher mammals, but it affects almost all the multicellular organisms — animals as well as plants. Nearly 175 years ago, the German microscopist, Johannes Müller, was the first to show that cancers were made up of cells. After this finding, an enormous amount of information has been amassed about this disease. Markedly, in the past two decades, rapid technological advancement has aided us as we dissever the cancer genomes, transcriptome, and proteome, in detail.

Classification of Cancer

The classification of cancer is highly complicated due to the presence of a wide variety of human cancers that arise in almost every tissue in our body. Oncologists and cancer biologists classify cancers based on the tissues of origin, regardless of organ location, focusing on similarities in cellular structure and function among tumors. A tumor is an abnormal mass of tissue that can be either benign (non-cancerous) or malignant (cancerous). Tumors can be either a solid mass comprised of epithelial or mesenchymal cells that are usually immobile, or they can be a liquid sac, which includes leukemias and lymphomas comprising neoplastic cells whose precursors are usually motile.[2] Further, pathologically, cancers are classified into four different types:

(1) Carcinoma: originates from epithelial cells in the skin or in other tissues that line or cover internal organ.

(2) Sarcoma: originates in bone, cartilage, fat, muscle, blood vessels, or other connective or supportive tissue.
(3) Leukemia: originates in blood-forming tissues of the body such as bone marrow, causing abnormal proliferation of blood cells usually, white blood cells (leukocytes).
(4) Lymphoma: originates in the cells of the immune system, also termed as cancers of the lymphoid organs such as the lymph nodes, spleen, and thymus, which produce and supply infection-fighting cells.[3]

Development of Cancer: Multi-Stage Carcinogenesis

Carcinogenesis, the process of cancer development, is a multi-stage process. Generally, cancer starts with a mutational event (i.e., genetic changes) in a single normal cell; then, it will develop into a multi-stage process through the acquisition of further mutations that are inherited by the progeny of that cell when it divides, thus cancer is also termed as clonal disease (Fig. 1.1). In higher animals or humans, the use of a cancer-causing agent (carcinogen) does not lead to the immediate production of a tumor. Rather, it will arise after a long latent period. Berenblum and Shubik in 1940[4] showed that there are three major stages involved in the process of carcinogenesis. The first is initiation, which involves the mutagenic effects of the carcinogen. The second stage is promotion, which may be induced by several agents that are not directly carcinogenic (promoters) and may be followed by the chronic treatment of the carcinogens. The third stage is progression in which benign tumors either spontaneously, or followed by additional treatment of the carcinogens, will progress to invasive tumors. The latent period between initiation and the appearance of tumors is very long. After exposure to carcinogens, it may take more than 20 years before tumors develop in humans. Even in animals, if given heavy doses of carcinogens, it may take up to one-third of the animal's total lifespan before tumors appear. Initiation and progression of cancer depend upon several external and internal factors such as tobacco use, exposure to infectious organisms, radiation, hormones, inherited mutations, and immune conditions. Uncontrolled mutations and selective expansion of cancer cells lead to tumor growth and progression,

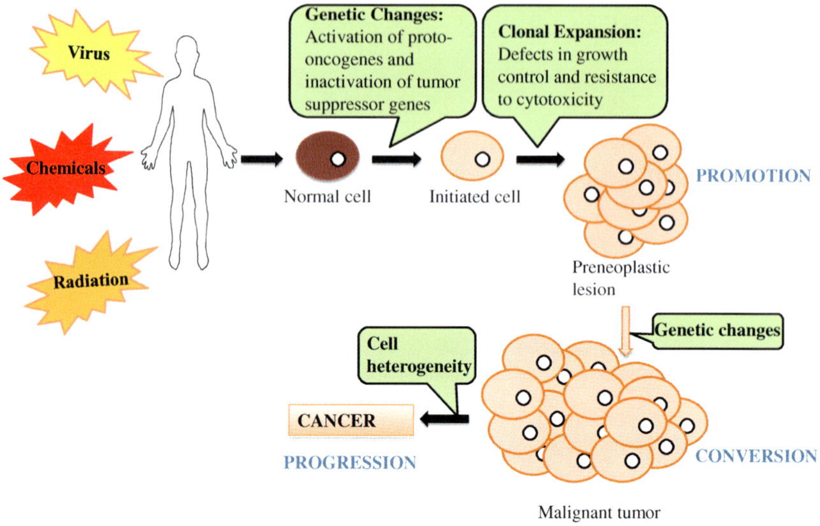

Figure 1.1: Progressive model for multi-stage carcinogenesis.

eventually spreading to other locations of the body. This proliferation of cancer cells is termed as metastasis.

Treatment Strategies for Cancer

Options for the treatment of cancer are expanding at a high rate. Current strategies for treating cancer involve surgery, radiation, or drugs — either singly or in combination.[5]

Surgery

Surgical treatment involves excision of tumor, the most frequently employed form of tumor therapy worldwide. In recent years, surgery combined with other treatment approaches such as chemotherapy and radiation therapy, has enhanced the effectiveness of cancer treatment. The side effects of the surgical treatment depend upon the location of the tumor, the patient's general health, type of operation, and other factors.

Radiation therapy

Radiation therapy involves the exposure of the body to ionizing radiations like X-rays and γ-rays to selectively target the cancer tissue. It includes the uptake of radioactive iodine, which travels in the blood to kill the cancer cells and is referred to as systemic radiation therapy. Additional types of radiation therapy include external beam radiation therapy (e.g., X-ray tubes, cobalt gamma rays, and linear accelerators), brachytherapy (caesium-137, iodine-125, or iridium-192), and radiopharmaceuticals that target specific tissues. Currently, much research focuses on radiosensitizers and radioprotectors. Radiosensitizers are drugs which make the cancer cells more sensitive to the radiation therapy, in addition to anti-cancer drugs like 5-fluorouracil and cisplastin. Natural radioprotectors like rutin and quercetin, among others, are drugs that protect the normal cells from damage and promote the repair of normal cells caused by radiation therapy.[6]

Chemotherapy

Chemotherapy is the use of chemicals to treat cancer. Research over the past several decades has developed many chemotherapeutic agents for the treatment of cancer. These include mustard gas, cyclophosphamide, vincristine, vinblastine, taxol, tyrosine kinase inhibitors, etc. The common side effects of chemotherapy include nausea and vomiting, hair loss (alopecia), suppression of white blood cells and production of platelets (myelosuppression), diarrhea, and decreased spermatogenesis/ ovarian follicle formation. Long-term toxicity and the risk of developing resistance to chemotherapy are formidable hindrances that could limit the chronic application strategy in the chemotherapy of several cancers.

Cancer Chemoprevention

Cancer chemoprevention is a relatively new area in the field of oncology that uses naturally occurring or synthetic agents to inhibit the process of carcinogenesis or to slow down the progression of cancer. Chemoprevention helps to lower the risk of developing invasive or clinically significant diseases. There are three different types of cancer chemoprevention: (1) primary prevention in high-risk healthy individuals; (2) cancer prevention in individuals who have developed pre-malignant lesions; and (3) prevention of secondary forms of cancers in patients already treated for a primary cancer. The final endpoint of all three aspects of chemoprevention is the attainment of clinical evidence for cancer reduction.[7] Cancer chemopreventive agents prevent the transformation of pre-malignant lesions to form malignant tumors by modulating cell proliferation and/or differentiation.[8] It has been recommended that these agents be administered over a long time period to individuals who have an increased risk of developing cancer; however, even minor adverse side effects would be unacceptable.[9] It is now well established that the compounds present in fruits and vegetables have fewer side effects and are, therefore, ideal for cancer chemoprevention.

Anticancer Properties of Fruits and Vegetables: Their Active Components

Research over the past several decades suggests that a high intake of fruits and vegetables decreases the risk of several cancers both in experimental animals and in humans. The information concerning common fruits and vegetables that are known to prevent cancer is extremely important for patients, nutritionists, medical practitioners, and individuals interested in following a healthy lifestyle. This section will discuss the common fruits and vegetables that are known to prevent cancer and their active ingredients (Figs. 1.2 to 1.4).

Fruits

Apple

Family: Rosaceae
Botanical name: *Malus domestica*
Apples are one of the most cultivated fruits in the world. It has been estimated that 69 million tons of apples were grown, worldwide, in 2010.

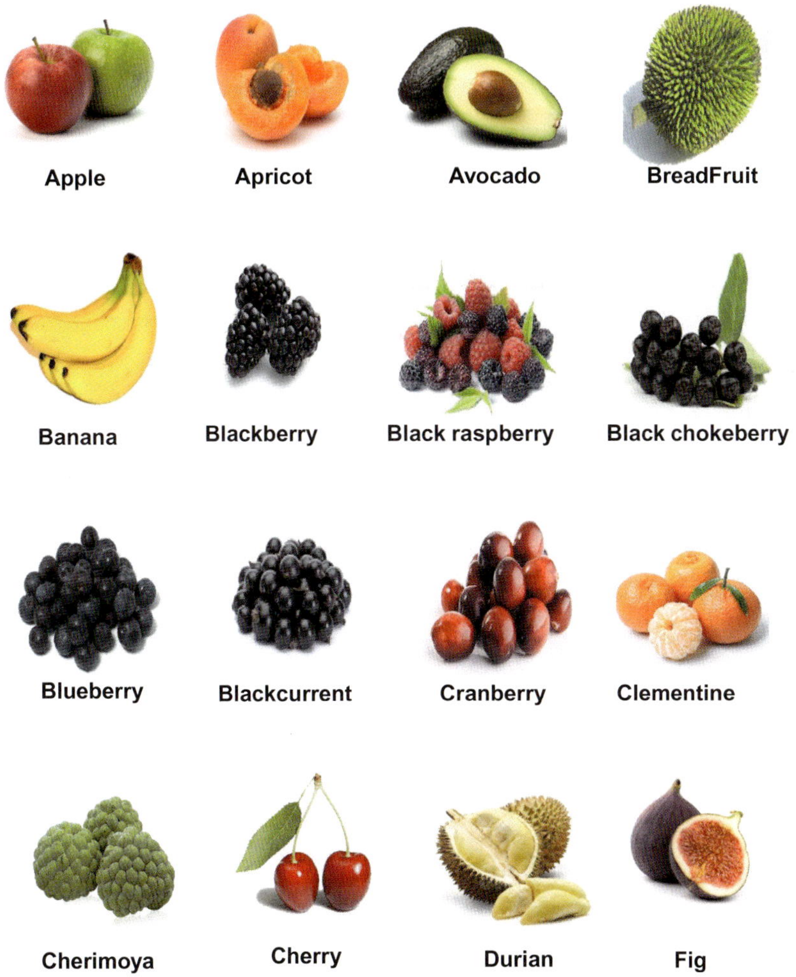
Apple
Apricot
Avocado
BreadFruit
Banana
Blackberry
Black raspberry
Black chokeberry
Blueberry
Blackcurrent
Cranberry
Clementine
Cherimoya
Cherry
Durian
Fig

Figure 1.2: Common fruits that have been shown to have anticancer properties.

China ranks first in apple production, followed by the United States, Iran, Turkey, Russia, Italy, and India. There are more than 7,500 different cultivars of apple. They are often consumed raw and are also important ingredients in many desserts such as apple pie, apple crumble, apple crisp, and apple cake. The saying "*An apple a day keeps the doctor away*" actually reflects the health benefits of this fruit. Studies have shown that the apple

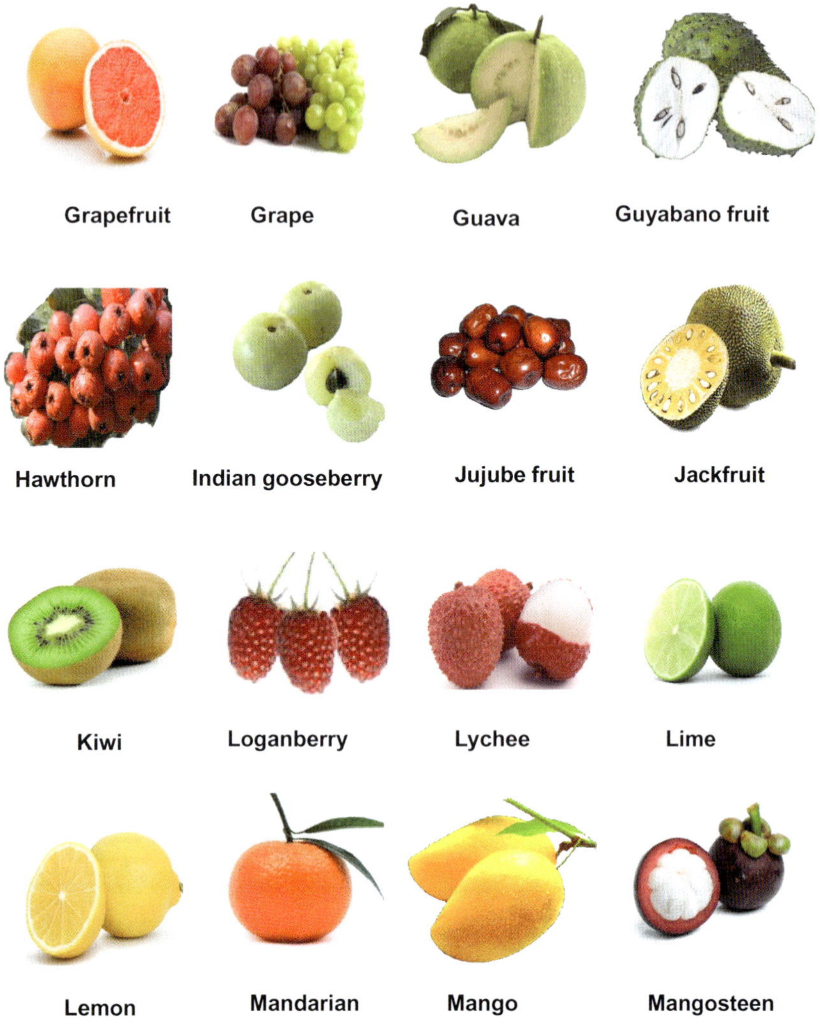
Grapefruit
Grape
Guava
Guyabano fruit
Hawthorn
Indian gooseberry
Jujube fruit
Jackfruit
Kiwi
Loganberry
Lychee
Lime
Lemon
Mandarian
Mango
Mangosteen

Figure 1.2 (*Continued*)

and its constituents possess anticancer properties in breast, colon, liver, skin, stomach, and prostate cancers. They contain many antioxidant phenolic compounds and triterpenoids such as quercetin, epicatechin, procyanidin B2, ursolic acid, phloretin, and maslinic acid.

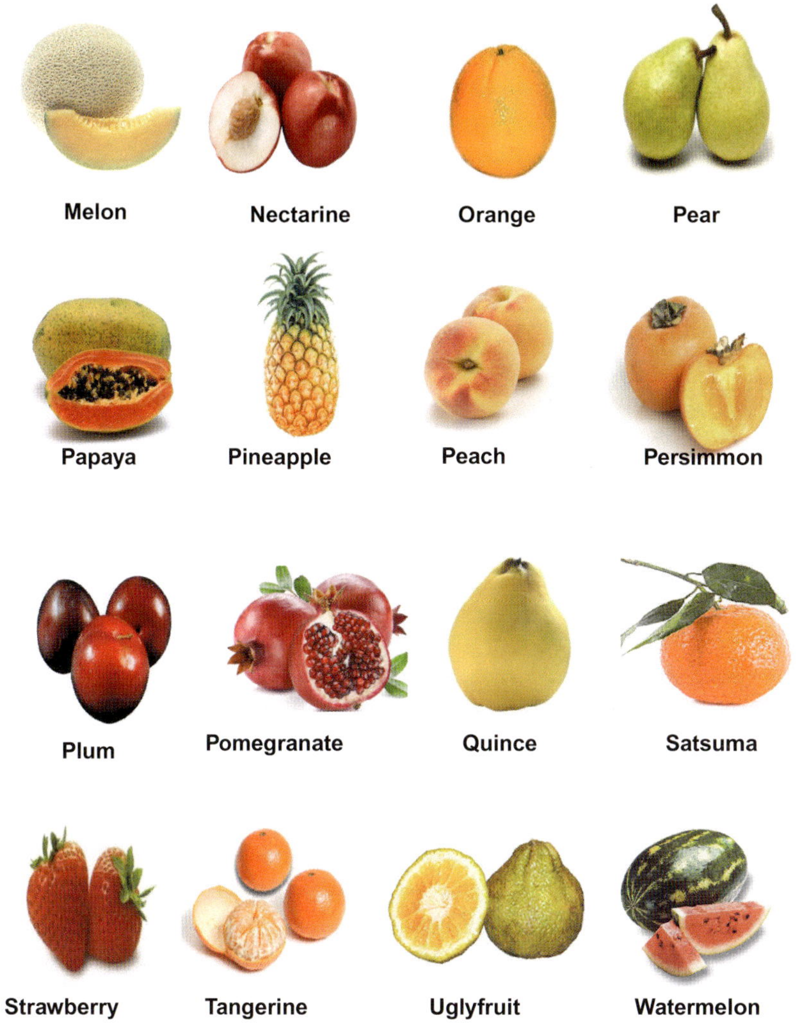
Melon
Nectarine
Orange
Pear
Papaya
Pineapple
Peach
Persimmon
Plum
Pomegranate
Quince
Satsuma
Strawberry
Tangerine
Uglyfruit
Watermelon

Figure 1.2 (*Continued*)

Apricot

Family: Rosaceae
Botanical name: *Prunus armeniaca*
Apricots are yellow- to orange-colored fruits ranging in taste from sweet to tart. The Vavilov Center of Origin believes that the apricot originated in

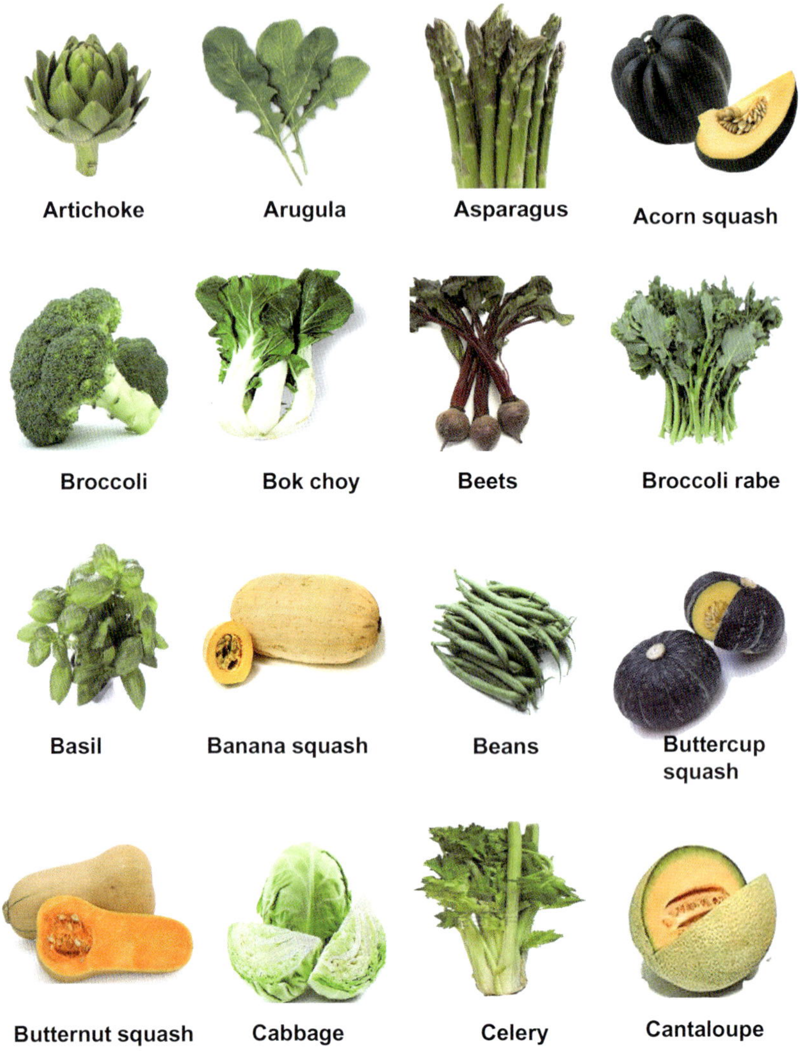

Figure 1.3: Common vegetables that have been shown to have anticancer properties.

China; however, many other sources hold that this fruit was first cultivated in India in about 3,000 B.C. There are more than 50 varieties of apricots in the world. Egyptians use this fruit to make a drink called *amar al-dīn*. Apricots seeds and oils were used to treat tumors in ancient medicine. This

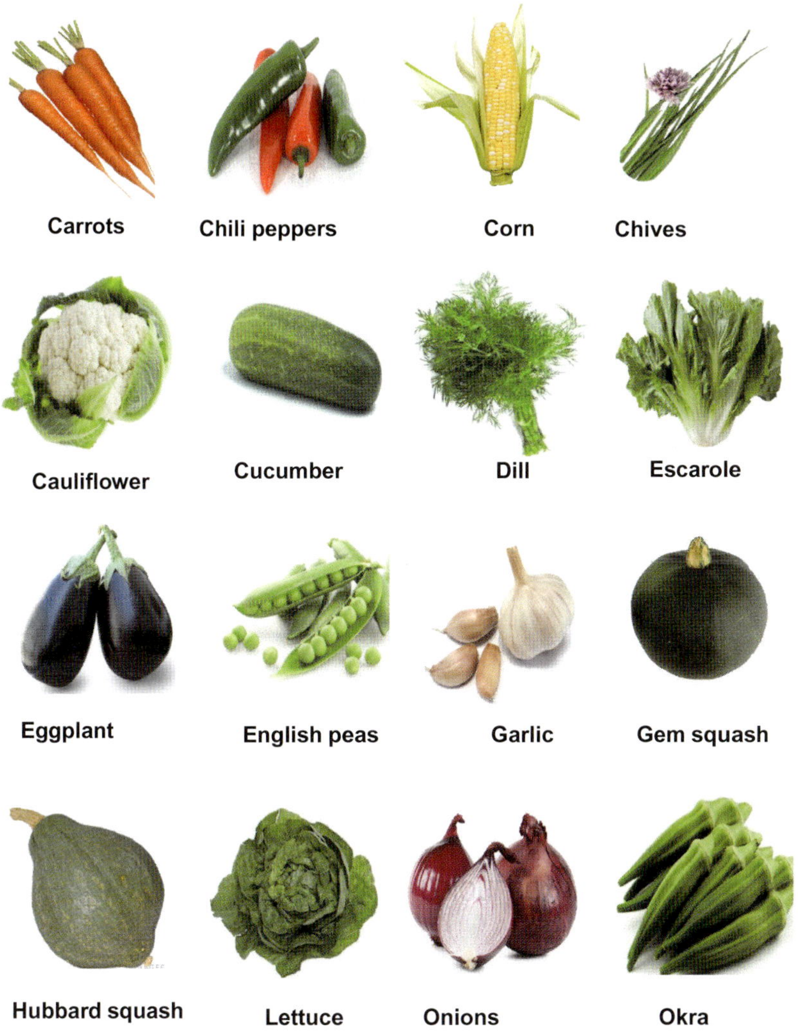
Carrots
Chili peppers
Corn
Chives
Cauliflower
Cucumber
Dill
Escarole
Eggplant
English peas
Garlic
Gem squash
Hubbard squash
Lettuce
Onions
Okra

Figure 1.3 (*Continued*)

fruit is rich in carotenes, vitamins A and C, dietary fibers, and cyanogenic glycosides. Amygdalin, a cyanogenic glycoside, and its semi-synthetic form, laterile, possess anticancer activities against breast, cervical, colon, and prostate cancers.

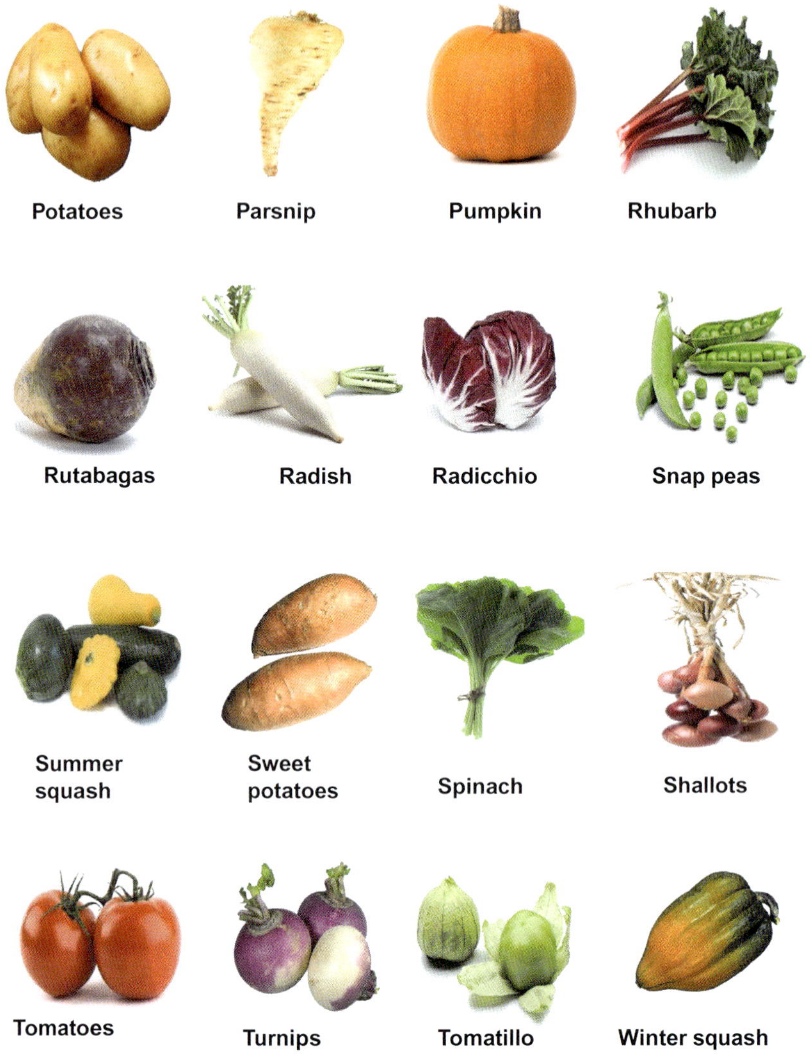
Potatoes
Parsnip
Pumpkin
Rhubarb
Rutabagas
Radish
Radicchio
Snap peas
Summer squash
Sweet potatoes
Spinach
Shallots
Tomatoes
Turnips
Tomatillo
Winter squash

Figure 1.3 *(Continued)*

Avocado

Family: Lauraceae
Botanical name: *Persea americana*
Avocados, also known as alligator pears, are native to the state of Puebla, Mexico. Cultivated in tropical and Mediterranean climates throughout the

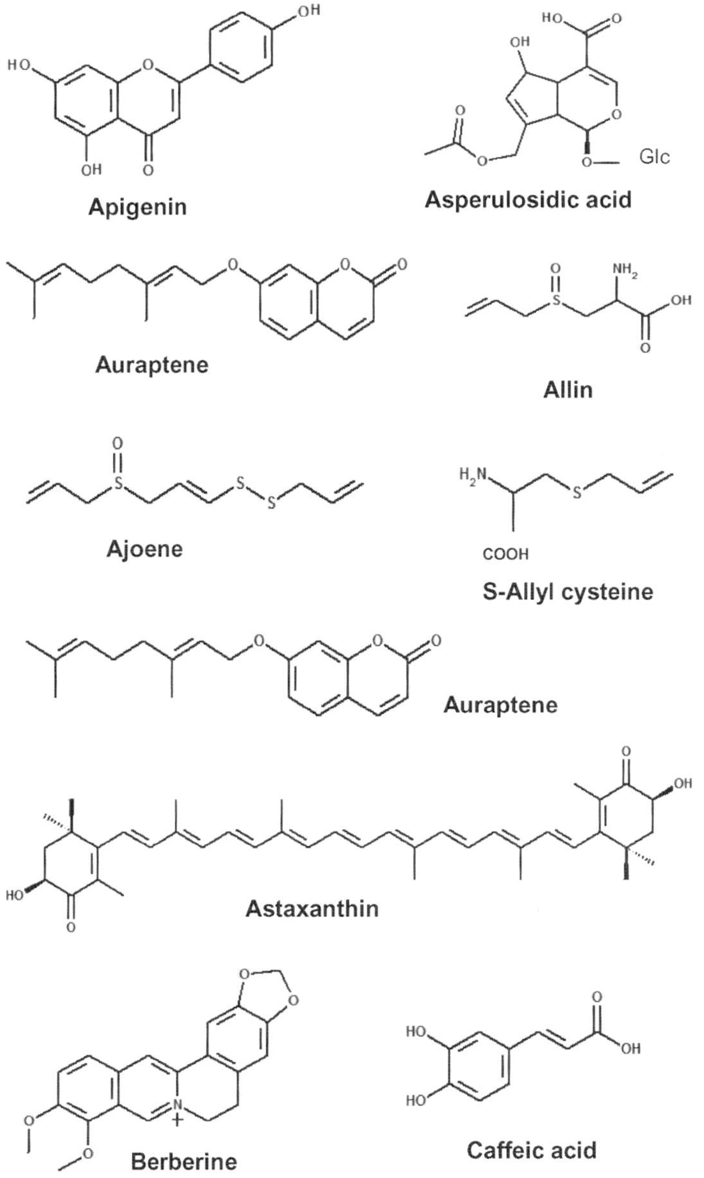

Figure 1.4: Anticancer compounds isolated from fruits and vegetables.

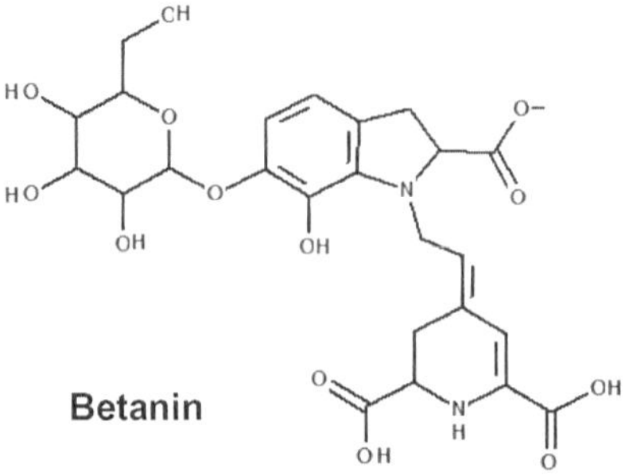

Betanin

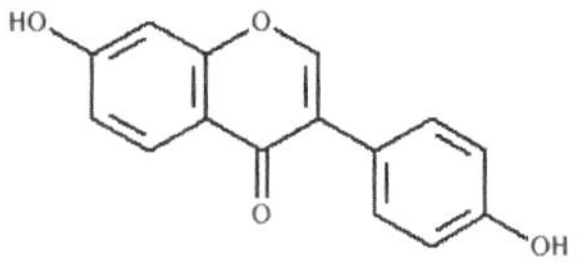

Daidzein

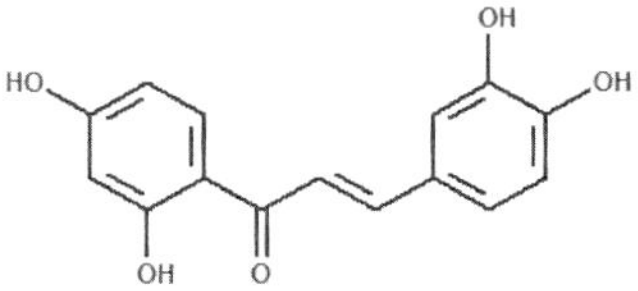

Butein

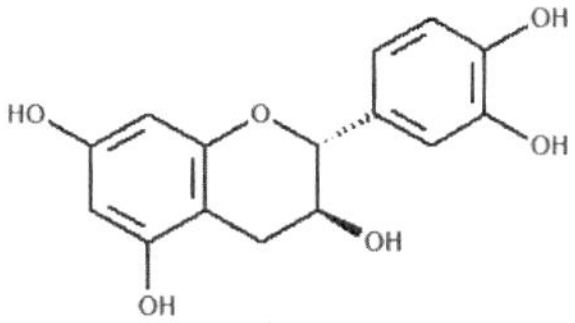

Catechin

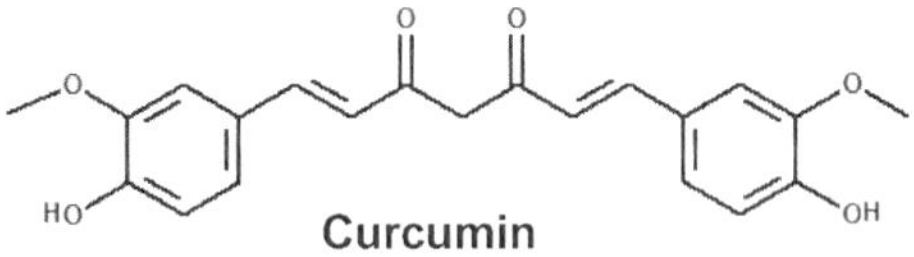

Curcumin

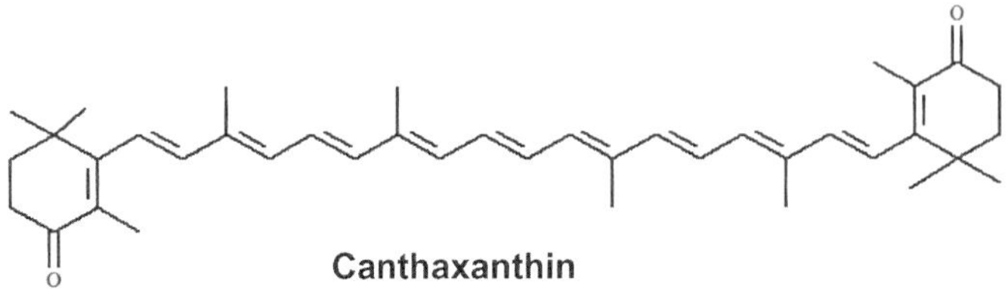

Canthaxanthin

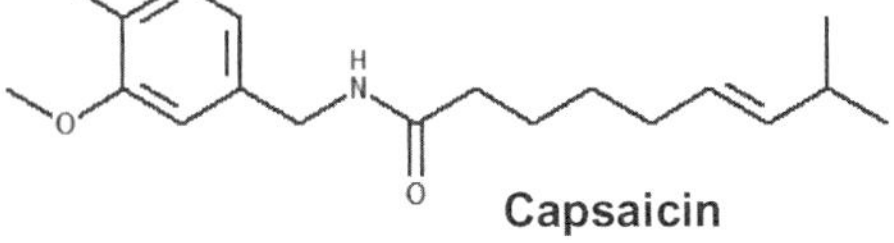

Capsaicin

Figure 1.4 (*Continued*)

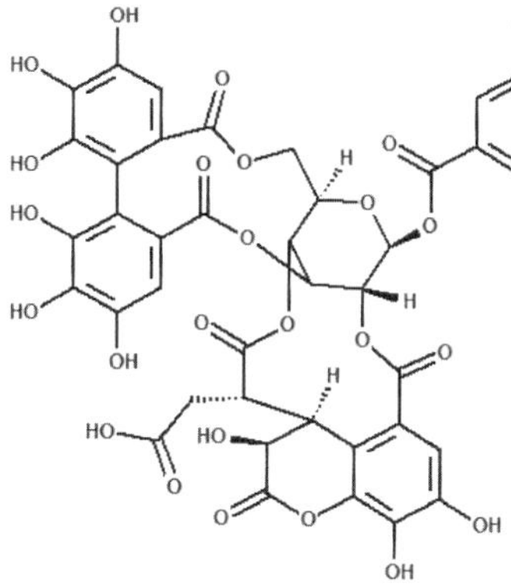

Chebulagic Acid

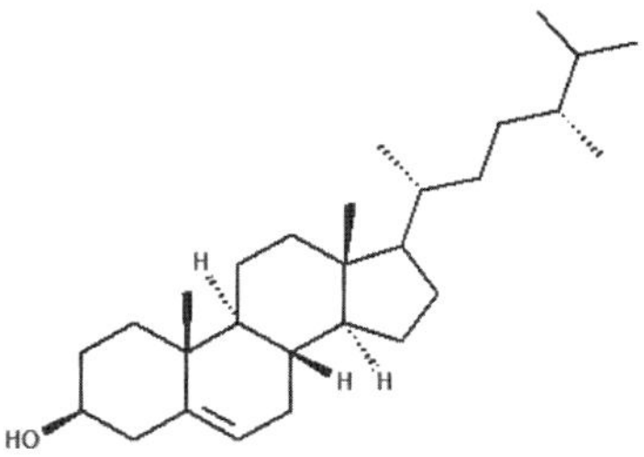

Campesterol

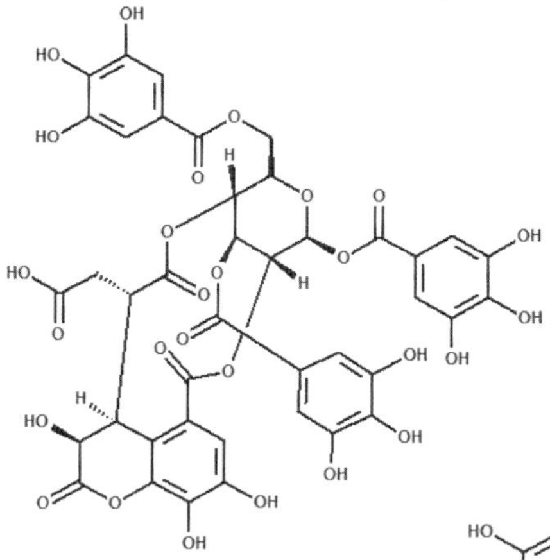

Chebulinic acid

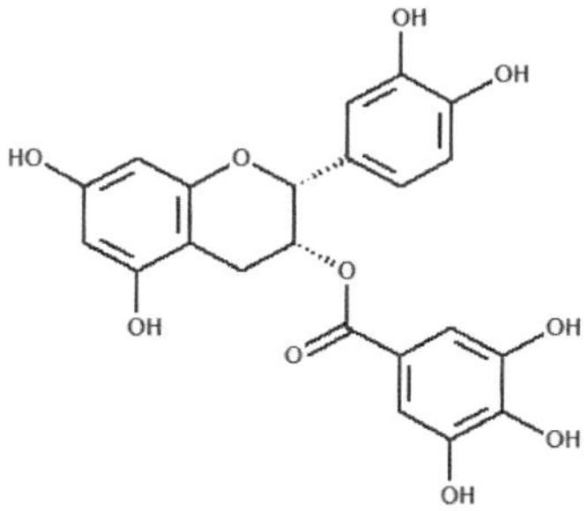

Catechin gallate

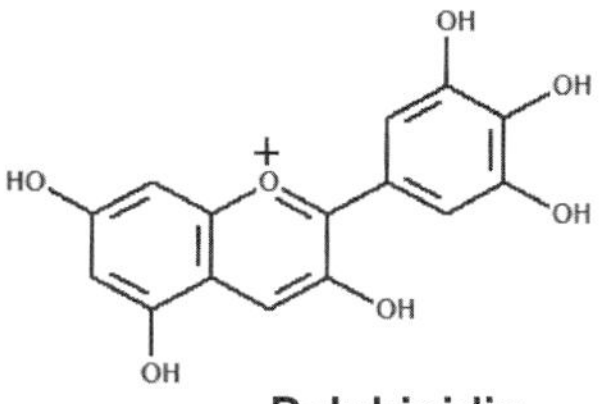

Delphinidin

Figure 1.4 (*Continued*)

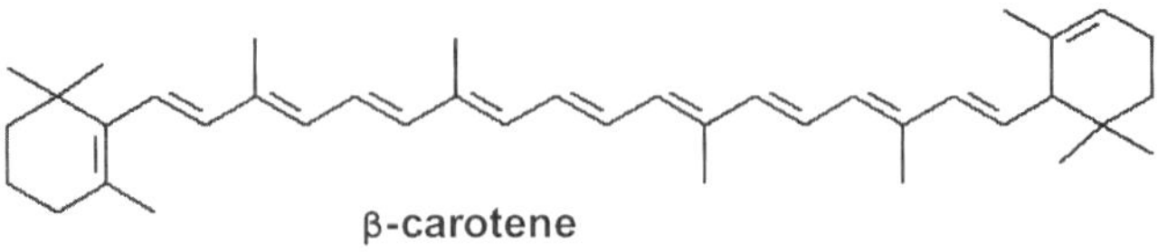

β-carotene

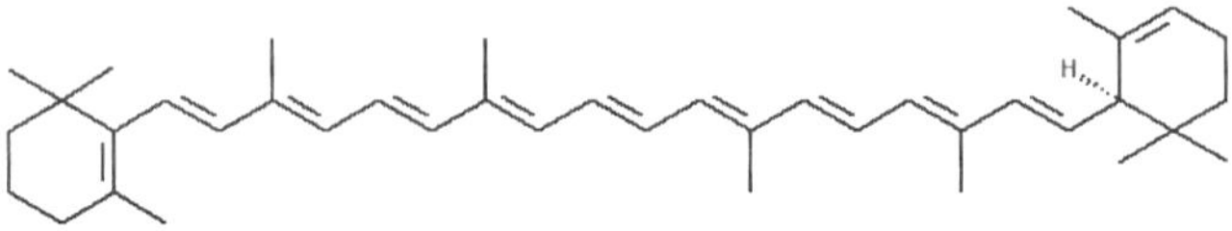

α-carotene

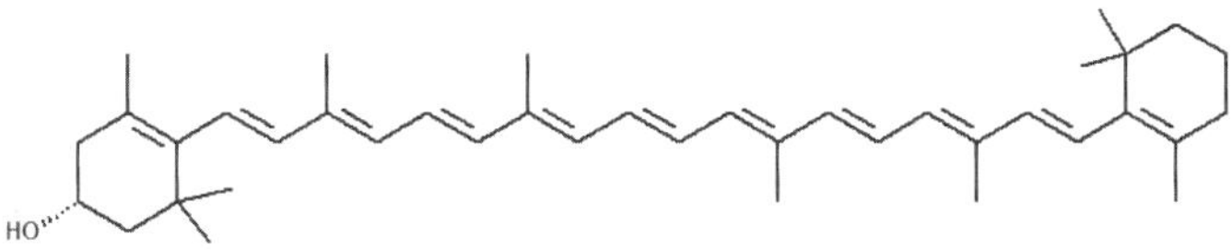

β-cryptoxanthin

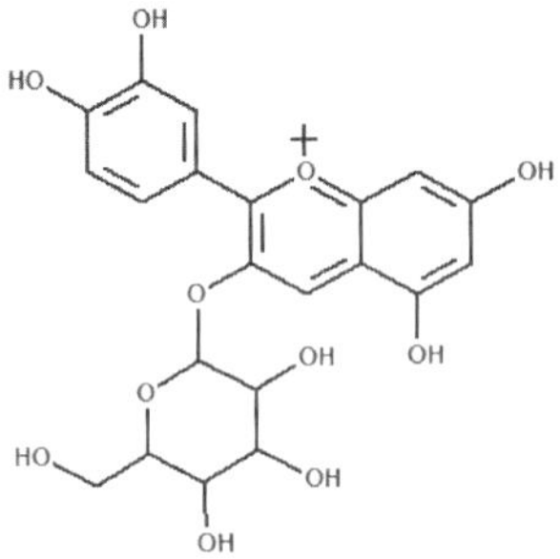

Cyanidin-3-O glucoside

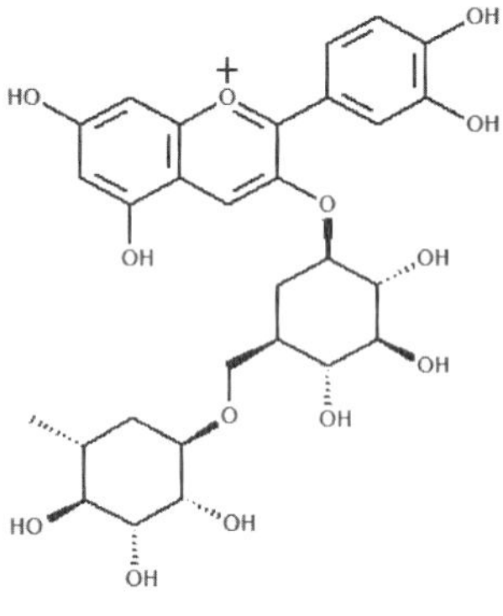

Cyanidin-3-O–rutinoside

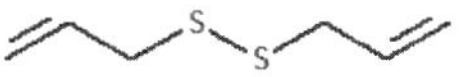

Diallyl sulfide

Figure 1.4 (*Continued*)

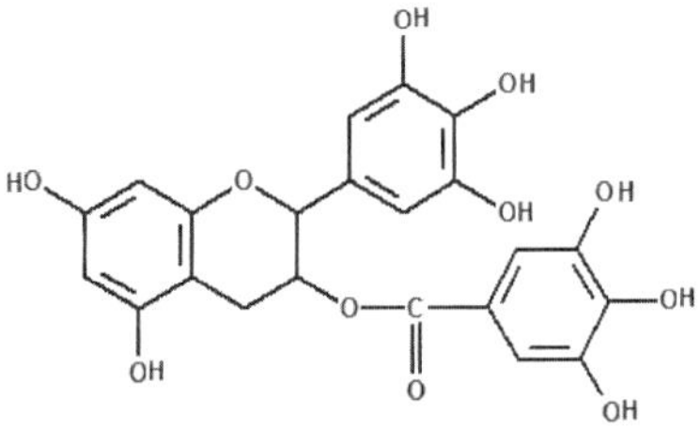

Epigallocatechin-3-gallate

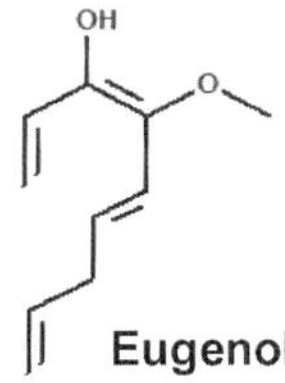

Eugenol

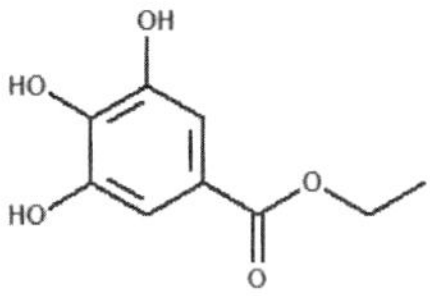

Ethyl gallate

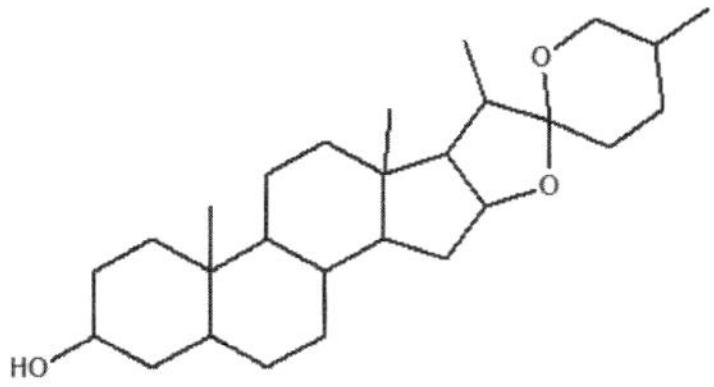

Delphinidin

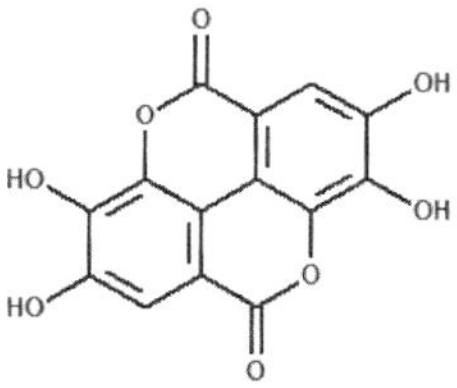

Ellagic acid

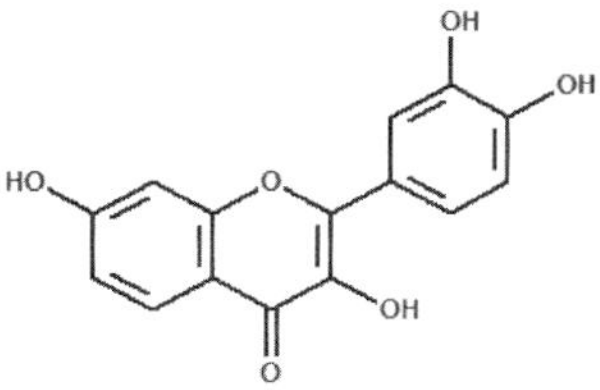

Fisetin

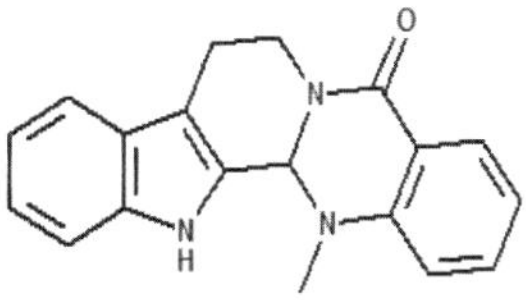

Evodiamine

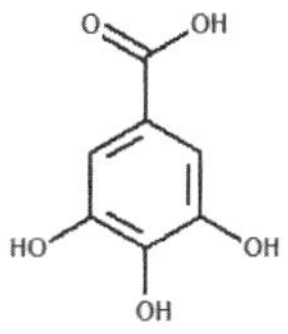

Gallic Acid

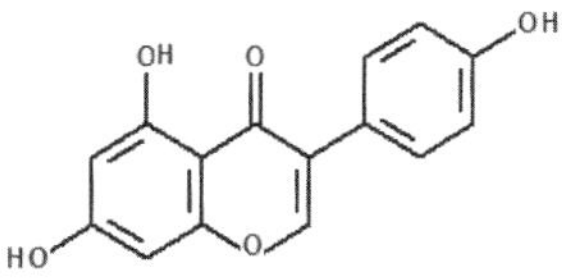

Genistein

Figure 1.4 (*Continued*)

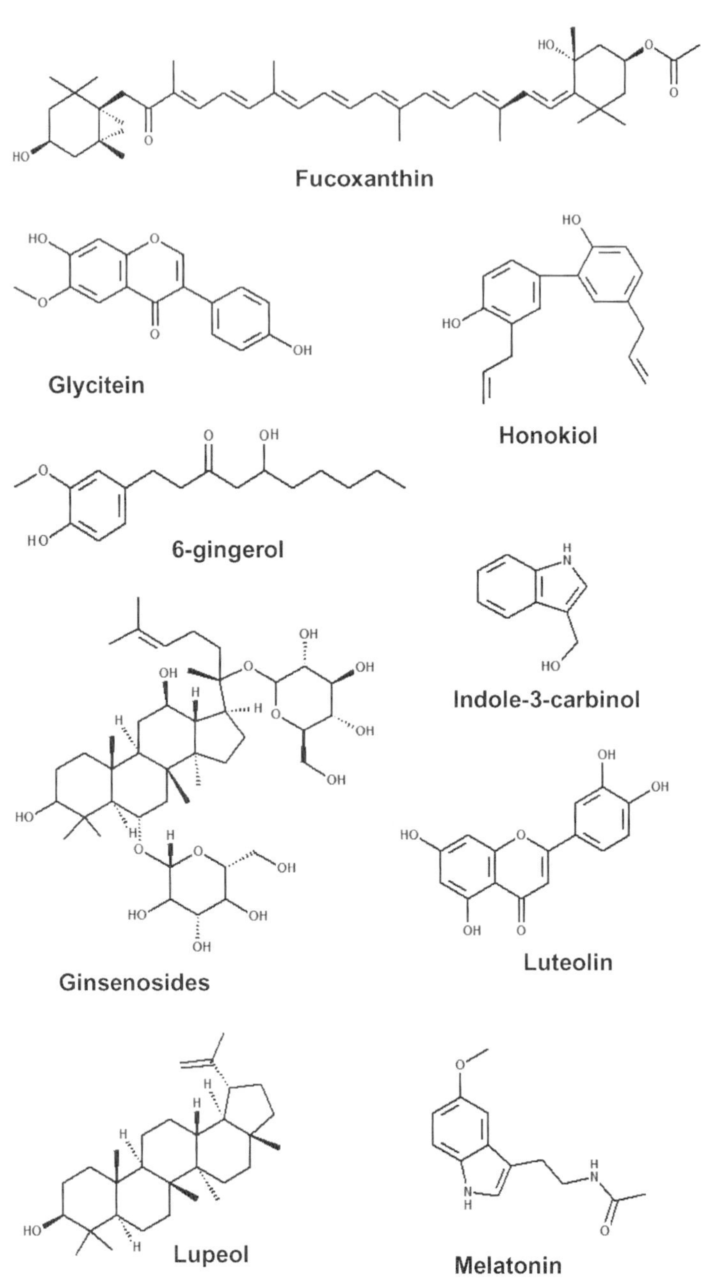

Figure 1.4 (*Continued*)

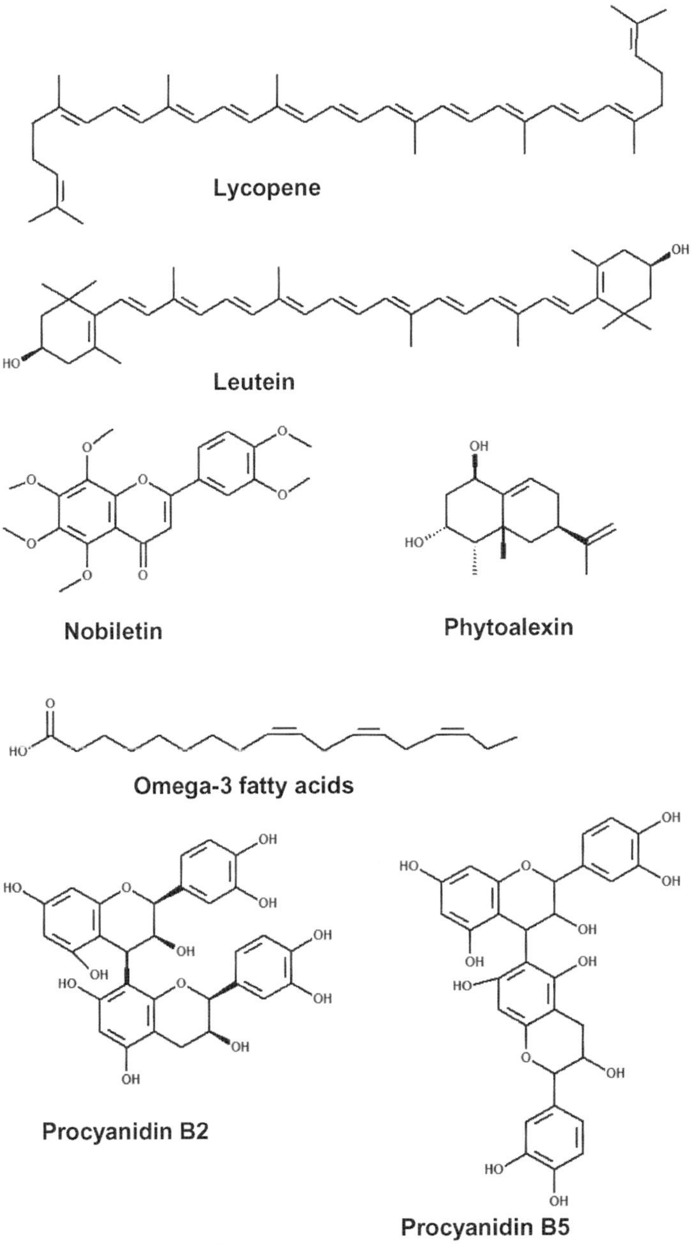

Figure 1.4 (*Continued*)

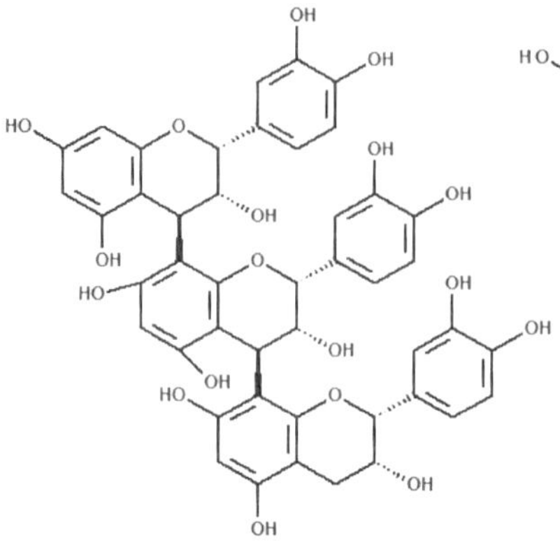

Procyanidin C1

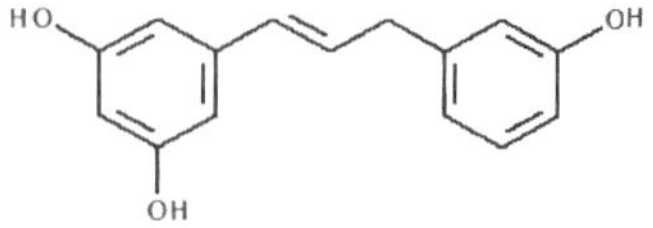

Resveratrol

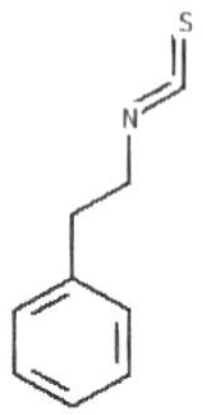

Phenethyl Isothiocynate

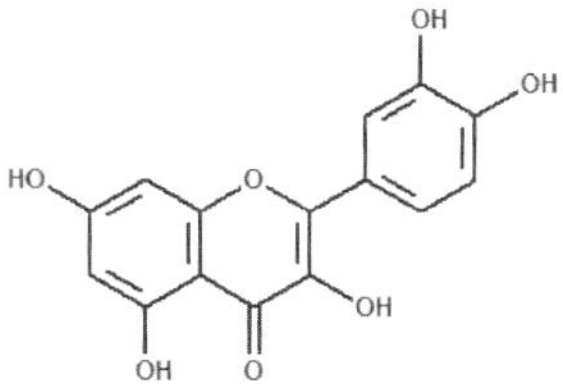

Quercetin

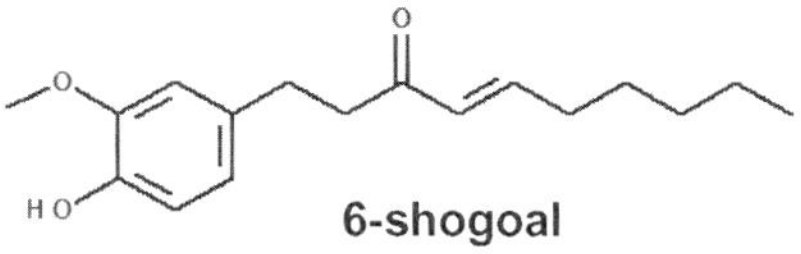

6-shogoal

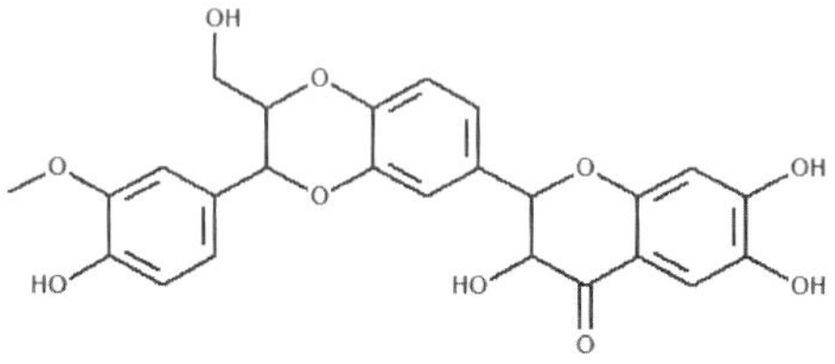

Silibinin

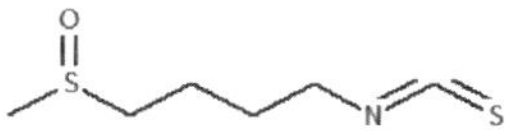

Sulforaphane

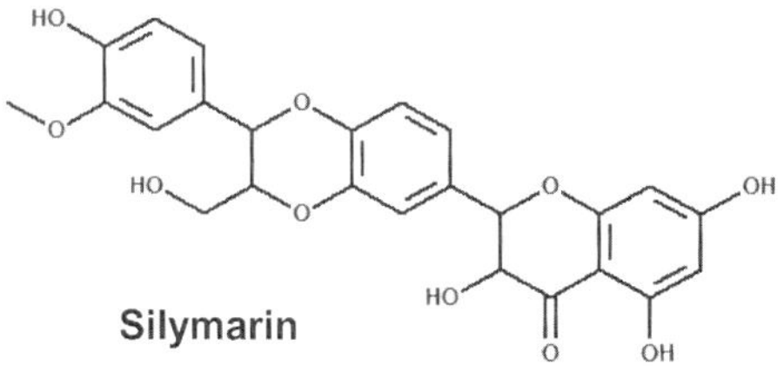

Silymarin

Figure 1.4 (*Continued*)

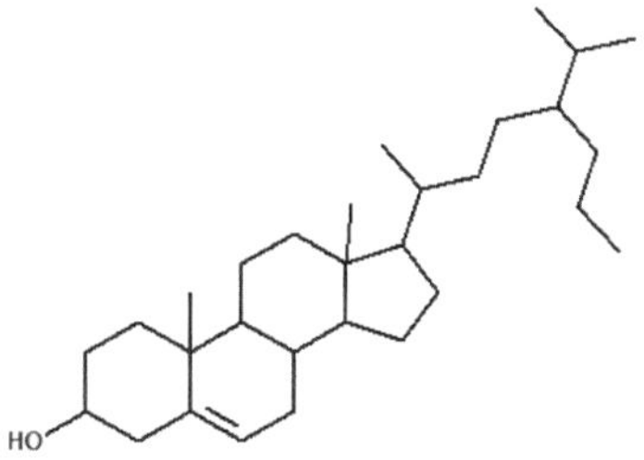

β-sitosterol

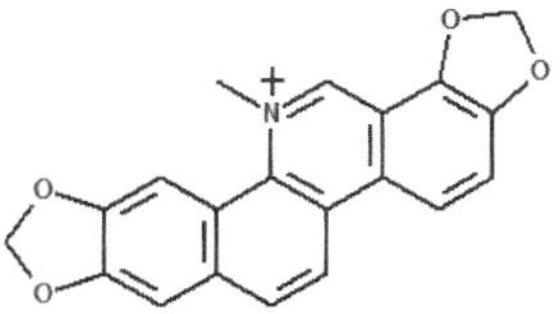

Sanguinarine

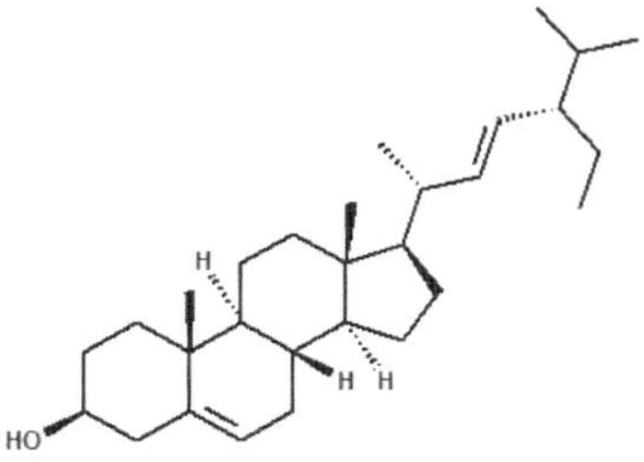

Stigmasterol

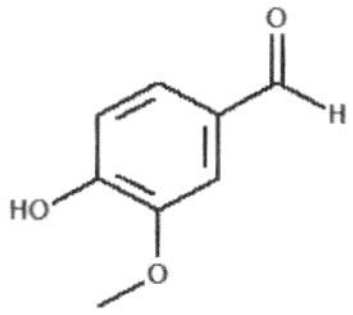

Vanillin

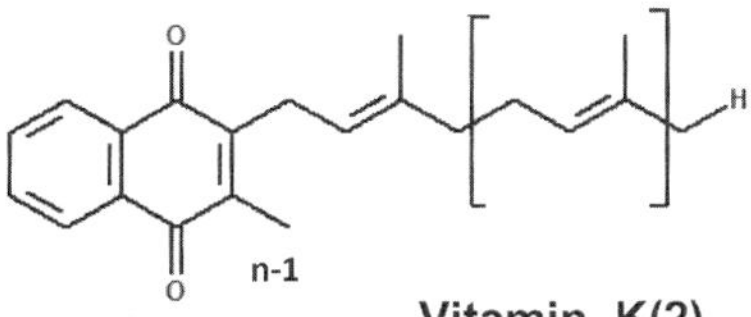

Vitamin K(2)

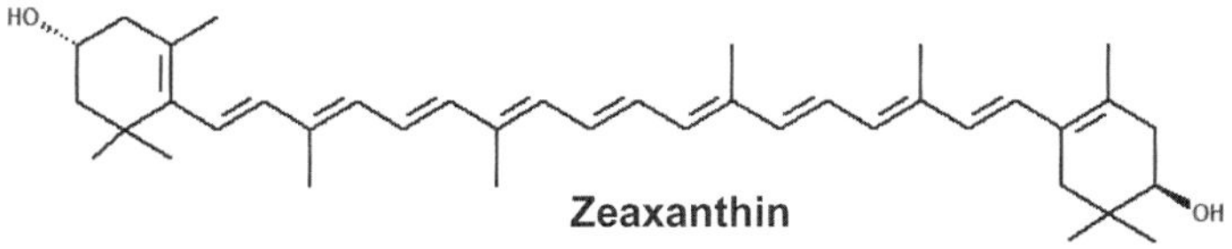

Zeaxanthin

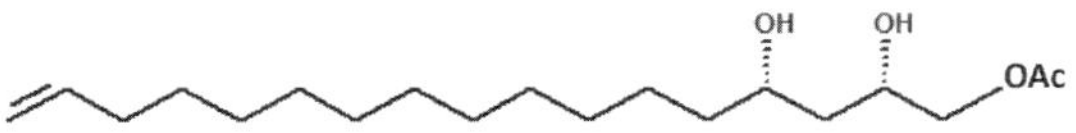

(2S,4S)-2,4-dihydroxyheptadec-16-enyl

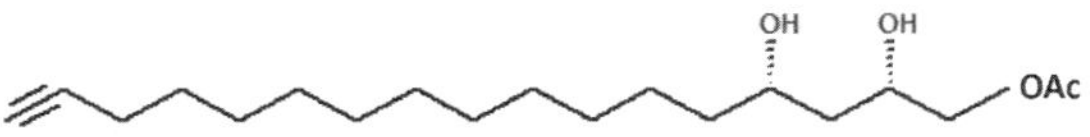

(2S,4S)-2,4-dihydroxyheptadec-16-ynyl acetate

Figure 1.4 (*Continued*)

world, avocados have been used as far back as 10,000 B.C. The avocado is the main ingredient in the Mexican dip, '*guacamole*', and is also used in '*California rolls*' and other '*makizushi*' (rolled sushi). Also frequently used in milkshakes, avocado intake has been shown to decrease blood low-density lipoprotein (LDL) and increase high-density lipoprotein (HDL) levels in humans. Laboratory experiments show that this fruit possesses anticancer activities against breast, oral, and prostate cancers. While avocados have a higher fat content than other fruits, they are mainly monounsaturated fats, and they are rich in vitamins B3, C, and E. The main biologically active compounds of this fruit are persin and persenone A.

Breadfruit

Family: Moraceae
Botanical name: *Artocarpus altilis*
Breadfruit, resembling jackfruit, is a staple food in many tropical regions. It is thought to originate in Northwest New Guinea. The world's largest collection of breadfruit varieties has been established by botanist Diane Ragone in Hawaii. In traditional medicine, this fruit is used to treat many ailments including blood pressure, asthma, and tumors. Breadfruit leaves are used to treat ear and skin infections and splenomegaly. The active components of this plant are dihydroxy chalcones, as well as geranyl and prenyl flavonoids. Geranyl flavonoids from the leaves of *Artocarpus altilis* have exhibited cytotoxicity against colon, liver, and lung cancer cells.

Banana

Family: Musaceae
Botanical name: *Musa acuminata* and *Musa balbisiana*
Southeast Asian farmers were the first to cultivate bananas. Evidence suggests that banana cultivation goes back to at least 5,000 B.C., and possibly to 8,000 B.C. in Papua New Guinea. Bananas are rich sources of carbohydrates, sugars, dietary fibers, and vitamin B6. The main biologically active compounds of this fruit are hydroxycinnamic acid, delphinidin, and naproxen. Studies have shown that banana consumption is associated with a reduced risk of colorectal and breast cancers, as well as renal cell carcinoma.

Berries

Blackberry

Family: Rosaceae
Botanical name: *Rubus fruticosus*
There are over 375 species of blackberries, mostly cultivated in Europe and the United States. The blackberry is an excellent source of dietary fiber, vitamins C and K, as well as folic acid. The biologically active compounds found in blackberries are ellagic acid, ellagitannins, quercetin, gallic acid, anthocyanins, and cyanidins. Studies have shown that blackberries can inhibit breast, colon, lung, prostate, and skin cancers under experimental conditions.

Black raspberry

Family: Rosaceae
Botanical name: *Rubus coreanus*, *Rubus leucodermis*, and *Rubus occidentalis*
The black raspberry, commonly known as wild black raspberry, black caps, black cap raspberry, thimbleberry, and scotch cap, is a native of Eastern North America. Black raspberries are rich in anthocyanins and ellagic acid. They possess high antioxidant and anti-inflammatory properties. Increasing lines of evidence suggest that black raspberries possess anticancer properties against colon, cervical, breast, esophageal, lung, oral, prostate, and skin cancers.

Black chokeberry

Family: Rosaceae
Botanical name: *Aronia melanocarpa* (Michx.) Ell, *Pyrus melanocarpa*, and *Photinia melanocarpa*
The black chokeberry is native to the Great Lakes Region and Northeastern United States. It is rich in vitamin C and antioxidants. The biologically active compounds isolated from these berries include cyanidin-3-galactoside, epicatechin, caffeic acid, quercetin, delphinidin, petunidin, pelargonidin, peonidin, and malvidin. Studies show that black chokeberries exhibit anticancer activities against breast, cervical, and colon cancers, as well as leukemia.

Blueberry

Family: Ericaceae
Botanical name: *Vaccinium* species
Blueberries are native to North America and are classified in the section of *Cyanoccocus* within the genus *Vaccinium*. They are now commercially grown in Australia, New Zealand, and South American countries. The biologically active compounds isolated from the blueberry mainly include anthocyanins such as delphinidin 3,7,3′,-5′-tetraglucosides, naphthalene glycoside, 2-acetyl-1,5-dihydroxy-3methyl-8-O(xylosyl-(1-6)-glucosyl) naphthalene, allylisothiocyanate (AITC), and resveratrol. Studies show that blueberries can inhibit selective tumor cell growth in prostate, lung, cervical, and colon cancers, as well as leukemia.

Cranberry

Family: Ericaceae
Botanical name: *Vaccinium erythrocarpum*, *V. macrocarpon*, *V. microcarpum*, and *V. oxycoccos*
Cranberries are primarily cultivated in the United States and Canada. Raw cranberries have been marketed as a "super fruit" due to their high nutritional content and antioxidant properties. They are used to make products such as juice drinks, sauce, and sweetened dried cranberries. The main bioactive components of this fruit include hydroxycinnamate, quercetin, myricetin, cyanidin, peonidin, and proantocyanidins. Studies have shown that cranberry possess anticancer activities against cancers of the breast, colon, lung, mouth, ovaries, and prostate.

Indian gooseberry

Family: Phyllanthaceae
Botanical name: *Phyllanthus emblica*
The Indian gooseberry is an edible fruit that possesses high medicinal value. It contains large amounts of vitamins C and E. It also contains phytochemicals such as emblicanin A, emblicanin B, punigluconin and pedunculagin, punicafolin, phyllanemblinin A, phyllanemblin, kaempferol, as well as ellagic and gallic acids. Gooseberries possess antiviral, antimicrobial,

antioxidant, antidiabetic, and anticancer properties. Studies have shown that this fruit prevents cervical, liver, lung, and oral cancers.

Strawberry

Family: Rosaceae
Botanical name: *Fragaria ananassa*
Strawberries are cultivated worldwide for their characteristic aroma, red color, juicy texture, and sweetness. They are used to make fruit juice, pies, ice cream, milkshakes, smoothies, yogurt, and chocolates. Strawberries are rich in vitamin C, flavonoids, dietary fiber, and fisetin. They have been shown to inhibit breast, cervical, colon, and prostate cancers under experimental conditions.

Blackcurrant

Family: Grossulariaceae
Botanical name: *Ribes nigrum*
The blackcurrant is native to Northern Europe and Asia. It is used in jams, jellies, ice cream, desserts, and sorbets. Rich in vitamins C, E, and B_5, the main chemical components of this fruit include delphinidin-3-O-glucoside, delphinidin-3-O-rutinoside, cyanidin-3-O-glucoside, and cyanidin-3-O-rutinoside. Experiments have shown that blackcurrants inhibit liver cancer in animals.

Cantaloupe

Family: Cucurbitaceae
Botanical name: *Cucumis melo*
Although a member of the squash family, and technically a vegetable, cantaloupe is considered a fruit because of the way it is used. Native to Central Asia, Europe, and Japan, it is commonly known as muskmelon and its fruit and peel have been used in traditional medicine. The major constituent of the cantaloupe is serine containing protease cucumisin. Cantaloupes possess anti-hyperlipidemia and laxative properties. Reports have shown that cantaloupe extract has enhanced differentiation in human colon cancer cell lines. See also section on Melon, below.

Cherimoya

Family: Annonaceae
Botanical name: *Annona cherimola*
Chirimoya is native to the Andes and is grown throughout South Asia, Central America, South America, Southern California, Southern Andalucia, and Southern Italy. The main bioactive phytochemicals from this fruit include annomolin, annocherimolin, and acetogenins. These chemicals are known to inhibit proliferation of breast, colon, and prostate cancer cell lines in experimental settings.

Cherry

Family: Rosaceae
Botanical name: *Prunus avium*
Approximately two million tons of cherries are produced every year, worldwide. Turkey stands number one in production followed by the United States and Iran. This fruit is rich in its content of dietary fiber, vitamins, and dietary minerals and is an excellent source of phenols, flavonoids, and anthocyanins. Cherries also possess antioxidant, immunomodulatory, and radioprotective properties.

Durian

Family: Malvaceae
Botanical name: *Durio zibethinus*
Durian is often referred to as the "king of fruits" in Southeast Asia. It contains high amounts of sugar, vitamin C, potassium, and the serotonergic amino acid tryptophan, carbohydrates, proteins, and fats. Reports suggest that the durian possesses antioxidant properties.

Fig

Family: Moraceae
Botanical name: *Ficus carica*
Native to the Middle East and Western Asia, the fig is widely grown throughout the temperate world, and is used to make jams and cookies.

Figs are a rich source of dietary fiber and vitamin K. The bioactive components of this fruit include gallic, chlorogenic, and syringic acids, as well as catechin, epicatechin, and rutin. Figs are known to inhibit breast, skin, and stomach cancers under experimental conditions.

Grapefruit

Family: Rutaceae
Botanical name: *Citrus paradisi*
The grapefruit, a citrus fruit, is known for its sour to semi-sweet flavor. It contains grapefruit mercaptan, a sulphur, which in turn contain sterpene, influencing its flavor. Grapefruit is an excellent source of vitamin C and pectin. It also contains polyamine, aspermidine compound, which is known to increase the lifespan of worms, fruit flies, yeast, and human immune cells. Studies have shown that grapefruit also contains compounds such as 4′-geranyloxyferulic acid, obacunone, and obacunoneglucoside. Experiments have shown that grapefruit inhibits colon cancer.

Grape

Family: Vitaceae
Botanical name: *Vitis vinifera*
Grapes are regarded as one of the most produced fruit crops. Large, seedless, thin-skinned commercial varieties of grapes are termed table grapes, while small, thick-skinned ones are referred to as wine grapes. Some of the grape's prime constituents are anthocyanins, polyphenols (resveratrol), catechins, phenolic acids (ferulic, gallic, caffeic, p-coumarics, and syringic acids), procyanidins, flavonoids, and sugars (glucose and fructose). Grape extract possesses antioxidant, anti-aging, anti-atherosclerotic, antiarrhythmic, vasorelaxation, anti-inflammatory, and antimicrobial properties. Many studies have shown that grape extract and its constituents inhibit numerous varieties of cancers including bladder, brain, breast, colon, head and neck cancers, as well as leukemia, lung, pancreatic, and skin cancers.

Guava

Family: Myrtaceae
Botanical name: *Psidium guajava*
Guavas are native to Mexico, Central America, and Northern South America. However, they are cultivated throughout the tropics and subtropics including Africa, South Asia, Southeast Asia, the Caribbean, North America, Hawaii, New Zealand, Australia, and Spain. Guavas are rich in dietary fiber and vitamins A and C. They also contain compounds such as (+)-gallocatechin, guaijaverin, leucocyanidin, amritoside, gallic acid, catechin, quercetin, and rutin. Guavas are known to inhibit lung and prostate cancers.

Guyabano fruit

Family: Annonaceae
Botanical name: *Annona muricata L.*
Commonly known as soursop, the guyabano fruit is native to Mexico, Cuba, Central America, the Caribbean, and Northern South America, primarily Colombia, Brazil, Peru, Ecuador, and Venezuela, as well as some parts of Africa, Southeast Asia, and the Pacific. Studies have reported that extracts from leaves of *Annona muricata* showed cytotoxic effects against hepatocellular carcinoma.

Hawthorn

Family: Rosaceae
Botanical name: *Crataegus pinnatifida* and *C. mexicana*
Also known as thornapple or hawberry, the hawthorn is commonly grown in the Northern Hemisphere in Europe, North America, and Asia. Used to produce jams, jellies, juices, and alcoholic beverages, the thornapple contains tannins, flavonoids, oligomeric proanthocyanidins (epicatechin, procyanidin, and particularly procyanidin B-2), flavone-C, triterpene acids (ursolic, oleanolic and crataegolic acids), and phenolic acids (caffeic, chlorogenic, and related phenolcarboxylic acids). The Chinese hawthorn fruit helps to lower blood cholesterol and the risk of cardiovascular diseases. Proanthocyanidins have exhibited cytotoxic effects on ovarian cancer cell lines.

Jackfruit

Family: Moraceae
Botanical name: *Artocarpus heterophyllus*
Native to South and Southeast Asia, the jackfruit is widely cultivated in the tropical regions of India, Bangladesh, Nepal, Sri Lanka, Vietnam, Thailand, Cameroon, Uganda, Tanzania, Malaysia, Indonesia, and the Philippines. Jackfruit is starchy, fibrous, and a rich source of dietary fiber. It contains various phytochemicals such as artocarpin, isobutyl isovalerate, 2-methylbutanol, jacalin, and butyl isovalerate. Jackfruit is known to inhibit breast and skin cancers.

Jujube fruit

Family: Rhamnaceae
Botanical name: *Ziziphus jujube*
Commonly known as the red Chinese, Korean, or Indian date, the jujube fruit is cultivated mainly in Southern Asia. The fruit and seeds have been used in Chinese and Korean traditional medicine for antifungal, antibacterial, antiulcer, anti-inflammatory, sedative, antispastic, antifertility, hypotensive, antinephritic, cardiotonic, antioxidant, immunostimulant effects as well as in wound-healing. The extracts from *Ziziphus jujube* have been shown to exert anti-proliferative effects against breast cancer cell lines as well as in liver carcinoma cell lines.

Kiwi

Family: Actinidiaceae
Botanical name: *Actinidia chinensis*
A native of Southern China, kiwifruit — a climacteric fruit — has been used as a prominent Chinese herbal medicine and is considered the "national fruit of China." Some of its prime constituents are anthraquinones, ascorbic acid, triterpenes, polyphenols, vitamins, minerals, protein (actinchinin), and dietary fiber. The kiwi also contains lutein and zeaxanthin. It is known for its antiangiogenic, anticancer, antifungal, antioxidant, and immunomodulatory properties. Kiwis also improve laxation, digestion, and cardiovascular health.

Lime and lemon

Family: Rutaceae
Botanical name: *Citrus limon*
These fruits, native to Asia, are used to make pickles, juices, and cocktails. They consist of flavonone (hesperetin and naringenin) and limonoids (obacunone, obacunone glucoside, limonin, limonin glucoside, nomilin, nomilinic acid glucoside, and deacetylnomilinic acid). The limonoids modulate the caspase-7-dependent pathways and may have the potential to combat breast cancer. They possess antiatherogenic, chemoprotective, anticancer effects in the cervix and colon and have anti-inflammatory, antihypertensive, and anti-aromatase properties.

Lychee

Family: Sapindaceae
Botanical name: *Litchi chinensis*
This delicious tropical fruit, native to Southern China, Taiwan, Bangladesh, and Southeast Asia, is cultivated around the globe, especially in semi-tropical areas. It contains vitamin C, cyanidin-3-glucoside, and malvidin-3-glucoside. The lychee may be used as a topical agent and anti-oxidant. Lychee seeds possess antitumor and anti-colorectal cancer properties and act as astringent, hyperlipidemic, anti-inflammatory, analgesic, and anti-hypoglycemic agents. This fruit's pericarp has been shown to inhibit breast and liver cancer cell growth.

Loganberry

Family: Rosaceae
Botanical name: Rubus (*Rubus ursinus*) × loganobaccus (*Rubus idaeus*)
The loganberry was derived accidentally by crossing blackberries and raspberries. The plant and fruit resemble blackberries, but the fruit is dark red in color. These berries are rich in soluble fiber and vitamins and minerals such as vitamins A and C, calcium, and iron, and also contain ellagic acid, known to inhibit cancer in humans.

Mandarin

Family: Rutaceae
Botanical name: *Citrus reticulate*
The mandarin, also known as the mandarin orange, is a juicy fruit, which resembles other oranges. In Chinese medicine, it has been used to enhance digestion and to reduce phlegm. The different cultivars and crosses of this fruit include satsuma, owari, clementine, tangerine, tangor, etc. Ugly fruit is a variety developed by hybridizing the mandarin orange (*Citrus reticulate*) × grapefruit (*Citrus paradise*). Mandarin oranges contain phytochemicals such as β-cryptoxanthin and hesperidin. Studies have shown that this fruit inhibits colon, lung, and stomach cancers in experimental models.

Mango

Family: Anacardiaceae
Botanical name: *Mangifera indica*
The mango is the national fruit of India and is native to South Asia. Mangoes are commonly cultivated in many tropical and subtropical regions. The fruit is used to prepare juice, jelly, jam, milkshakes, pickles, etc. It contains chemicals such as provitamin A, α-carotene, β-carotene, lutein, quercetin, kaempferol, catechins, mangiferin, as well as caffeic and galllic acids. The mango has been shown to inhibit cancers of the breast, colon, lung, skin, and prostate in experimental settings.

Mangosteen

Family: Clusiaceae
Botanical name: *Garcinia mangostana*
Mangosteen trees are found in all over the world, especially in the Southeast Asian rainforests. The mangosteen has been used as a therapeutic agent, especially in Chinese and Ayurvedic medicine. It possesses oxygen-containing heterocyclic compounds, i.e., xanthones (mangostingone, cudraxanthone G, 8-deoxygartanin, garcimangosone B,

garcinone D, tovophyllin A, α-mangostin, γ-mangostin, smeathxanthone, and 8-hydroxycudraxanthone G). Moreover, α-mangostin is a competitive antagonist of the histamine (H1) receptor. This fruit shows antifungal, anti-inflammatory, antibacterial, antiviral, anti-tuberculosis, neuroprotective, cardioprotective, immunomodulatory, anti-allergic, and antitumor effects. Studies have shown that this fruit inhibits proliferation and growth of bladder, breast, brain, colon, prostate, and skin cancer cells as well as leukemia.

Melon

Family: Cucurbitaceae
Botanical name: *Benincasa hispida* (winter melon), and *Cucumis metuliferus* (horned melon), *Cucumis melo* (different varieties: muskmelon, canary melon, honeydew, and hami melon)
A group of fleshy fruits belonging to the family Cucurbitaceae, melons contain compounds such as cucurbitacin A & B, and lycopene. Although the flesh of wild melon, Egusi is inedible, the seeds rich in fat and protein are a wildly used food source in Africa. Horned melon also known as African horned cucumber is a culinary fruit. Its peel is rich in vitamin C and dietary fiber. Winter melon, belonging to the genus *Benincasa,* is a culinary vegetable which helps to increase appetite. Moreover, its fresh juice has the ability to cure kidney stones. Various studies have shown that phytochemicals present in melon prevent cancers of the brain, breast, colon etc.

Orange

Family: Rutaceae
Botanical name: *Citrus sinensis*
Orange trees, considered to have originated in Southeast Asia, are widely grown in tropical and subtropical regions for their sweet fruit. There are many different varieties, including Valencia, Hart's Tardiff Valencia, Hamlin, caracara, navel, blood, and acidless oranges. They provide a rich source of vitamin C and the dietary fiber, pectin. Oranges contain compounds such

as chitooligosaccharides, cyanidin 3-O-glucoside, hesperidin, narirutin, didymin, sinensetin, nobiletin, tangeretin, and ferulic acid. Studies have shown that this fruit inhibits breast, colon, and skin cancers.

Papaya

Family: Caricaceae
Botanical Name: *Carica papaya*
Papaya, alternately referred to as pawpaw, is a tropical fruit native to Central America, Southern Mexico, and Northern South America, and is cultivated in Africa, Malaysia, and the West Indies. Some of its chemical constituents are benzyl glucosinolate, ferulic acid, tocopherols, alkaloids, p-coumaric acid, vitamin C, caffeic acid, β-carotene, etc. The papaya is used in the conventional treatment of ringworm and malarial episodes. It also possesses antioxidant, anti-atherosclerotic, cardioprotective, hypolipidemic, wound-healing, hepatoprotective, neuroprotective, anticancer (colon), and anti-hypertensive properties. The hydroloysis product of benzyl glucosinolate of this fruit is postulated to have anticancer properties.

Peach (Nectarine)

Family: Rosaceae
Botanical name: *Prunus persica*
Peaches and nectarines are the same species of edible, juicy fruits native to Northwest China and are cultivated in Ecuador, Colombia, Ethiopia, India, and Nepal. Peaches contain high amounts of carbohydrates and vitamins A and C. They are known to contain mandelic acid glycosides (β-gentiobioside and β-D-glucoside) and benzyl alcohol glycosides (β-gentiobioside and β-D-glucoside) that are responsible for this fruit's anticancer properties. Phenolic compounds derived from peach are chlorogenic acid, (+)-catechin and (−)-epicatechin, gallic acid, neochlorogenic acid, procyanidin B1 and B3, procyanidin gallates, and ellagic acid. The fleshy extracts of peach have been shown to improve the efficiency of cisplatin and protected cisplatin-treated mice against nephrotoxicity. Peach extract also inhibited cell-derived allergic inflammation.

Pear

Family: Rosaceae
Botanical name: *Pyrus* species
Pears are edible fruits, native to Western Europe and North Africa as well as across Asia. Pears are rich in vitamins A, C, and K and in dietary fiber. They also contain quercetin and hydroxycinnamic acid, and pears are known to lower the risk of breast, lung, and stomach cancers.

Pineapple

Family: Bromeliaceae
Botanical name: *Ananas comosus*
The pineapple is a tropical fruit indigenous to South America. It is used in juices, jams, curries, etc. Known to enhance digestion in traditional medicine, pineapples have also been used to treat inflammatory disorders. Pineapples contain a chemical, bromelanin, which is known to inhibit the proliferation of breast and skin cancer cells.

Persimmon

Family: Ebenaceae
Botanical name: *Diospyros* species
Persimmons are edible fruits, which range in color from yellowish-orange to dark reddish-orange, depending on the species and variety. These fruits are cultivated in South Asia, Europe, Japan, and America. The persimmon contains a high amount of dietary fiber and also compounds like betulinic acid, catechin, gallocatechin, and shibuol. Studies have shown that it reduces ear diseases and cancer.

Plum

Family: Rosaceae
Botanical name: *Prunus* species
Plums are cultivated all over the globe and China stands as the world's largest producer. Some of the different cultivars used today are damson,

greengage, mirabelle, and yellowgage. The plum is rich in antioxidants and contains dietary fiber, sorbitol, isatin, and amygdalin. Plums are known to prevent a number of cancers including those of breast, colon, liver, and skin.

Pomegranate

Family: Lythraceae
Botanical name: *Punica granatum*
Its use in folk medicine in various cultures and its presence in the Garden of Eden, attests to the pomegranate's long history. The fruit consists of polyplenolic flavonoids like anthocyanins (such as delphinidin-3-glucoside, cyanidin-3-glucoside, and cyanidin-3,5-diglucoside) and anthoxanthins (such as gallic acid, ellagic acid, catechins, and ellagic tannins). It possesses antioxidative, cardioprotective, antiosteoarthritic, and antiatherogenic, properties. Pomegranate seed oil comprises several conjugated fatty acids, such as punicic acid, having anticancer effects. Its extract down-regulates homologous recombination and hence sensitizes breast cancer cells to drug therapy. It may emerge as a potential treatment for cancer, especially for colon and prostate cancers.

Quince

Family: Rosaceae
Botanical name: *Cydonia oblonga*
Native to Southwest Asia, Turkey, and Iran, quince is cultivated in many countries such as Turkey, China, Uzbekistan, Morocco, and Iran. Used to make jam, jelly, quince pudding, and wine, the fruit contains 5-O-caffeoylquinic acid and is known to inhibit the proliferation of colon, kidney, liver, and lung cancer cell lines.

Watermelon

Family: Cucurbitaceae
Botanical name: *Citrullus lanatus*
Watemelons originated from Southern Africa, and are considered a good source of vitamin C and glutathione, carotenoids such as lycopene,

β-carotene, and β-cryptoxanthin, as well as L-citrulline (an effective precursor of L-arginine) and a small fraction of cucurbitacins, all of which have been shown to have cancer chemopreventive properties. The watermelon also has been shown to possess anti-inflammatory and antimicrobial properties and to reduce cardiovascular risk factors by improving glycemic control and ameliorating vascular dysfunction in laboratory animals with type 2 diabetes. Cucurbitacin E and cucurbitacin B are associated with a lower risk of breast cancer according to a recent study.

Vegetables

Artichoke

Family: Asteraceae
Botanical name: *Cynara scolymus*
Artichokes were believed to have originated in the Mediterranean Region, the state of Virginia (in the United States), and Southern Europe. Used to make "Tisane" (artichoke tea), some of its vital constituents are hydrolysable tannins (chlorogenic acid, cynarin), flavone glycosides (luteolin), phenylpropanoids (caffeic acid), sesquiterpene lactones (cynaropicrin), volatile oils (caryophyllene), and phytosterols (taraxasterol). The extract of this vegetable possesses anticancer properties against breast, liver, and skin cancers. The artichoke's medicinal importance lies in its ability to inhibit angiogenesis, inflammation, and cancer cell proliferation.

Arugula

Family: Brassicaceae
Botanical name: *Eruca sativa*
Arugula is an edible annual plant, commonly known as salad rocket, native to Central Asia, South Europe, Morocco, and Portugal in the West, and to Lebanon and Turkey in the East. Its leaves and seeds were mainly used in traditional medicine. Arugula has acted as an astringent, aphrodisiac, diuretic, digestive, and emollient. It also has been utilized to encourage hair growth and as a depurative and laxative with potential use as an alternative to mineral oil. Additionally, it has industrial applications in soap-making

and as a lubricant. Moreover, arugula possesses anti-inflammatory properties for the treatment of colitis. The active ingredients include fatty acids such as erucic, oleic, palmitic, linoleic, and linolenic acids, as well as flavonoids and glucosinolate (4-mercaptobutyl glucosinolate). Arugula contains two cancer-fighting agents, namely, kaempferol and quercetin, which have been reported to reduce the risk of lung cancer.

Asparagus

Family: Liliaceae
Botanical name: *Asparagus officinalis*
Asparagus is a spring vegetable that is native to the temperate regions of the Himalayas and Spain. In traditional medicine, the roots, leaves, bark, and fruit of the asparagus were used frequently. The chemical constituents of asparagus include vitamins, kaempferol, quercetin, rutin, asparagine, sarsasapogenin and shatavarin I–IV, asparagamine, curillins G and H, and spirostanosides. Asparagus is well known for its antioxidant, anti-inflammatory, antioxytocic, antibacterial, antifungal, hypocholesterolemic, hepatoprotective, and immunostimulant properties. Studies have shown that this plant possesses anticancer activities against breast, colon, liver, and skin cancers.

Basil

Family: Lamiaceae
Botanical name: *Ocimum sanctum*
Basil, or sweet basil, is a common name for the herb *Ocimum basilicum*. The plant is found in Asia, East Anatolia in Turkey, and Africa. The whole plant is used in traditional medicine. It has been reported that the essential oil of basil contains carvacrol, methylchavicol, caryophyllene, nerol, camphene, geraniol, linalool, camphor, citral, eugenol, ursolic acid, oleanolic acid, quercetin, isoquercetin, kaempferol, rosmarinic acid, catechin, caffeic acid, ferulic acid, rutin, rutiniside, and apigenin. Carnosol has been shown to inhibit carcinogenesis in human prostate cancer cells. Basil leaf extract has been found highly effective in inhibiting carcinogen-induced lung tumors in experimental mice. Basil oil and its components

have been shown to have significant anti-proliferative activity in mouse leukemia and kidney cells. In addition, basil oil has been found to significantly inhibit carcinogen-induced squamous cell carcinomas in the stomachs of mice.

Beans

Family: *Fabaceae*
Botanical name: *Phaseolus vulgaris*
A bean is a type of legume and 'bean' is the common name for plant seeds used for human food or animal feed of several genera belonging to the family Fabaceae. Dry beans and other legumes contain dietary fiber and folate. Several studies link higher consumption of legumes with lower risk of colon cancer or the benign adenomas (polyps) that are the beginning of most colon cancers. Beans, rich in the B vitamin folate, can contribute to a diet that helps lower the risk for pancreatic cancer. Beans contain mainly peptides namely cyclotides and exhibit antimicrobial, anti-proliferative, antioxidative, and anti-HIV activities.

Beet

Family: Chenopodiaceae
Botanical name: *Beta vulgaris*
Commonly known as sugar beet, red beet, or beetroot, beets were believed to be natives of California. Leaves and roots were used as medicines in traditional practice. The active components of the beet include α-tocopherol, β-carotene, betanin, polyphenols, and fiber. Beets also contain betacyanins (red-violet pigments) and betaxanthins (yellow pigments). Several reports about the effect of *Beta vulgaris* show an improvement in the quality of life of metastatic prostate cancer patients. The cytotoxic effect of red beetroot extract, compared to doxorubicin (Adriamycin), in human prostate and breast cancer cell lines has also been reported. It has also been reported that extract of beet has significant antiproliferative effects against colon cancer cells.

Bok choy

Family: Brassicaceae
Botanical name: *Brassica chinensis (Chinese cabbage)*
The geographical distribution of bok choy, commonly known as Chinese white cabbage, has mostly been in Asia, particularly in China. Bok choy contains glucosinolates as its main constituents, which in turn contain a sulfur group. Once ingested, bok choy is broken down into oxazolidines, thiocyanates, and nitriles. It also contains myrosinase, which increases glucosinolate hydrolysis and sulforaphane, which exhibit antioxidant and anti-inflammatory activities. Scientific reports have shown the preventive effect of *Brassica chinensis* against colon carcinogen 2-amino-1-methyl-6-phenylimidazo [4,5-b]pyridine (PhIP)-induced PhIP-DNA] adduct formation in Sprague–Dawley rats, and the mechanism is likely to involve the induction of detoxification enzymes.

Broccoli

Family: Bracicaceae
Botanical name: *Brassica oleraceae* var. *italica* and *Brassica rapa*
Broccoli belongs to the cabbage family native to California. The parts of broccoli include its stem, leaves, and inflorescences, and they were used in traditional medicine. The chemical constituents of broccoli include glucoraphanin, glucoiberin, sulforaphane, carotenoids, vitamins, particularly vitamin C, and myrosinase. Many reports have shown broccoli extracts' anticancer activity including cancers of the breast, bladder, colon, and lung.

Broccoli rabe or rapini

Family: Bracicaceae
Botanical name: *Brassica rapa*
Broccoli rabe, also called rapini, resembles broccoli and is a green cruciferous vegetable. It is a source of vitamins C and K and also contains compounds such as brassicaphenanthrene A, 6-paradol, and trans-6-shogaol. These compounds are known to inhibit the growth of colon and breast cancer cell lines.

Brussels sprouts

Family: Bracicaceae
Botanical name: *Brassica oleracea*
Brussels sprouts are native to Belgium and Brazil. They have been used extensively in Brazilian traditional medicine to treat gastric ulcers. The constituents of Brussels sprouts include caffeic, ferulic, sinapic and p-coumaric acids, methylsulfanylalkyl glucosinolate, isothiocyanates, sulforaphane, and indoles that are involved in inhibition of procarcinogen activation. The immunomodulatory activity of sulforaphane, a naturally occurring isothiocyanate from *Brassica oleracea*, has been reported recently. Many scientific reports have evidenced that Brussels sprout extracts inhibit the cell proliferation of colon cancer cell lines. A number of recent epidemiological studies have pointed out that high intake of Brussels sprouts may be associated with a lower risk of cancers of the pancreas, breast, prostate, stomach, and lungs.

Cabbage

Family: Bracicaceae
Botanical name: *Brassica oleracea*
Another cultivar of the species '*oleracea*,' the cabbage was most likely domesticated in Europe before 1,000 B.C. Cabbages have been used to prepare dishes such as sauerkraut and kimchee. This vegetable is a good source of β-carotene, vitamin C, and dietary fiber, and also contains anticancer compounds such as sulforaphane and indole-3-carbinol. The cabbage is known to prevent certain cancers, including breast, gastric, liver, lung, and prostate cancers.

Carrot

Family: Apiaceae
Botanical name: *Daucus carota*
The carrot is an orange-colored, horn-like root vegetable. Its dietary use renders the body with inadequate amounts of vitamin A, whereas carrot juice imparts considerable amounts of therapeutic provitamin A. The active compounds reported in carrots include myristicin, pectin, falcarinol, β-carotene, and α-terpineol. Recent research performed on rats fed raw carrots or merely falcarinol — an antioxidant extracted from carrots — demonstrated a delay

in the growth of colon tumors. The compound falcarinol is a polyacethylene and hence its efficacy is greatly reduced during cooking. A study found that drinking carrot juice increases the levels of carotenoids in the blood of breast cancer survivors, which help to prevent the cancer from recurring. Carrots contain much beta carotene, which may help reduce a wide range of cancers including those of the lung, mouth, throat, stomach, intestine, bladder, prostate, and breast.

Cauliflower

Family: Brassicaceae
Botanical name: *Brassica oleracea* var. *botrytis*
Cauliflower is originally from Italy, Northeast Europe, and Asia, and is commonly known as green or white curd cauliflower. Its inflorescence is most often used. The major compounds present in cauliflower are glucosinolates, sulforaphane, peroxidases, isalexin, S-(−)-spirobrassinin, 1-methoxybrassitin, brassicanal C, indole-3-carbinol, and caulilexins A, B, and C. A high intake of cauliflower has been associated with reduced risk of aggressive prostate cancer; hence, it is also called a *cancer-killing crucifier.* Reports on sulforaphane, a compound released when cauliflower is chopped or chewed, has shown protection against many cancers. Indole-3-carbinol has been reported to prevent the growth of different cancer cells.

Celery

Family: Apiaceae
Botanical name: *Apium graveolens*
Apium graveolens is used either for its crisp leaf stalk or fleshy taproot. The leaves are strong-flavored and are included in soups and stews or as a dried herb. The essential oil of celery contains d-limonene, p-mentha-2,8-dien-1-ol, p-mentha-8(9)-en-1,2-diol, 3-n-butyl phthalide, sedanolideβ-pinene, β-phellendrene, α-thuyene, camphene, cumene, sabinene, and terpinolene. Celery exhibits antiulcerogenic, antimicrobial, antifungal, hepatoprotective, anti-hyperlipidemic, and larvicidal activities, and can also serve as a mosquito repellent. Celery seed extracts exhibit anti-proliferative effects on human gastric cancer cells. Celery is also known to inhibit liver cancer and stomach cancer in animals.

Chili pepper

Family: Solanaceae
Botanical name: *Capsicum baccatum*, *Capsicum annuum*, and *Capsicum pubesceis*
The chili pepper is the fruit of a plant that belongs to the genus *Capsicum*, members of the nightshade family, Solanaceae. This vegetable originated in the Americas, more specifically in Culiacan, Sinaloa in Mexico, and also in Asia. The reported active ingredients of *C. pubescens* include 2-methoxypyrazines, 2-nonenals, and 2,6-nonadienal. *C. baccatum* contains guaiacol, 2-heptanethiol, α-pinene, 1,8-cineol, linalool, and 3-isobutyl-2-methoxypyrazine. Chili pepper extract has evidenced cytotoxic impacts on human cervical cancer cells. Capsanthin and capsanthin 3′-ester and capsanthin 3,3′-diester, isolated from the fruits of red paprika (*C. annuum*) have exhibited potent antitumor-promoting activity in an *in vivo* mouse skin two-stage carcinogenesis model.

Chives

Family: Amaryllidaceae
Botanical name: *Allium schoenoprasum*
Chives are bulb-forming herbaceous plants used for culinary purposes as flavoring herbs. Used as an ingredient for fish, potatoes, soups, and other dishes, chives' medicinal properties are similar to those of garlic and contain organosulphur compounds. The compounds from chive are known to inhibit the growth of colon cancer cells.

Corn

Family: Poaceae
Botanical name: *Zea mays*
Corn, also called maize, is a rich source of starch and is used as an important excipient in the pharmaceutical industry. Two grades of corn starch are available — 'Maizena' and 'Mondamin.' It has been reported that the main constituents of corn lutein are gluten and starch. Corn oil is rich in vitamin E. Lutein prevents the *in vivo* oxidation of vitamin A, and may

exert chemopreventive effects against colon cancer. It is also known to inhibit N-nitrosodiethylamine-induced hepatocellular carcinoma. Lutein is non-toxic and will be one of the prime compounds in the cancer chemoprevention trials of the future.

Cucumber

Family: Cucurbitaceae
Botanical name: *Cucumis sativus*
The cucumber is native to India. The important phytochemicals of this vegetable include cucurbitacins, vitexin, cucumerin A and B, divinyl reductase proteins, cucumegastigmanes I and II, orientin, and glucosides. Cucumbers scavenge, *in vivo,* unwanted wastes and toxic substances, and they also combat irritation and inflammation. This vegetable exhibits antidiabetic, hemostatic, lipid-lowering, tonic, and antioxidant activities. The cucumber is known to inhibit skin cancer in animals.

Dill

Family: Apiaceae
Botanical name: *Anethum graveolens*
Dill, also known as Lao coriander, is a native of the Mediterranean region, Central Asia, countries in the southern areas of the former USSR, and Japan. Dill grows easily from seed, is delicious in a variety of dishes, and attracts beneficial insects to the garden with its tiny flowers. The major components present in dill are quercetin, isorharmentin, umbelliferone, myristicin, anethofuran, carvone, and limonene. The oil of dill was found to contain anethofuran, carvone, and limonene, all of which have shown strong antioxidant and chemopreventive properties.

Eggplant

Family: Solanaceae
Botanical name: *Solanum melongena*
Eggplant, also known as brinjal or guinea squash, is native to the Indian subcontinent and is a widely used vegetable in a variety of dishes. Eggplant

contains low amounts of fats, proteins, and carbohydrates, and is found to reduce weight and lower plasma cholesterol levels and aortic cholesterol content in hypercholesterolemic rabbits. Eggplant extracts inhibit the growth of human fibrosarcoma cell lines.

English peas

Family: Fabaceae
Botanical name: *Pisum sativum*
English peas, also known as garden, smooth, or field peas, are traditionally eaten without the pods. Copper-containing amine oxidases, isolated from the seedling of this vegetable, are known to metabolize biogenic amines *in vivo* and thus combat several allergic reactions. Peas also exhibit selenium accumulation properties. The major active compounds present are flavonoids, polyphenols, and starch. Additionally, peas are rich in protein and possess strong antioxidant, hypocholesterolaemic, and anticarcinogenic properties. Scientific evidence shows that peas inhibit the proliferation of colon cancer cells.

Endive

Family: Asteraceae
Botanical name: *Cichorium endivia*
Escarole, popularly known as endive or chicory, is used in salads or cooked in olive oil with garlic. The active components from this vegetable are scyllo-inositol, carotenoids, phenols, kaempferol, and its conjugates. Endive possesses strong antioxidant and anticancer activities *in vitro* against cervix epithelial adenocarcinoma, skin epidermoid carcinoma, and breast epithelial adenocarcinoma cell lines.

Garlic

Family: Liliaceae/Alliaceae
Botanical name: *Allium sativum*
Garlic is a species in the onion genus, *Allium,* native to central Asia. Garlic has been traditionally used to fight bacterial infections. The active ingredient diallyltrisulfide (DATS) present in garlic oil significantly reduces liver injury

caused by carbon tetrachloride (CCl_4) in rats. Other medicinal uses of garlic include prevention against heart disease, including atherosclerosis, high cholesterol, and high blood pressure. The medicinal use of garlic is mainly attributed to its protective role against colorectal and stomach cancers.

Kohlrabi

Family: Brassicaceae
Botanical name: *Brassica oleracea*
Kohlrabi, a low and stout cultivar of cabbage, is an important part of the Kashmiri diet. It can be eaten raw as well as cooked. It is a rich source of vitamin C and contains chemicals that are known to possess anti-inflammatory and anticancer properties.

Lettuce

Family: Asteraceae
Botanical name: *Lactuca sativa*
Lettuce is a leafy vegetable first cultivated by the ancient Egyptians. The therapeutic proteins isolated with lettuce inhibit dengue and hepatitis B infections. Freeze-dried lettuce cells are used to produce vaccines. The water extracts of lettuce are known to inhibit the growth of human leukemia and breast cancer cell proliferation.

Okra

Family: Malvaceae
Botanical name: *Abelmoschus esculentus*
Okra, commonly known as lady's finger, is cultivated in tropical, subtropical, and temperate regions around the world. Okra originated in Africa and spread to several tropical countries including Brazil and Nigeria. Okra's chemical constituents include polysaccharides, lectin, flavonoids, and phenols. This vegetable has strong antioxidant properties and is used to treat numerous maladies like cancer, constipation, hypoglycemia, hemagglutination, inflammation, microbial infections, and urine retention. Okra extracts are known to inhibit the proliferation of colon cancer and retinoblastoma cells.

Onion

Family: Amaryllidaceae
Botanical name: *Allium cepa*
Onions, also known as bulb onions, are cultivated worldwide. The leading onion-producing countries are, in descending order, China, India, the United States, Turkey, and Pakistan. The chemical constituents present in onions are allyl methyl trisulfide (AMT), allyl methyl disulfide (AMD), diallyltrisulfide (DAT), and diallyl sulfide (DAS). Onions possess antitumor, schistosomicidal, immunomodulatory, and radioprotective effects. The onion also inhibits platelet aggregation. The consumption of onions is consistently associated with a reduced risk of stomach cancer. Epidemiologic and laboratory studies suggest that allium vegetables, including onions and their constituents, reduce the risk of prostate cancer.

Radicchio

Family: Asteraceae
Botanical name: *Cichorium intybus*
Radicchio is an Italian salad plant that looks lovely in the garden with its red foliage. Radicchio is also called leaf chicory and its chemical constituents include terpenoids, chicoric acid, caftaric acid, inulin, and β-sitosterol. Traditionally, radiccio is used as a liver tonic, cardiotonic, diuretic, cholagogue, depurative, and an emmenagogue. Radicchio also serves in the treatment of hepatomegaly, cephalalgia, inflammations, anorexia, dyspepsia, jaundice, and splenomegaly. It possesses antibacterial, antiplaque, hypercholesterolemic, hepatoprotective, and anti-inflammatory properties, and wound-healing effects.

Parsnip

Faily: Apiaceae
Botanical name: *Pastinaca sativa*
The parsnip, a root vegetable resembling white carrots, is native to Eurasia. Parsnips are used in soups and stews and are often roasted. The active ingredients present in the parsnip include falcarinol, falcarindiol, myristicin, psoralen, bergapten, xanthotoxin, isopimpinellin, and umbelliferone.

Parsnips exhibit anti-proliferative activity in human leukemia and colon cancer cells.

Potato

Family: Solanaceae
Botanical name: *Solanum tuberosum*
The potato is a starchy edible tuber native to the Andes of South America and now cultivated in more than 160 countries. Potatoes are rich in starch, steroids, alkaloidal glycosides (solanine), vitamins C and B, and potassium. Potatoes alleviate pain when applied topically in the form of packs. Raw potatoes are used for gastrointestinal disorders. The glycoalkaloids (α-chaconine and α-solanine) from potatoes are shown to inhibit the proliferation and growth of human cervical, liver, lymphoma, and stomach cancer cells.

Pumpkin

Family: Cucurbitaceae
Botanical name: *Cucurbita moschata* and *Cucurbita moschata*
The pumpkin is a gourd-like squash, indigenous to North America as well as Argentina, China, India, Mexico, Brazil, Korea, and Iran, and is now found all over the world. Its chemical constituents are polysaccharides, sterols, β-carotene, α- and β-moschins, and ryonolic acid. Pumpkin exhibits analgesic, anti-hypertension, antidiabetic, antitumor, antibacterial, antifungal, immunomodulatory, and anti-inflammatory activities. β-carotene reduces skin damage from the Sun and acts as an anti-inflammatory agent. α-carotene is thought to slow the aging process, reduce the risk of developing cataracts, and prevent tumor growth. Studies have reported that the pumpkin can be used for the treatment of benign prostate hyperplasia because of its high β-sitosterol content.

Radish

Family: Brassicaceae
Botanical name: *Raphanus sativus*
The radish, which belongs to the cruciferae family, is a common edible leafy vegetable largely consumed in Korea as well as in Asia and Japan. The chemical

constituents present in the radish are glucoraphenin, glucoerucin, 4-methylthio-3-butenyl glucosinolate, 4-hydroxyglucobrassicin, glucobrassicin, and 4-methoxy-glucobrassicin. It possesses antioxidant, hypolipidemic, anticancer, and anti-hypertensive effects. The polyphenols and flavonoids present in radishes inhibit cell proliferation and induce, apoptosis in cancer cells.

Rhubarb

Family: Polygonaceae
Botanical name: *Rheum officanale* and *Rheum rhabarbarum*
Rhubarb is native to Tibet, South East China, and Asia. The chemical constituents reported in rhubarb are rhein-8-glucoside, piceatannol, emodin, gallic acid, d-catechin, and epicatechin. The anthroquinone, emodin, and aloe-emodin, present in rhubarb have the potential to inhibit cancer cell proliferation and apoptosis induction, as well as the possible prevention of metastasis. Rhein is the other major rhubarb anthraquinone that has the property to inhibit the uptake of glucose in tumor cells, which causes changes in membrane-associated functions leading to cell death.

Rutabaga

Family: Brassicaceae
Botanical name: *Brassica napus*
Rutabaga, also known as Swedish turnip, rapeseed, or yellow turnip (*Brassica napobrassica*, or *Brassica napus* var. *napobrassica*, or *Brassica napus* subsp. *rapifera*) is a root vegetable that originated as a cross between the cabbage and the turnip. The active components present in rutabagas are tocopherol, brassinolide, cerebroside, and ceramide. Brassinolide is a plant sterol first isolated from the rape pollen of *Brassica napus* L. and has been shown to induce apoptosis in human prostate cancer cells, thereby acting as promising candidate for the treatment of prostate cancer.

Spinach

Family: Amaranthaceae
Botanical name: *Spinacia oleracea*
Spinach is an edible flowering plant, thought to have originated in ancient Persia. Spinach is an excellent dietary source of folate vitamins A, B6, C, D,

and vitamin K, as well as iron, manganese and magnesium. Spinach contains various carotenoids such as β-carotene and lutein, as well as flavonoids such as kaempferol, and a variety of lignans, chlorophylls, and glycolipids with demonstrated cancer-fighting properties. Dietary intake of spinach has been found to be associated with lower risks of head and neck, lung, gallbladder, stomach, liver, bladder, prostate, and ovarian cancers in population-based studies.

Shallot

Family: Amaryllidaceae
Botanical name: *Allium cepa* var. *aggregatum*
Shallots originated in Central or Southeast Asia and are extensively cultivated for culinary uses. The chemical constituents present in the shallot are allyl methyl trisulfide, allyl methyl disulfide, diallyltrisulfide, and diallyl sulfide. Shallots have been shown to possess antitumor, immunomodulatory, and radioprotective effects in laboratory animals.

Snap pea

Family: Fabaceae
Botanical name: *Pisum sativum* var. *macrocarpon*
The snap pea is a cool-season vegetable belonging to the group of edible-podded peas. Snap peas contain porphyrins and lectins and are known to inhibit colon, gastric, and liver cancers.

Sweet potato

Family: Convolvulaceae
Botanical name: *Ipomoea batatas*
The sweet potato is a tuber crop, native to Jamaica and other Caribbean countries. Its active constituents are starch, phenols, β-carotene, and ascorbic acid. Sweet potatoes possess hypoglycemic, anti-proliferative, and antiradical activity. Known to inhibit liver and lung cancers, sweet potatoes have also been found to exert a protective effect against leukemia, kidney, gallbladder, and breast cancers.

Summer squash

Family: Cucurbitaceae
Botanical name: *Cucurbita pepo*
Summer squash, varieties of *Cucurbita pepo*, include cousa, pattypan, yellow crookneck, and yellow summer squash, as well as astromboncino and zucchini. Summer squash are rich in vitamin A and folate and are known to inhibit human liver and colon cancer cells. See also section on 'Winter Squash,' below.

Tomatillo

Family: Solanaceae
Botanical name: *Physalis philadelphica*
Tomatillo, a plant of the nightshade family, is native to the Mesoamerican population and Mexico. According to scientific reports, 14 new compounds were isolated from the wild tomatillo, including withaphysacarpin, ixocarpanolide, philadelphicalactone-A, C, D, and ixocarpalactone. These compounds these have potent anticancer effects in melanomas, thyroid, head and neck squamous cell cancers, breast cancer, glioblastoma brain tumors, and certain leukemias.

Tomato

Family: Solanaceae
Botanical name: *Solanum lycopersicum*
The tomato is an edible fruit that is consumed in diverse ways — raw or as an ingredient in many dishes, sauces, salads, and drinks. The major chemicals present in tomatoes are rubijervine, solanine, lycopene, and strigolactones. Lycopene is an antioxidant that has been found to prevent prostate malignancies. Many scientific reports have shown that tomato consumption is associated with a decreased risk of breast and head and neck cancers, as well as an agent against neurodegenerative diseases.

Turnip

Family: Brassicaceae
Botanical name: *Brassica rapa* var. *rapa*
Turnip is a root vegetable that is rich in vitamins A, C, and K. It is rich in lutein, which is known to inhibit colon, gastric, and liver cancers, as well

as leukemia. It is also known to inhibit gastric ulcers in experimental animals.

Winter squash

Family: Cucurbitaceae
Botanical name: *Cucurbita* species
Winter squash is harvested and eaten in the mature fruit stage. It contains high amounts of carbohydrates, dietary fiber, and vitamins A and C. The different varieties of winter squash include ambercup, banana, buttercup, hubbard, mooregold, cushaw, butternut, acorn, gem, and gold nugget squash. Winter squash contains compounds such as cucurbitacins and is known to prevent different cancers.

CONCLUSION

Above-mentioned are some of the important fruits and vegetables that have shown potential in the prevention and treatment of cancer. However, there are many edible fruits and vegetables found in the nature that have not been studied for cancer prevention and treatment. Therefore, more scientific studies are required for exploring their anticancer potential.

REFERENCES

1. Jemal, A., F. Bray, M.M. Center, J. Ferlay, E. Ward, and D. Forman, Global cancer statistics, *CA Cancer J Clin* **61**(2): 69–90 (2011).
2. Reson, M., Wilms' tumor and other pediatric renal masses, *Magn Reson Imaging Clin N Am* **16**(3): 479–497 (2008).
3. Morandeira, R., A.S. Marín, F. Pereferrer, H. Gonzalez, and E. Dejardin, Solid pseudopapillar tumour of the pancreas, *Cir Esp* **84**(1): 47–49 (2008).
4. Berenblum, I. and P. Shubik, The role of croton oil applications, associated with a single painting of a carcinogen, in tumour induction of the mouse's skin, *Br J Cancer* **1**(4): 379–382 (1947).
5. Stoppler, M.C., Lung cancer, causes, types, and treatment, retrieved from Medicine Net Inc., 2009. [Online] URL http://www.medicinenet.com/lung cancer, 2009.
6. Gavhane, Y.N., A.S. Shete, A.K. Bhagat, V.R. Shinde, K.K. Bhong, G.A. Khairnar, and A.V Yadav, Solid tumors: Facts, challenges and solutions, *IJPSR* **2**(1): 1–12 (2011).

7. Tsao, A.S., E.S. Kim, and W.K. Hong, Chemoprevention of cancer, *CA Cancer J Clin* **54**(3): 150–80 (2004).
8. Hong, W.K. and M.B. Sporn, Recent advances in chemoprevention of cancer, *Science* **278**(5340): 1073–1077 (1997).
9. Wattenberg, L.W., What are the critical attributes for cancer chemopreventive agents?, *Ann NY Acad Sci* **768**: 73–81 (1995).

2

Phytochemicals Safeguard the Genome: Tiny Molecules, Big Role

*Sanjit Dey**, *Nilanjan Das, Debdutta Ganguli, Mahuya Sinha, Kunal Sikder, Swaraj Bandhu Kesh, Dipesh Kr Das, Amitava Khan, Ujjal Das, Krishnendu Manna, Sushobhan Biswas, Anirban Pradhan and Rakhi Sharma Dey*

INTRODUCTION

The genome, the inner core of the organism, is guarded and cared for by Mother Nature by all means. However, the fact is that the genome encounters a huge number of threats from both exogenous as well as endogenous agents. A healthy genome translates to a healthy life for an organism. DNA and chromosomal breaks lead to a multitude of chaos like aging, cancer, neurodegenerative disorders. Therefore, safeguarding the genome is a big challenge for all organisms. The physiological systems present the best machineries to keep the genome intact, stable, and protected from most endogenous and exogenous threats.

Historical Aspects and Background

The human beings have adopted a wonderful balance with their habitat and availability of their diet. The prehistoric humans were more acquiescent with nature and they assumed a fruits and vegetables based diet. These diets

*Corresponding author: Sanjit Dey, Ph.D., Associate Professor, Department of Physiology, University of Calcutta, West Bengal-700009, India.

have shown benefits toward the health of the individual where physiological harmony is achieved. With the adoption of agriculture and advancements of industrial civilization, human beings have developed novel food habits. A large part of the modern human society is susceptible to unhealthy food habits, and humans are facing unwanted chemical exposure which is the byproduct of the detrimental lifestyle. Nevertheless, society has now realized the dangers due to widespread risk of disease due to the so-called flavorsome diet. In many occasions, these delicious diets lack essential micronutrients and phytonutrients. These tiny molecules or phytochemicals are a gift from Mother Nature to keep our genomes healthy against any challenge. These molecules play a big role due to their chemical structure.

Now, with growing consumer awareness and greater support from contemporary and state-of-the-art techniques that analyze the bioactive components of foods and their cellular targets, phytochemicals have been shown to prevent, delay, or even reverse diseases.

This chapter will review three different aspects of development of disease and its prevention strategies and remedy methods based on the current elucidation of the role of phytochemicals.

An overview of the current scientific developments of threats against genome structure and function will be given, along with an update of the current status of the biochemical potential of the wide variety of phytochemicals, with emphasis on their chemical basis in the metabolic process, leading to the safeguarding of the intricate harmony between the cell and organism as a whole.

THREATS AGAINST THE GENOME

Nature has taken all measures to safeguard its genomic template during the evolution process. In spite of that, the genome cannot completely escape hits from the physical, chemical, or biological weapons. Sometimes, the cell's own molecules may pose a threat and become a weapon. For example, the deficiency of micronutrients can mimic radiation which damage DNA by causing single- and double-strand breaks (SSBs and DSBs, respectively), oxidative lesions, or both since other balancing molecules are absent.[1] This decade-old observations in favor of micronutrients and vitamins are still pertinent. The most authenticated link between the lack of lifestyle issues and cancer and genome instability came from the

Professor Bruce Ames. In that order, he advocated chiefly on micronutrients such as minerals, vitamins, and phytochemicals, which actually can reverse, prevent, or delay the onset of chronic diseases. Professor Ames, the pioneering scientific campaigner of the benefits of consumption of fruits and vegetables in daily servings, identified that deficiencies of certain vitamins are of greatest threat to the human genome, which can result in a multitude of diseases.[2] On the other hand, with increasing interest in the field of clinical pathology and advancements of state-of-the-art technology in biomedical engineering, the beneficial role of fruits, vegetables, and their components have shown tremendous potential in combating our lifestyle disorders.[2–4]

There is evidence that an inadequate supply of nutrients can cause sizeable levels of genome mutation and alter the expression of genes required for genome maintenance. Thus, deficiencies in one or several micronutrients have been shown to cause DNA damage,[1] and are thought to be associated with a number of serious chronic or acute symptoms leading to fatal diseases; e.g., folic acid, niacin, and vitamins B_6 and B_{12} deficiencies may increase the risk of colon cancer, heart disease, and neurological dysfunction due to chromosomal breaks and faulty DNA repair mechanisms.[5] Chromosomal aberrations such as DSBs are a strong predictive factor for human cancer.[6]

In this regard, there are two major issues to be addressed: (1) do we know our enemies within?, and (2) are we prepared to counter these threats?

The direct threats to nucleotides and DNA are as causal as indirect threats. Therefore, we first need to identify the threats. We can classify these threats as follows:

(1) Single lesions: single pyrimidine and purine base lesions, intrastrand cross-links, purine cyclo-nucleosides, DNA-protein adducts, and interstrand cross-links;
(2) Tandem base lesions (OH• and one-electron oxidation); and
(3) DNA interstrand cross-links.

Hydroxyl Radicals

Hydroxyl radicals are one of the major causes of single base lesions. A hydroxyl radical efficiently reacts with nearby biomolecules. The most likely source of OH• in cells is the result of the Fenton reaction, which involves the reaction of reduced redox active metal ions, such as ferrous and cuprous ions, with H_2O_2 generated as metabolic byproduct. Thus, the chelators of the physiological system play a crucial role for this defense mechanism against reactive oxygen species (ROS) by aerobic organisms. Many phytochemicals are efficient metal-binding chelators and some proteins in mammalian system (e.g., ferritin) are excellent chelators to minimize the concentration of labile metal ions. In this mechanism, catalase and peroxidases are also involved to minimize the concentration of H_2O_2.

Singlet Oxygen

Singlet oxygen ($^1O_2$) is a major contributor of the UV radiation-mediated oxidation reactions to cellular DNA.[5,6] It reacts selectively with guanine components at the exclusion of other nucleobases and the 2-deoxyribose moiety.[7] In the latter case, this is consistent with the inability of singlet oxygen to induce DNA strand breaks in cells in significant amounts.[7]

Superoxide Radicals

DNA and its associated structures and other biomolecular structures are subject to attack by oxidation products due to the generation of superoxide radical ($O^{2\bullet-}$) during mitochondrial respiration and other pathways. The superoxide release is aggravated under the stress conditions such as mitochondrial dysfunction, inflammatory response, iron overload, or activation of xanthine oxidoreductase. The reasons for the excess oxidative species productions are multiple such as ischemia–reperfusion,[8] aging, diabetes mellitus,[9,10] obesity,[11] infertility,[12] neurodegenerative diseases,[13–15] and malignant tumors.[16] There are numerous exogenous chemical sources of $O^{2\bullet-}$ that include ultrafine particles,[16] cigarette smoke, and xenobiotics. Spontaneous or enzymatically driven dismutation of $O^{2\bullet-}$ gives rise to poorly reactive H_2O_2 that is converted upon reduction by transition metals according to the so-called Fenton reaction to highly reactive hydroxyl radicals.

One-Electron Oxidants

Several biologically relevant systems are able to induce one-electron reactions of nucleobases whose one-electron ionization potentials decrease in the following order: guanine, adenine, cytosine, and thymine. Ionizing radiation and high-intensity 266 nm-ns laser photolysis are able to ionize all of the five main DNA bases with similar efficiency; whereas most type I photosensitizers including 6-thioguanine mainly target guanine.

Hypochlorous Acid

Hypochlorous acid (HOCl) is generated in neutrophils during inflammation upon activation of myeloperoxidase, which triggers the reaction of chloride anion with H_2O_2 as one of the main cellular systems for eradicating microorganisms. Major achievements have been made in the quantitative and accurate measurement of several oxidatively generated single base lesions in cellular DNA resulting from the exposure to OH•, one-electron oxidants, $^1O_2$, and HOCl. It appears that the levels of base damage are much lower, by about two orders of magnitude, compared to those estimated at the end of the 1990s. It remains to be established what is the biological relevance of most of the single oxidized bases, which in most cases are efficiently removed through base excision repair.

Oxidative intermediates formed may lead to the development of lesions in DNA in the presence or absence of oxygen. DNA interstrand cross-links, and photo-induced DNA damage in the presence or absence of sensitization may also cause serious consequences and render the genome unstable. Some studies have provided more than a simple association between these harmful agents leading to the neurodegeneration,[15] aging, and/or enhancement of carcinogenesis. In most cases, these agents are responsible for oxidative DNA damage either by causing SSBs or DSBs.

Other Intermediates

There is recent information concerning the formation of DNA-protein and interstrand DNA cross-links caused by the one-electron oxidation of guanine bases. Efforts should now be made to search for the formation of these two types of complex damage in cellular DNA whose biological role remains to be assessed. It is now possible to propose comprehensive mechanisms of DNA damage arising from ionizing radiation and the damaging effects of solar radiation on DNA in the human skin.

Epigenetic Modification

Epigenetic changes are inherited alterations in DNA that affect gene expression and function without altering the DNA sequence. DNA methylation is one of the epigenetic processes implicated in human disease that is influenced by diet. DNA methylation involves the addition of a 1-C moiety to cytosine groups in DNA. The threat to the genome is not only to the nucleic acid itself, but to the protein component as well. DNA wraps around an octameric complex of core histones H2A, H2B, H3, and H4, which form nucleosomes built by several amino acids which are methylated or acetylated by specific enzymes at specific signals. Reactive species such as ROS generated either by radiation, metabolic processes, or replication stress can cause SSBs or DSBs and create DNA-protein cross-links, adducts, or other non-functional structures which prove useless or pose a burden to the machineries responsible for normal cellular milieu. Thus, endogenous as well as by exogenous agents like UV radiation, radiotherapy, or other genotoxic agents are thought to be the cause of most dangerous lesions threatening genomic integrity.

MOLECULES THAT SAFEGUARD THE GENOME

The Food Elements: Fruits and Vegetables

Mother Nature is very kind to all her creatures. She has presented a wonderful gift from her own garden. Human beings and even all the living beings have learned to sustain their lives based on the elements provided by her. Based on the *in vitro* studies and extrapolation of the epidemiological data, the crucial role of phytochemicals from fruits, vegetables, and spices is now well-known. The overall beneficial aspect leading to the reversal of multitude of diseases is increasingly endorsed with the insight from sophisticated experimental validation. The research results are consistent with the strong correlation between a high intake of fruits and vegetables, which are the principal source of dietary antioxidants, and reduction in cancer risk by as much as half.[1,7,17]

In the context of prevention, the word most widely discussed is 'antioxidant.' The literal meaning of antioxidant is a substance which prevents oxidation. This definition is especially relevant in biological systems. Other functions of antioxidants include peroxide decomposition, singlet oxygen quenching, and inhibition of enzymes such as NADH oxidase, succinoxidase, ATPase, and nitric oxide synthase (NOS). On the other hand, these antioxidants are usually strong reducing agents which when in proximity with reactive species take up the electron or oxidizing groups. These reactions actually prevent further reaction of electrons of important structural and functional molecules of the cell or subcellular structures. The antioxidant activity of the group of compounds is predominantly determined by their structures, in particular the electron delocalization over an aromatic nucleus, as in a phenolic structure. There is delocalization of the gained electron over the phenolic antioxidant when these compounds react with free radicals, and the stabilization by the resonance effect of the aromatic nucleus prevents the continuation of the free radical chain reaction. This phenomenon is often called radical scavenging, but polyphenolic compounds inhibit oxidation through a variety of mechanisms.[17–23] Gutteridge and Halliwell[24] defined an antioxidant as any substance that, when present at low concentrations relative to that of an oxidizable substrate, significantly delays or prevents the oxidation of that substrate.

Antioxidants can be classified into two groups, namely chain-breaking (primary) antioxidants and preventative (secondary) antioxidants.[23] Chain-breaking antioxidants act by scavenging free radicals and donating hydrogen atoms. Preventative antioxidants are generally metal chelators and reductants capable of sparing other antioxidants *in vivo*. The anticancer activity of flavonoids has been attributed to a large variety of different mechanisms.[24–26]

In general, these food components are not essential elements of food. However, the causal role of these bioactive elements against dysfunctional metabolism leading to DNA and biomolecular damage is gaining more attention with their mechanisms of actions being elucidated.[22,24] In the current review, we will analyze how some well-established structured phytochemicals participate in defending attacks against the genome.

Flavonoids

These are the major bioactive group of food phenolic compounds, capable of preventing or reversing a range of events leading to human metabolic or lifestyle disorders. In their support, several *in vitro* or animal experiments have documented that flavonoids possess antioxidant and antimutagenic activities.[1,2,24] In many ways, flavonoids confer protection against chronic diseases such as atherosclerosis and cancer and other physiological management. This ability of reducing the burden of ROS is inherent to their chemical structure, where they can exchange the electrons from the reactive species mentioned above. They have also been implicated to reduce the risk of cardiovascular disease and stroke.[9] Isoflavonoids too perform a range of hormonal and non-hormonal activities in animals or *in vitro*,[25–28] suggesting potential human health benefits of diets rich in these compounds. Flavonoids act as antioxidants to inhibit free radical mediated hepatotoxicity and lipid peroxidation.[15–17] Now, the question is how do they mediate their effects? The antioxidant mechanisms of flavonoids fall under free radical chain breaking, metal chelating, singlet oxygen quenching, or with the inhibition of enzymatic activity. Flavonoids including naringenin, hesperetin, and apigenin were also found to form pro-oxidant metabolites that oxidize NADH and glutathione upon oxidation by peroxidase/hydrogen peroxide. Flavonoids have been reported to chelate iron and copper and this may partly explain their antioxidant effects. The chemical structure of flavonoids is crucial and explains why these compounds are vital in food and health maintenance.

Let us now have a look at what are the major plant-derived phytochemicals and why these are being established as potential saviors of human health disorders.

Carotenoids

Carotenoids, including xanthophylls (oxygen-containing carotenoids) are naturally occurring colored pigments in plants. About 600 specific carotenoids have been identified, mostly from plants and algae.

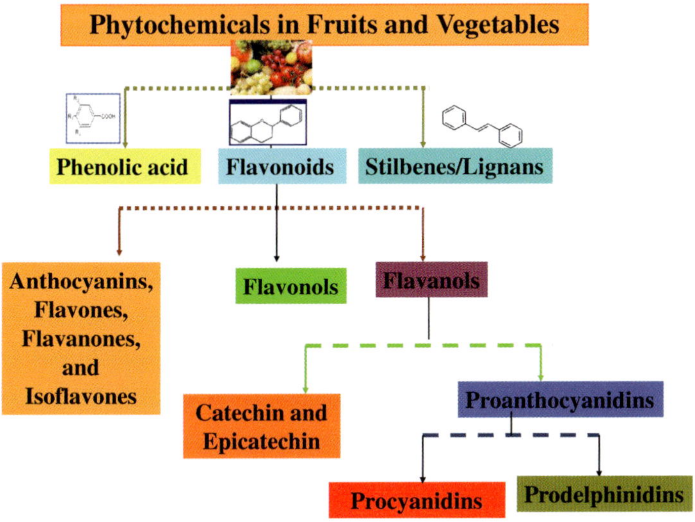

Figure 2.1: Phytochemicals in fruits and vegetables — the major chemicals that participate in safeguarding the genome.

Carotenoids have the capacity to trap not only lipid peroxyl radicals, but also singlet oxygen species.[29] The essential role of carotenoids as a major dietary source of vitamin A has been known for many years. Although all carotenoids contain extensive conjugated double bonds, individual carotenoids differ in their antioxidant potential in humans.

Polyphenolics

Polyphenolics is a general term that covers many different subgroups of phenolic acids and flavonoids. More than 5,000 polyphenolics, including over 2,000 flavonoids have been identified, and the number is still growing.[29] Polyphenolics vary in structure; hydroxybenzoic acids and hydroxycinnamic acids have a single-ring structure. Flavonoids can be further classified into anthocyanins, flavan-3-ols, flavones, flavanones, and flavonols. Some of the flavonoids such as flavan-3-ols can be found in dimmers, trimmers, and polymers.

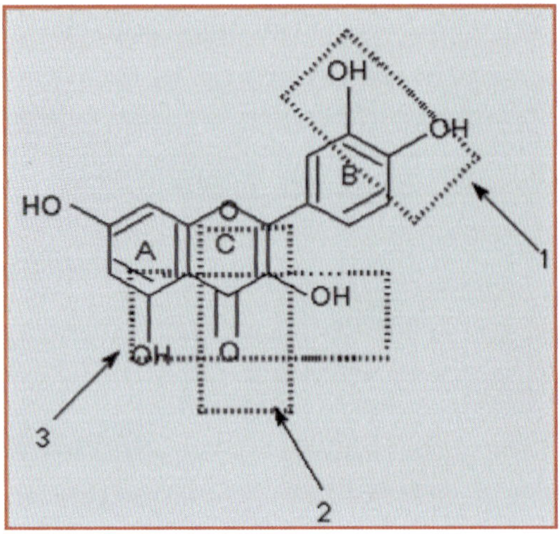

Figure 2.2: Structural characteristics of flavonoids conferring maximum antioxidant activity: (1) the ortho-3′ 4′-dihydroxy moiety in the B-ring; (2) the 2,3-double bond in combination with the 4-keto group; (3) the 3- and 5-hydroxyl groups in the C- and A-ring, respectively, in combination with the 4-keto group in the C-ring.

Polyunsaturated Fatty Acids, Plant Sterols, and Phytoestrogens

These are three different groups of phytoelements with potential to participate in a multitude of biological processes. Polyunsaturated fatty acids are essential components of our diets having either n-3 or n-6 PUFAs. The n-3s are elements with most potential that lower the risks of chronic diseases. There are several experimental and observational data showing the physiological benefits of using PUFA.[29]

More than 200 sterols or stanols have been identified. The most abundant sterols are β-sitosterol, stigmasterol, and campesterol. We have shown that β-sitosterol is capable of reducing the high fat diet induced oxidative stress and inflammatory developments which are one of the leading cause of DNA metabolism disorders (unpublished data).

Dietary phytoestrogens are plant-derived dietary components that exhibit structural and functional similarities which mimic the effects of estrogen and its groups of derivatives. The dietary phytoestrogens belong to four subclasses of the polyphenolics: isoflavonoids, isoflavones, lignans, and stilbenes (e.g., resveratrol).

Isothiocyanates

This group of compounds, derived from cruciferous vegetables, take part in many unique mechanisms. These are highly bioavailable electrophilic compounds that participate in anti-inflammatory as well as mitochondrial metabolism.[29] At subtoxic doses, they act as chemoprotective agents against chemically induced carcinogens by blocking the initiation of tumors in a variety of mammalian tissues. They exhibit their effect by inducing phase I and phase II enzymes, inhibiting enzyme activation, modifying steroid hormone metabolism, and protecting against oxidative damages.[30]

Micronutrients

Micronutrients, which are minerals including the trace elements, play a major role in defining good genome health. It is increasingly evident that the risk for developing degenerative diseases increases with greater DNA damage, which in turn is dependent on micronutrient status.[31,32]

A damaged genome has huge repercussions on the cell, and an organism has to pay the price for it at all stages of life. An ongoing prospective cohort studies in European countries showed that the causative factor of cancer, neurodegenerative diseases, as well as accelerated aging was the higher incidence of chromosomal damage. It has also been suggested that an individual with suboptimal intake of micronutrients can be more prone to the effects of genome damage. There is a clear correlation between accelerated aging syndrome with suboptimal DNA repair or imbalance redox potential.[28,32]

Our laboratory is currently engaged with elucidating preventive mechanisms against cellular challenges developed due to reactive species. We have documented the cellular threats using different model systems in terms of protection of DNA in cell-free conditions, in single cells, in SSBs or DSBs, and in membrane damage. To protect these indispensible biomolecular structures, we introduced assays which gave us proof of the concept that signaling routes leading to DNA breakage or signaling events after DNA breakage leading to apoptosis or disruption of cell cycle occurs after reactive species-mediated damage (unpublished data). Subsequently, our laboratory has also assessed the potential of several substances: the leaf and seed extracts of *Moringa oleifera*, also known as drumstick tree; Sea Buck throne, an indigenous flora of the Himalayan belt; coconut water concentrate or green and black tea (extract concentrate); and some of their vital components like quercetin, ferulic acid, and epicatechin which are either common vegetables and/or fruit components. We have shown that the leaf extract of *Moringa oleifera* not only prevents DNA damage, it also effectively prevents inflammation originated from reactive species regulating NF-κB, a crucial transcription factor.[18–22] The individual components of this plant are also responsible for the development of any damage if they are administered together with a high-fat diet. A high-fat diet triggers the production of ROS; the former also induces mitochondrial processes and an array of signaling cascades, leading to inflammation, steatohepatitis, apoptosis, and insulin resistance, which are the hallmarks of a disorder called metabolic syndrome. The recent guidelines by the National Cancer Institute promote the regular consumption of vegetables and fruits, encouraging plant-based diets and discouraging the intake of high-fat food and alcohol, if at all in the beverage list. Hence, DNA or genome protection is not mediated by any single mechanism. The whole cellular milieu is responsible for maintaining the delicate balance to safeguard the genome. Vegetables, fruits, and a healthy lifestyle can greatly minimize the risk of these threats.

Among the 40 different micronutrients required in our daily diet for healthy living, many micronutrients like vitamins and minerals are necessary as enzyme cofactors and also part of proteins (or enzymes) involved in DNA synthesis and repair, prevention of oxidative damage, and maintenance of genome stability.[1,2] As already mentioned, one of the causes of DNA damage is micronutrient deficiency, which ultimately leads to serious human diseases such as cancer and neurodegenerative diseases. The level of genome damage caused by exposure to sizeable doses of environmental factors such as chemical carcinogens and UV radiation are similar to that caused by moderate micronutrient deficiency, which is of increasing concern today.[17]

Optimal intakes of individual micronutrients can ensure a healthy and harmonious quality of life. The deficiencies may lead to many disorders as a result of DNA damage.[3] However, there exist great variations in the intake among individuals due to physiological or other lifestyle demands like cultural and religious issues. Here lies a demand of personalized nutritional status for individuals with unique mitochondrial and chromosomal DNA composition. There is no single amount of micronutrients and phytoelements to guarantee the protection of the genome from damage. The issues also change with aging and other consequences. Thus, the sustenance of health for a long life span will vary among the individuals and among different situations.[4,29]

PHYTOCHEMICAL AND GENOME/DNA STABILITY: A FRUITFUL SOLUTION

The Role of HAT/HDAC, Fruits, and Vegetables

The octameric core complex of histones H2A, H2B, H3, and H4 protects the DNA in a robust way. However, there are several endogenous agents or physical phenomena such as reactive species, replication stress, or exogenous agents (e.g., UV irradiation, radiotherapy, or other genotoxic agents) that may prove fatal in terms of genomic integrity if there are DSBs. The DSBs are critical and their repair is also a complex phenomenon.[17,33–37] There is growing interest and evidence that the epigenetic mechanisms which affect DNA methylation and histone status contribute to genomic instability. The DNA damage response, for example, is modulated by the acetylation status of histone and non-histone proteins, and by the opposing activities of histone acetyltransferase (HAT) and histone deacetylase (HDAC) enzymes. Many HDACs which are overexpressed in cancer cells have been implicated in protecting such cells from genotoxic insults. Thus, HDAC inhibitors, in addition to unsilencing tumor suppressor genes, also can silence DNA repair pathways, inactivate non-histone proteins that are required for DNA stability, and induce ROS production and DSBs.

Currently, elucidating the role of HDACs in maintaining genome stability is a popular area of research among epigenesists. Histone hyperacetylation induced by HDAC inhibitors causes structural alterations in the chromatin. This can open up regions of DNA that are normally protected among the nucleosomes in the heterochromatin enabling DNA-damaging agents to gain access to the exposed template. Importantly, HDAC inhibitors have been shown to decrease the expression of a number of DNA repair proteins.[38] There are validations using *in vitro* and *in vivo* experiments involving clinical trials to establish whether transcription mediates HDAC inhibitor activities or whether non-transcriptional targets of HDAC inhibitors are playing the role. HDAC inhibitors can wreak havoc by targeting multiple signaling and repair mechanisms in DNA damage pathways and histones and non-histone proteins to regulate genomic structure and function.[39–42]

CHROMOSOMAL DNA AND TELOMERE STABILITY: ROLE OF VITAMINS AND PHYTOCHEMICALS

Nutrigenomics refers to the effect of diet on DNA stability and gene expression.[43] Suboptimal nutrient supplies can cause considerable levels of genome mutation and alter the expression of genes required for genome maintenance, which are in turn unique to individuals. However, deficiencies in several micronutrients and phytonutrients which are potent in causing DNA damage and are thought to be associated with a number of serious human diseases are reversed or delayed by appropriate administration of folic acid, niacin, and vitamins B6 and B12. In many cases, they prevent the risk of colon cancer, heart disease, and neurological dysfunction due to chromosomal breaks and dysfunctional DNA repair. Vitamin C deficiency increases cataract and cancer risks due to DNA oxidation. Insufficient vitamin E levels may have a role in increasing the risk of colon cancer, heart disease, and immune dysfunction via DNA oxidation. Zinc deficiency is associated with memory loss due to chromosome breaks.[32]

Telomeres are nucleoprotein structures which basically protect the ends of chromosomes and hence, maintain chromosome stability. These structures are also responsible for the prevention of end-to-end fusion of chromosomes during cell division. Degradation of telomeres has been shown to lead to whole chromosomal instability, an important risk factor for cancer.[33,34] These structures are sensitive to folate and nicotinic acid deficiencies, and together with increased oxidative stress, may accelerate telomere dysfunction. Such metabolic imbalances may possibly explain the observed associations between telomere shortening and a number of conditions including obesity, psychological stress, immune dysfunction, cancer, and cardiovascular disease.[44–46]

Under folate-deficient conditions, the base uracil is incorporated into DNA instead of thymidine, leading to chromosomal breakage. In addition, folate and vitamin B12 play a critical role in the maintenance of DNA methylation which, apart from its importance for transcriptional control of gene expression, determines the structural stability of important regions of the chromosomes. There is strong evidence that defects in the DNA methylation process can cause excessive telomere dysfunctions.[46,47] It is therefore possible that a deficiency of folate and other methyl donors may also result in telomere instability by causing the poor maintenance of methylation. Nicotinic acid (niacin) is another dietary micronutrient that is known to play a fundamental role in chromosome integrity and reduction of cancer risk.[48]

Damage to DNA, lipids, and proteins induced by ROS or reactive nitrogen species (RNS) or their active end products are mostly managed by antioxidants (e.g., phytochemicals, vitamins A, C, and E, and others) as well as enzymatic mechanisms such as superoxide dismutase and catalase.[47,48] Under the conditions of increased levels of free radicals and/or low levels of antioxidants, there would be an imbalance, leaning toward lack of prevention amd repair. In *in vitro* studies, antioxidant treatment has been found to prevent telomere abrasion and thus increase cellular lifespan;[1,25,27,43,44] however, whether similar effects can be achieved *in vivo* remains uncertain.

Micronutrients and Polymorphisms

Some cases of micronutrient deficiencies along with certain polymorphisms can worsen existing DNA damage.[45,46] The reasons are mainly due to poor diet and that the variant genes are not able to process the nutrients appropriately.[45] Approximately 50 human genetic diseases have been attributed to these so-called enzyme polymorphisms. Such common genetic variations may alter the activity of genes that affect the bioavailability of micronutrients and/or the affinity for micronutrient cofactors in key enzymes involved, for example, in DNA metabolism or repair.[46,47] Supplementation of a diet enriched with phytochemicals, vitamins, and minerals could, in some cases, help to overcome the inherited metabolic blocks in key DNA maintenance pathways, potentially decreasing cancer risk.[43] A plausible clue is that the enhanced concentration of a cofactor or providing phytochemicals in the diet by supplementation is expected to be particularly effective when a mutation (polymorphism) in a gene decreases the binding affinity for its cofactor resulting in a lower reaction rate.[48–52]

Studies on the common mutations in methylenetetrahydrofolate reductase (MTHFR) gene polymorphisms have been implicated in modulating the effects on the risk of developmental defects and cancer. There are significant interactions between MTHFR C677T, its cofactor riboflavin, and folic acid in relation to chromosomal and genome instability; high riboflavin concentration increases instability under low folic acid conditions.[48,50]

In addition to cancer, a number of genetic variations have been shown to increase the susceptibility to micronutrient-related diseases, such as type 2 diabetes mellitus, obesity, cardiovascular diseases, and some autoimmune disorders. The vitamin D3 receptor (VDR) gene, which encodes the nuclear hormone receptor for vitamin D3, belongs to the family of transcriptional regulatory factors.[51,52] Targets of this receptor are principally involved in mineral metabolism though the receptor regulates a variety of other metabolic pathways, such as those involved in immune response and cancer. Polymorphism of the *VDR* gene has been linked to bone mineral density, and also to multiple chronic diseases such as cancer — mainly breast cancer,[24] prostate cancer and malignant melanoma,[22–25] type 2 diabetes mellitus, Parkinson's disease, lung diseases, gastrointestinal diseases, multiple sclerosis, and periodontal disease.[51,52]

It is evident that micronutrients play an important role in genome maintenance. Damage to the genome is the most critical event that can lead to dysfunction. It is essential that greater attention is given to the nutritional requirements for genome-health maintenance. Development of dietary patterns, functional foods, and supplements that are designed to improve genome-health maintenance in humans with specific genetic backgrounds may provide an important contribution to a new cost-effective health strategy based on the diagnosis and individualized nutritional prevention of genome instability (e.g., chromosomal and telomere aberrations) and neurodegenerative diseases.[52,53] Although it is not yet possible to make distinct dietary recommendations for the prevention of

DNA damage based solely on an individual's genetic background, it is feasible to use current diagnostics to determine whether dietary patterns or supplement recommendations actually result in benefit or harm to the genome of an individual.

CONCLUSION

The physiological, biochemical, and chemical roles of phytochemicals have been identified and defined. These findings are illuminating new strategies for therapy. These compounds can either be used as supplements as inhibitors of certain signaling molecules or as activators of protection molecules. On the other hand, the pro-oxidant role of some structurally potent phytochemicals as potential drug targets might be fruitful. The key idea is to destabilize the genome of pathologic cells over normal cells by keeping the latter genome intact.

ACKNOWLEDGMENT

Sanjit Dey acknowledges the funding from DBT, DST, CSIR, UGC, UGC-DAE, NTRF Government of India and WB DBT, Government of West Bengal, and Rakhi Sharma Dey acknowledges UGC, Government of India for a minor grant.

REFERENCES

1. Ames, B.N., DNA damage from micronutrient deficiencies is likely to be a major cause of cancer, *Mutation Res* **475**: 7–20 (2001).
2. Ames, B.N., M.K. Shigenaga, and T.M. Hagen, Oxidants, antioxidants, and the degenerative diseases of aging, *Proc Natl Acad Sci* **90**(17): 7915–7922 (1993).
3. Ames, B.N., Delaying the mitochondrial decay of aging, *Ann NY Acad Sci* **1019**: 406–411 (2004).
4. Ames, B.N., L.S. Gold, and W.C. Willett, The causes and prevention of cancer, *Proc Natl Acad Sci* **92**: 5258–5265 (1995).
5. Cadet, J., T. Douki, and J.L. Ravanat, Oxidatively generated damage to the guanine moiety of DNA: Mechanistic aspects and formation in cells, *Acc Chem Res* **41**: 1075–1083 (2008).

6. Cadet, J., T. Douki, J.L. Ravanat, and P. Di Mascio, Sensitized formation of oxidatively generated damage to cellular DNA by UVA radiation, *Photochem Photobiol Sci* **8**: 903–911 (2009).
7. Ravanat, J.L., S. Sauvaigo, S. Caillat, G.R. Martinez, M.H.G. Medeiros, P. Di Mascio, A. Favier, and J. Cadet, Singlet oxygen-mediated damage to cellular DNA determined by the comet assay associated with DNA repair enzymes, *Biol Chem* **385**: 17–20 (2004).
8. Bonassi, S., L. Hagmar, U. Strömberg, A.H. Montagud, H.A. Tinnerberg, P. Forni, S. Heikkilä, P. Wanders, I.L. Wilhardt, L.E. Hansteen, and H.N. Knudsen, Chromosomal aberrations in lymphocytes predict human cancer independently of exposure to carcinogens. European study group on cytogenetic biomarkers and health, *Cancer Res* **60**: 1619–1625 (2000).
9. Allen, C.L. and U. Bayraktutan, Oxidative stress and its role in the pathogenesis of ischaemic stroke, *Int J Stroke* **4**: 461–470 (2009).
10. Monteiro, R. and I. Azevedo, Chronic inflammation in obesity and the metabolic syndrome, *Mediators Inflamm* **2010**: 1–10 (2010).
11. Takayanagi, R., T. Inoguchi, and K. Ohnaka, Clinical and experimental evidence for oxidative stress as an exacerbating factor of diabetes mellitus, *J Clin Biochem Nutr* **48**: 72–77 (2011).
12. Zhang, H., C. Xie, H.J. Spencer, C. Zuo, M. Higuchi, G. Ranganathan, P.A. Kern, M.W. Chou, Q. Huang, B. Szczesny, S. Mitra, A.J. Watson, G.P. Margison, and C.Y. Fan, Obesity and hepatosteatosis in mice with enhanced oxidative DNA damage processing in mitochondria, *Am J Pathol* **178**: 1715–1727 (2011).
13. Aitken, R.J. and B.J. Curry, Redox regulation of human function: From the physiological control of sperm capacitation to the etiology of infertility and DNA damage in the germ line, *Antioxid Redox Signal* **14**: 367–381 (2011).
14. Martin, L.J., Mitochondrial and cell death mechanisms in neurodegenerative diseases, *Pharmaceuticals* **3**: 839–915 (2010).
15. Gille, G. and H. Reichmann, Iron-dependent functions of mitochondria — relation to neurodegeneration, *J Neural Transm* **118**: 349–359 (2011).
16. Lawless, M.W., K.J. O'Byrne, and S.G. Gray, Targeting oxidative stress in cancer, *Expert Opin Ther Targets* **14**: 1225–1245 (2010).
17. Bidlack, W.R. and R.L. Rodriguez, *Nutritional Genomics*, CRC Press, Taylor and Francis, Florida, USA (2012).
18. Reuter S., S.C. Gupta, M.M. Chaturvedi, and B.B. Aggarwal, Oxidative stress, inflammation, and cancer: How are they linked, *Free Radic Biol Med* **49**: 1603–1616 (2010).
19. Das, D.K., M. Sinha, A. Khan, K. Das, K. Manna, and S. Dey, Radiation protection by major tea polyphenol, epicatechin, *Int J Hum Genet* **13**(1): 59–64 (2013).

20. Sikder, K., M. Sinha, N. Das, D.K. Das, S. Datta, and S. Dey, *Moringa oleifera* leaf extract prevents *in vitro* oxidative DNA damage, *Asian J Pharm Clin Res* **6**(2): 92–96 (2013).
21. Das, N., K. Sikder, S. Ghosh, B. Fromenty, and S. Dey, *Moringa oleifera* Lam. leaf extract prevents early liver injury and restores antioxidant status in mice fed with high-fat diet, *Indian J Exp Biol* **50**(6): 404–412 (2012).
22. Sinha, M., D.K. Das, K. Manna, S. Datta, T. Ray, A.K. Sil, and S. Dey, Epicatechin ameliorates ionizing radiation-induced oxidative stress in mice liver, *Free Radic Res* **46**(7): 842–849 (2012).
23. Das, N., K. Sikder, S. Bhattacharjee, S.B. Majumdar, S. Ghosh, S. Majumdar, and S. Dey, Quercetin alleviates inflammation after short term treatment in high fat fed mice, *Food Funct* **4**(6): 489–498 (2013).
24. Gutteridge, J.M. and B. Halliwell, Free radicals and antioxidants in the year 2000. A historical look to the future, *Ann NY Acad Sci* **899**: 136–147 (2000).
25. Ames B.N., Low micronutrient intake may accelerate the degenerative diseases of aging through allocation of scarce micronutrients by triage, *Proc Natl Acad Sci* **103**: 17589–17594 (2006).
26. Fenech, M., Nutritional treatment of genome instability: A paradigm shift in disease prevention and in the setting of recommended dietary allowances, *Nutr Res Rev* **16**: 109–122 (2003).
27. Fenech, M., P. Baghurst, W. Luderer, J. Turner, S. Record, M. Ceppi, and S. Bonassi, Low intake of calcium, folate, nicotinic acid, vitamin E, retinol, beta-carotene and high intake of pantothenic acid, biotin and riboflavin are significantly associated with increased genome instability–results from a dietary intake and micronucleus index survey in South Australia, *Carcinogenesis* **26**: 991–999 (2005).
28. Ames, B.N., A role for supplements in optimizing health: The metabolic tune-up, *Arch Biochem Biophys* **423**: 227–234 (2004).
29. Fenech, M., The role of folic acid and vitamin B12 in genomic stability of human cells, *Mutat Res* **475**: 56–67 (2001).
30. Jeffery, E.H., Diet and detoxification enzymes, *Altern Ther Health Med* **13**(2): S98–S99 (2007).
31. Bull, C. and M. Fenech, Genome-health nutrigenomics and nutrigenetics: Nutritional requirements or 'nutriomes' for chromosomal stability and telomere maintenance at the individual level, *Proc Nutr Soc* **67**: 146–156 (2008).
32. Ames, B.N. and P. Wakimoto, Are micronutrient deficiencies a major cancer risk? *Nat Rev Cancer* **2**: 694–704 (2002).
33. Callen, E. and J. Surralles, Telomere dysfunction in genome instability syndromes, *Mutat Res* **567**: 85–104 (2004).

34. Brouilette, S., R.K. Singh, J.R. Thompson, A.H. Goodall, and N.J. Samani, White cell telomere length and risk of premature myocardial infarction, *Arterioscler Thromb Vasc Biol* **23**: 842–846, (2003).
35. Cawthon, R.M., K.R. Smith, E. O'Brien, A. Sivatchenko, and R.A. Kerber, Association between telomere length in blood and mortality in people aged 60 years or older, *Lancet* **361**: 393–395 (2003).
36. Epel, E.S., E.H. Blackburn, J. Lin, F.S. Dhabhar, N.E. Adler, J.D. Morrow, and R.M. Cawthon, Accelerated telomere shortening in response to life stress, *Proc Natl Acad Sci* **101**: 17312–17315 (2004).
37. Valdes, A.M., T. Andrew, J.P. Gardner, M. Kimura, E. Oelsner, L.F. Cherkas, A. Aviv, and T.D. Spector, Obesity, cigarette smoking, and telomere length in women, *Lancet* **366**: 662–664 (2005).
38. Rajendran, P., E. Ho, D.E. Williams, and R.H. Dashwood, Dietary phytochemicals, HDAC inhibition, and DNA damage/repair defects in cancer cells, *Clin Epigenet* **3**(4): 1–23 (2011).
39. Robert, T., F. Vanoli, I. Chiolo, G. Shubassi, K.A. Bernstein, R. Rothstein, O.A. Botrugno, *et al.*, HDACs link the DNA damage response, processing of double-strand breaks and autophagy, *Nature* **471**: 74–79 (2011).
40. Putiri, E.L. and K.D. Robertson, Epigenetic mechanisms and genome stability, *Clin Epigenet* **2**: 299–314 (2010).
41. Purrucker, J.C. and U. Mahlknecht, Targeting the epigenome: Effects of epigenetic treatment strategies on genomic stability in healthy human cells, *Clin Epigenet* **1**: 45–54 (2010).
42. Lichtenstein, A.V., Cancer: Evolutionary, genetic and epigenetic aspects, *Clin Epigenet* **1**: 8–100 (2010).
43. Gonzalo, S., I. Jaco, M.F. Fraga, T. Chen, E. Li, M. Esteller, and M.A. Blasco, DNA methyltransferases control telomere length and telomere recombination in mammalian cells, *Nat Cell Biol* **8**: 416–424 (2006).
44. Kirkland, J.B., Niacin and carcinogenesis, *Nutr Cancer* **46**: 110–118 (2003).
45. Evans, M.E., M. Dizdaroglu, and M.S. Cooke, Oxidative DNA damage and disease: induction, repair and significance, *Mutat Res* **567**: 1–61 (2004).
46. Kimura, M., K. Umegaki, M. Higuchi, P. Thomas, P and M. Fenech, MTHFR C677T polymorphism, folic acid and riboflavin are important determinants of genome stability in cultured human lymphocytes, *J Nutr* **134**: 48–56 (2004).
47. Raimondi, S., H. Johansson, P. Maisonneuve, and S. Gandini, Review and meta-analysis on vitamin D receptor polymorphisms and cancer risk, *Carcinogenesis* **30**(7): 1170–1180 (2009).

48. Hossein-nezhad, A., K. Mirzaei, P. Shabani, A. Najmafshar, S. Emamgholipour, M. Rahmani, and B. Larijani, Association of VDR gene polymorphism with insulin resistance in diabetic patients, *Iran J Diabetes Lipid Disord* **8**: 18 (2009).
49. Butler, M.W., A. Burt, T.L. Edwards, S. Zuchner, W.K. Scott, E.R. Martin, J.M. Vance, and L. Wang, Vitamin D receptor gene as a candidate gene for Parkinson disease, *Ann Hum Genet* **75**(2): 201–210 (2011).
50. Sharma, P.R., S. Singh, M. Jena, G. Mishra, R. Prakash, P.K. Das, R.N. Bamezai, and P.K. Tiwari, Coding and non-coding polymorphisms in VDR gene and susceptibility to pulmonary tuberculosis in tribes, castes and Muslims of Central India, *Infect Genet Evol* **11**(6): 1456–1461 (2011).
51. Ramagopalan, S.V., N.J. Maugeri, L. Handunnetthi, M.R. Lincoln, S.M. Orton, D.A. Dyment, G.C. Deluca, B.M. Herrera, M.J. Chao, A.D. Sadovnick, G.C. Ebers, and J.C. Knight, Expression of the multiple sclerosis-associated MHC class II allele HLA-DRB1*1501 is regulated by vitamin D, *PLoS Genet* **5**(2): e1000369 (2009).
52. Lonergan, R., K. Kinsella, P. Fitzpatrick, J. Brady, B. Murray, C. Dunne, R. Hagan, M. Duggan, S. Jordan, M. McKenna, M. Hutchinson, and N. Tubridy, Multiple sclerosis prevalence in Ireland: Relationship to vitamin D status and HLA genotype, *J Neurol Neurosurg Psychiatry* **82**(3): 317–322 (2011).
53. Aggarwal, B.B., H. Kumar, and S. Dey, Prevention and treatment of neurodegenerative diseases by spice-derived phytochemicals, Packer, L., H. Sies, M. Eggersdorfer, and E. Cadenas (Eds.), in *Micronutrients and Brain Health*, CRC Press (2010).
54. Kunnumakkara, A.B., C. Kocha, J.G. Chung, and S. Dey, The mint (Menthol), Aggarwal, B.B. and A. Kunnumakkra (Eds.), in *Molecular Targets and Therapeutic Uses of Spices*, World Scientific Publishing (2009).

3

Phytonutrients from Fruits and Vegetables in Breast Cancer Control

Madhumita Roy, Apurba Mukherjee,*
Sutapa Mukherjee and Jaydip Biswas

INTRODUCTION

The overall burden of cancer in the world continues to rise with the increase in population as well as changes in lifestyle and dietary habits of the people. The most common types of cancer cases today involve the lung, breast, cervical, colorectal, and stomach. Breast cancer is one of the leading cancer types diagnosed in women today. This cancer is of importance as early detection and treatment of this disease can lead to significant prognosis. Although survival rates of breast cancer have improved considerably in the last decade, efforts are still needed to reduce the burden of this disease.

Breast cancer is a malignant (cancerous) growth that begins in the tissues of the breast. Breast cancer is the most common cancer in women, but it can also appear in men. It can be invasive or non-invasive. In invasive breast cancer, the cancer cells spread from inside the lobules or ducts to invade nearby tissue, thereby reaching the lymph nodes and eventually

*Corresponding author: Madhumita Roy, Ph.D., Department Environmental Carcinogenesis and Toxicology, Chittranjan National Cancer Institute. 37, S P Mukherjee Road, Kolkata, West Bengal, India. Tel: (+91) 33-2746-5101, Fax: (+91) 33-2475-7606, Email: mitacnci@yahoo.co.in.

leading to metastasis to the bones, liver or lungs. In non-invasive breast cancer, the cancer cells do not spread and remains confined to its place of origin. Breast cancer can originate in different areas of the breast like the ducts, the lobules, and the tissue in between. Cancer developing inside the lobules is termed lobular carcinoma *in situ*, whereas that in the milk ducts is called ductal carcinoma *in situ*. Women suffering from these forms are at high risk of developing invasive breast cancer. The forms of invasive breast cancer include invasive ductal carcinoma and invasive lobular carcinoma. Other forms of breast cancer which are less commonly seen are inflammatory breast cancer, triple-negative (ER, PR, and HER2-negative) breast cancer, Paget's disease of the nipple, phyllodes tumor, and angiosarcoma.

INCIDENCE AND MORTALITY OF BREAST CANCER

Breast cancer is the second most common cancer diagnosed in women worldwide. An estimated 1.38 million women across the world were diagnosed with breast cancer in 2008. This accounts for nearly a quarter (23%) of all cancers diagnosed in women. The highest incidence rates are observed in the United Kingdom and the United States (together with the rest of North America and Australia/New Zealand), making these countries a priority for breast cancer awareness. Female breast cancer incidence rates vary nearly five-fold across the regions of the world. In 2008, rates ranged from around 20 per 100,000 in Eastern and Middle Africa to 90 per 100,000 in Western Europe. The countries with the highest incidence rates in 2008 were Belgium and Denmark (109 and 101 per 100,000, respectively). Breast cancer is estimated to have caused almost 460,000 deaths in 2008. There is less variation in female breast cancer mortality across regions around the world, largely due to better survival in the developed countries (where rate of incidence is high), with rates ranging from 6 per 100,000 in Eastern Asia to 19 per 100,000 in Southern and Western Africa in 2008.[1] The incidence of breast cancer is high (greater than 80 per 100,000) in developed regions of the world (except Japan) and low (less than 40 per 100,000) in most of the developing regions. The number of deaths as a percentage of incident cases in 2008 was found to be 48% in low-income, 40% in low-middle-income, and 38% in high-middle-income countries, while it was 24% in high-income countries according to Globocan/IARC data.

The age-standardized incidence rate for breast cancer in India is 22.9 per 100,000, one-third that of Western countries and the mortality rates are disproportionately higher.[2,3] The rates of breast cancer in women of Indian origin living in Western countries are intermediate to their Western counterparts (who have much higher rates) and their Indian counterparts (who have much lower rates).[4] Breast cancer accounts for 22.2% of all new cancer diagnosed and 17.2% of all cancer deaths among women in India.

RISK FACTORS

Risk factors of breast cancer include age and family history. The chances of having breast cancer have been found to increase with age. Women whose blood relatives have suffered from breast cancer are at higher risk of developing the disease. Race and ethnicity of the women also affect the chances of having mammary cancer. It is seen that white women are more likely to develop the disease than African women. Inherited gene mutations account for a very small fraction of breast cancer cases. Mutations of the *BRCA1*, *BRCA2*, *CDH1*, *STK11*, and *TP53* genes contribute to the development of breast cancer. Variations of *AR*, *ATM*, *BARD1*, *BRIP1*, *CHEK2*, *DIRAS3*, *ERBB2*, *NBN*, *PALB2*, *RAD50*, and *RAD51* genes are also associated with breast cancer. Exposure to radiation and harmful chemicals increases the risk of breast cancer. Early puberty, late pregnancy, prolonged use of oral contraceptives, late menopause, and use of hormone therapy after menopause can be considered as causative factors for breast cancer. Obesity, lack of exercise, smoking, and excessive consumption of alcohol are also contributory factors.

SYMPTOMS

Breast cancer in its early stages usually does not cause pain and may exhibit no noticeable symptoms. As the disease progresses, signs and symptoms can include a lump or thickening in or near the breast; a change in the size or shape of the breast; nipple discharge, tenderness, or retraction (turning inward); and skin irritation, dimpling, or scaliness.

STAGES OF BREAST CANCER

Staging of breast cancer is done to detect the extent of cancer in the patient's body after the cancer is diagnosed. The various stages of breast cancer are determined using the TNM staging system. This system is based on three characteristics: size of tumor ('T' stands for tumor), involvement of lymph nodes ('N' stands for node), and whether the cancer has metastasized to other parts of the body ('M' stands for metastasis).

T Stage

This stage is denoted by the letter T followed by a number from 0 to 4. Higher numbers of T indicate a larger tumor size and spread of tissues near the breast.

N Stage

This stage, denoted by the letter N followed by number from 0 to 3, is used to determine whether the cancer has spread to the lymph nodes.

M Stage

This stage is used to detect if the cancer has spread to distant parts of the body. It is denoted by the letter M followed by number 0 or 1.

DIAGNOSIS AND TREATMENT

Blood tests, mammogram, ultra-sonography, fine needle aspiration cytology, surgical biopsies, breast MRI, chest X-rays, bone scans, CT scans, and PET scans are major diagnostic tools for the detection of breast cancer. The treatment modalities for breast cancer include surgery (lumpectomy, lymphectomy, or mastectomy), radiation therapy, immunotherapy (using the body's natural defense system to fight the disease, as for example Herceptin) and systemic therapy. Systemic therapy includes chemotherapy and hormone therapy. Adjuvant systemic therapy is used to destroy any undetected cancer cells, after removal of the offending growth by surgery. However, these treatments are not free from adverse side effects. Some of the commonly observed side effects of these treatment modalities are soreness, tenderness, lymphedema, scarring, and pain at the incision site (in the case of surgery), fatigue, irritation, hair loss (alopecia), insomnia, heart problems (in the case of radiation therapy and chemotherapy). Hormonal therapy using tamoxifen may affect functioning of the ovaries and may even cause cancer of the endometrium. Immunotherapy also results in certain side effects like fever, nausea, pain, weakness, and loss of appetite.

PROGNOSIS

Early diagnosis and treatment of breast cancer can significantly improve the survival rates. A study conducted by Coleman *et al.* in 2008[5] showed that the five-year survival rate for women diagnosed with the breast cancer vary greatly worldwide, ranging from 80% or over in North America, Sweden, and Japan; about 60% in middle-income countries; and below 40% in low-income countries. The prognostic factors to determine the likelihood of recurrence are as follows:

1. Location of the tumor: The location and size of tumor within the breast is an important predictor. Tumors developing toward the outside of the breast tend to be less aggressive than those occurring toward the middle of the breast.
2. Hormone receptor: Breast cancer cells may contain receptors for the hormones estrogen and progesterone. Cells containing these binding sites are known as hormone receptor-positive cells. If cells lack these, they are called hormone receptor-negative cells. Women tend to have a better prognosis if their tumors are hormone receptor-positive because these cells grow slowly compared to receptor-negative cells.
3. Tumor markers: The markers relevant for prognosis of breast cancer include:

   a. HER2: Breast cancer cells containing amplification of the gene for human epidermal growth factor receptor type 2 (HER2) or its product have a lower 10-year overall survival proportion.
   b. Other tumor markers include cancer antigen 15-3 (CA 15-3), cancer antigen 27.29 (CA 27.29), carcinoembryonic antigen (CEA), estrogen receptor (ER), progesterone receptor (PR), urokinase

plasminogen activator (uPA), and plasminogen activator inhibitor type-1 (PAI-1).

4. Gene expression profiling: Gene expression profiling tests (Oncotype DX, MammaPrint) are another prognostic factor; they carried out to examine a set of genes in tumor tissue to determine the chances of recurrence of the disease. These tests also help to decide whether post-surgery patients can be given adjuvant therapy.

DIET AND CANCER

The World Health Organization (WHO) has predicted that by 2020 the incidence of breast cancer cases will become alarming and one in every eight women would have the chance of developing the disease. Early detection and regular medical check-ups are always advisable, but it is important to be careful about the diet.

Foods and Breast Cancer

A study conducted by Doll and Peto[6] concluded that about 35% of all cancer mortality is attributable to diet. Various studies conducted in the first decade of the twenty-first century have highlighted the possible contribution of food habits to the development of breast cancer. The primary ingredients of diet that increases breast cancer risk are alcohol, caffeine, and foods rich in saturated fat, grilled foods and red meat. A high-fat diet leads to obesity which increases the risk of breast cancer. Fat cells contain the enzyme aromatase, which converts testosterone to estrogens. Thus, the higher the amount of fat cells in a woman's body, more estrogen is formed, thus stimulating breast cell growth. This can increase chances of getting breast cancer.[7] Foods rich in carbohydrates have also been found to increase chances of breast cancer. It has been observed that women having high carbohydrate intake (62% or more of their diet) are more susceptible to develop breast cancer than those with a lower carbohydrate intake (52% or less).[8]

On the other hand, foods do not only contribute to carcinogenesis, but also reduce the risk of cancer. A healthy diet has been found to be intricately linked to cancer prevention. Diets rich in fruits and vegetables have shown to limit the risks of cancer and certain other diseases. Some of the major breast cancers-fighting foods are fruits, vegetables, whole grains, nuts, seeds, and legumes. These foods are rich in vitamins like vitamins A (β-carotene), C, and E, and folic acid; minerals, dietary fibers, and plant-derived chemicals called phytochemicals. They are also low in fat content, salt, and sugar. Thus, a daily diet rich in these foods help to prevent obesity and maintain a healthy body weight, thus lowering the risks of breast cancer. Therefore, attention needs to be given to good lifestyle and healthy dietary habits to reduce the risk of breast cancer.

PHYTOCHEMICAL IN BREAST CANCER

The term phytochemical refers to a wide variety of compounds which are produced by plants. These are active compounds present in fruits, vegetables, grains, and other plant products that can be used to combat the occurrence of chronic diseases including cancer.

Phytochemicals are the major components responsible for the protection conferred by fruits and vegetables against various diseases. Nearly 5,000 different varieties of phytochemicals have been identified in plants. Therefore, this area demands significant attention for the scientists.

Phytochemicals present in fruits and vegetables have various health-promoting properties that act in conjunction with vitamins and nutrients to prevent, halt, and lessen diseases. They have antioxidant, antiestrogen, and chemopreventive properties that may prevent breast cancer. Experimental evidences reveal that these dietary compounds may prevent the formation of active carcinogens, prevent action of carcinogens on their target cells, and retard the development of cancer. The major chemopreventive phytochemicals identified from fruits and vegetables that have the potential to fight breast cancer include carotenoids, phenolic acids, flavonoids, and organosulfur compounds. These phytochemicals act as antioxidants to protect against damage to cells and repair them. Cruciferous vegetables, rich in phytochemicals, help fight breast cancer by converting a cancer-promoting estrogen into a more protective hormone. They are also a good source of vitamin C and soluble fiber, which help control body weight. They occupy the estrogen receptors on the surface of breast cells to block normal estrogen activity, thereby reducing the risk of breast cancer.[9]

Breast Cancer Chemoprevention

The concept of chemoprevention took root back in 1966 when Lee Wattenberg found that active compounds in fruits and vegetables could restrict development of cancer including breast cancer. It was only after a decade that the term chemoprevention was coined by Michael Sporn. The properties of an ideal chemopreventive agent are:

- Little or no toxicity;
- Effective at multiple sites;
- Consumable orally;
- Have known mechanism of action; and
- Cost-effective.

Phytochemicals present in fruits and vegetables behave as chemopreventive agents. Chemopreventive phytochemicals retard, block, and suppress the progression of breast cancer. They aim to prevent the process of carcinogenesis at early stages by inhibiting one or more steps in the process. These phytochemicals inhibit, delay, or reverse the process of carcinogenesis by inducing detoxifying and antioxidant enzymes, by regulating inflammatory/proliferative signaling pathways, by inducing antiestrogenic activity, and by triggering apoptosis of breast cancer cells. Numerous studies suggest that chemoprevention by dietary phytochemicals is an important means for breast cancer prevention for the general population and for individuals who are at high risk of developing the disease. Chemoprevention has thus emerged as an important subject of cancer research and a new medical strategy for breast cancer prevention.

Selective estrogen receptor modulators (SERMs) are a class of agents that possess the ability to block the effects of estrogen on the tissues of the breast. Tamoxifen is one such SERM that is highly recommended for lowering the chances of breast cancer among high-risk women. It was concluded from a study that the breast cancer risk in women receiving tamoxifen for five years was lowered by 50%. Raloxifene shows effects similar to tamoxifen. The NSABP Study of Tamoxifen and Raloxifene (STAR) trial was conducted in 2006 to compare the effects of tamoxifen and raloxifene in post-menopausal high risk women. This study concluded that raloxifene could reduce invasive breast cancer risk as effectively as tamoxifen. Aromatase inhibitors (anastrozole, letrozole, and exemestane) are used as adjuvant therapy for prevention of breast cancer recurrence in women with cancers that are hormone receptor-positive. The ATAC (Arimidex, Tamoxifen, Alone or in Combination) trial was conducted to evaluate the efficacy of anastrozole as an adjuvant treatment for women with breast cancer, and it was apparent that the risk of developing cancer in the other breast can be efficiently reduced by 58%.[10] A study carried out in women diagnosed with breast cancer in 2006 showed that chances of developing a second breast cancer was decreased in those who received fenritinide (a synthetic retinoid derivative) for five years.[10]

There are various phytochemicals that act as potent chemopreventive agents. Chemopreventive phytochemicals not only block initiation or reverse the promotion stage of multi-step carcinogenesis, but they can also stall or retard the progression of the disease process.

Agents having chemopreventive potential target some upstream signals leading to genotoxic damage, redox imbalances, and some form of cellular stress. A rational strategy in chemoprevention is to target malfunctioning molecules in the signal transduction pathway leading to cancer. Chemoprevention by phytochemicals involves modulation of proteins that play a key role in cellular signaling pathways like apoptosis, cell cycle, cell proliferation, cell growth, metastasis, angiogenesis, and so on.[11] The uniqueness of dietary phytochemicals lies in the fact that they differentially modulate the various signal transduction pathways in cancer, vis-à-vis, they can induce antioxidant defense enzymes in normal cells to protect them against carcinogenesis.[12]

Some of the primary targets of these phytochemicals in signaling pathways that cause breast cancer are shown in Fig. 3.1.

FRUITS AND VEGETABLES IN BREAST CANCER

Oxidative stress and gene-environment interactions play a significant role in the development of cancer. Prolonged lifetime exposure to estrogen is associated with several kinds of DNA damage. Oxidative stress and estrogen receptor-associated proliferative changes are suggested to play important roles in estrogen-induced breast carcinogenesis. BRCA1, a tumor suppressor against hormone responsive cancers such as breast cancer, plays a

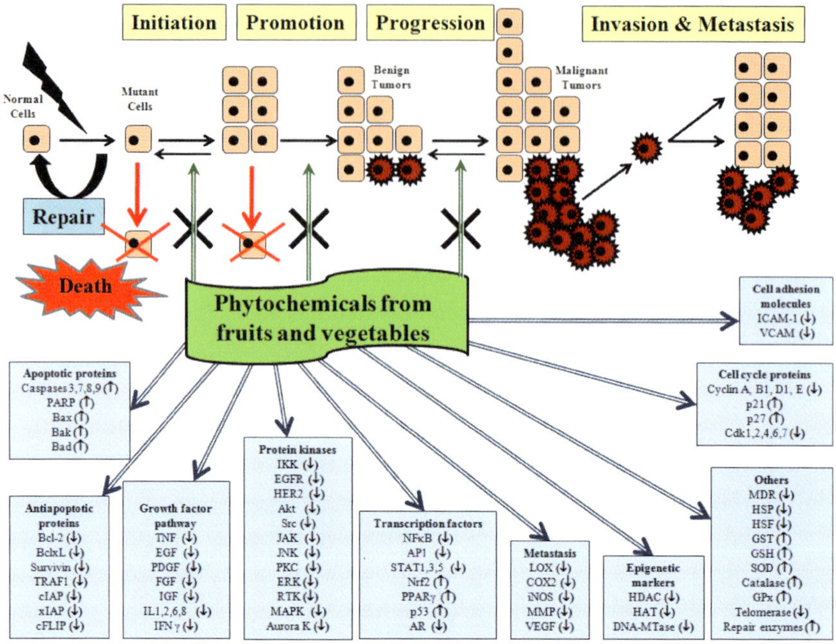

Figure 3.1: Molecular targets of phytochemicals isolated from fruits and vegetables for Breast cancer prevention. Phytochemicals inhibit all the three stages of carcinogenesis, i.e., initiation, promotion, and progression by altering the levels of various proteins involved in key signaling pathways. Modulation of various targets include apoptotic proteins, anti-apoptotic proteins, growth factors, protein kinases, transcription factors, metastasis-related proteins, epigenetic markers, cell-adhesion molecules, cell cycle regulatory proteins, and some other important proteins involved in carcinogenesis.

significant role in inhibiting reactive oxygen species (ROS) and estrogen-mediated DNA damage, thereby regulating the redox homeostasis of the cells. Several transcription factors and tumor suppressors are involved during stress response such as Nrf2, NF-κB, and BRCA1. A promising strategy for targeting redox status of the cells is to use readily available natural substances from vegetables, fruits, herbs, and spices. Many of the phytochemicals have already been identified to have chemopreventive potential, capable of intervening in carcinogenesis.

Some of the most important fruits and vegetables that can combat breast cancer are cruciferous vegetables (broccoli, cabbage, cauliflower, radish, turnip, watercress), umbelliferous vegetables (celery, parsley, fennel, carrots, parsnip), leafy green vegetables (lettuce, spinach), alliums (garlic, onion, shallots), solanaceous vegetables (tomato, peppers), soy foods, berries, citrus foods, pomegranate, and grapes.

Vegetables that Help Fight Breast Cancer

Cruciferous vegetables

These vegetables are part of the Brassica genus of plants. They contain vitamins (C, E, and K), folate, minerals, fiber, and phytochemicals. The major phytochemicals present in these vegetables are glucosinolates (sulfur-containing compounds), which are broken down during chewing and digestion to form indoles (indole-3-carbinol), nitriles, thiocyanates, and isothiocyanates (sulforaphane, PEITC).[13] Isothiocyanates containing the –N=C=S group detoxify and remove carcinogens, cause apoptosis of cancer cells, and prevent tumor growth, metastasis, and angiogenesis. The chemopreventive effects of sulforaphane, an isothiocyanate, have been proven in various preclinical studies. The mechanisms of action of this phytochemical include inhibition of phase I enzymes, induction of phase II enzymes to detoxify carcinogens, cell-cycle arrest, apoptosis induction, inhibition of histone deacetylase, modulation of the MAPK pathway, inhibition of NF-κB, and production of ROS.[14]

Umbelliferous vegetables

The major phytochemicals found in these vegetables are flavones, carotenoids, phthalides, and polyacetylenes. Carrots are an excellent source of carotenoids, falcarinol, luteolin, sulfoquinovosyl, diacylglycerol, and various lignans, all of which have been shown to have anticancer activities.[15] Celery contains apigenin, apiuman, luteolin, chrysoeriol, coumarin, several polyacetylenes, phthalides, and perillyl alcohol, which has been found to have chemopreventive activity. These phytochemicals have the ability to inhibit aromatase activity (the synthesis of estrogen from androgens within the body), which is important for reducing growth-stimulatory effects in estrogen-dependent breast cancer.

Green leafy vegetables

Vegetables such as spinach and lettuce contain fibers, vitamin B, and carotenoids like lutein, xeaxanthin, chlorophyll, glycolipids, etc. that can help fight breast cancer. It has been revealed from various studies that consumption of spinach is associated with lower risks of breast cancer due to its antioxidant and anti-inflammatory effects. Lettuce is a dietary source of vitamins A, K, and C, folate, manganese, and various flavonoids like quercetin and luteolin that have protective activity against breast cancer.

Alliums

The major active ingredients of these vegetables are organosulfur compounds and mainly allyl derivatives, which inhibit carcinogenesis. Various mechanisms have been proposed to explain the cancer-protective effects of *Allium* vegetables and related organosulfur compounds. These effects include inhibition of mutagenesis, modulation of enzyme activities, inhibition of DNA adduct formation, free-radical scavenging, and effects on cell proliferation and tumor growth.[16] Onions are also reported to contain the flavonoids kaempferol, myricetin, and quercetin, all of which possess antioxidant properties. Quercetin exhibits anti-proliferative activity *in vitro* and inhibits various signal transduction targets such as tyrosine kinases, protein kinase C, and phosphatidyl inositol-3 kinase.[17]

Solanaceous vegetables

These vegetables belong to the family Solanaceae. The main phytochemicals found in these vegetables are lycopene, capsaicin, and anthocyanins. Lycopene, a major carotenoid component of tomato, has potential anticancer activity. It acts as an antitumor agent by arresting cell proliferation and/or by inducing apoptosis.[18] It has been seen that capsaicin, a significant pungent ingredient in a variety of red peppers of the genus *Capsicum*, exerts anticarcinogenic, antimutagenic, and chemopreventive properties in breast cancer.[19]

Soy foods

The active components of soy foods that help in prevention of cancer are isoflavones (genistin and daidzein), saponins, triterpenes, phytosterols, and lignans. Isoflavones exert their effect through their estrogenic activity. The molecular structures of isoflavones, especially genistein, are similar to that of 17-β-estradiol.[20] Genistein is also a protein tyrosine kinase (PTK) inhibitor. Isoflavones exert antioxidant activities. The anticarcinogenic properties of soyasaponins and soyasapogenols are via direct cytotoxicity, induction of apoptosis, antiestrogenic activity, and inhibition of tumor cell metastasis, antimutagenic activity effect, and normalization of carcinogen-induced cell proliferation.[21] Phytosterols are believed to act through multiple mechanisms such as the inhibition of cancer-cell growth, angiogenesis, invasion, and metastasis, and through the promotion of apoptosis of cancerous cells.

Fruits that Help Fight Breast Cancer

Berries

Flavonoids, anthocyanins, and phenolic acids are some of the bioactive substances present in berries that exert anticancer effects such as the inhibition of cell proliferation, induction of apoptosis, and modulation of cell signaling, thereby affecting expression of various genes. Cranberries are a rich source of phenolics, which are powerful antioxidants. They are known to possess strong anticarcinogenic properties.[22,23]

Citrus foods

These fruits contain various phytochemicals which can help fight breast cancer. Some of them are limonoids, vitamin C, coumarins, and limonene. Vitamin C, an antioxidant, protects cell membranes and DNA from oxidative damage. It also helps to combat cancer via its ability to scavenge and reduce nitrite, thereby reducing substrate for the formation of nitrosamines. These phytochemicals play a role in increasing the activity of certain detoxifying enzymes like glutathione transferase.[24] Apart from the above mentioned groups, there are various other fruits that are of prime importance in fighting breast cancer.

Pomegranates

It has been reported that pomegranates possess various chemopreventive properties due to the presence of components such as ellagic acid, punicic acid, ursolic acid, luteolin, and several anthocyanin pigments. Pomegranate juice is rich in antioxidant tannins and flavonoids that help prevent breast cancer.[25]

Grapes

Grapes contain polyphenols (resveratrol, quercetin, and catechin) that act as antioxidants, antiangiogenic agents, and SERMs. Grapes also contain lupeol and fisetin, which also have anticancer properties. Red grapes and grape seeds are a good source of resveratrol, which suppresses the proliferation of breast cancer cells and promotes cell apoptosis. Resveratrol inhibits aromatase (responsible for the synthesis of estrogen from androgens within the body), which is important for reducing growth-stimulatory effects in estrogen-dependent breast cancer. Resveratrol has effects on all the stages of carcinogenesis (initiation, promotion, and progression) by modulating signal transduction pathways that control cell division and growth, apoptosis, inflammation, angiogenesis, and metastasis.[26] Other polyphenols present in grapes like quercetin and catechin have also been shown to have chemopreventive effects.

Guavas

Guavas contain vitamins A and C, folic acid, potassium, copper, manganese, fiber, flavanoids, and carotenoids (lycopene, β-carotene, lutein, and cryptoxanthin). Lycopene has antioxidant properties that can combat breast cancer by combating free radicals.

Apples

Apples, members of the Rosaceae family, contain various phytochemicals that are effective against breast cancer. Some examples are quercetin, catechin, phloridzin, and chlorogenic acid, all of which have antioxidant properties. The phytochemicals present in apples have also been found to inhibit cell proliferation.[27]

Thus, in a nutshell, the active components (phytochemicals) present in fruits and vegetables help to reduce the risk of breast cancer by preventing

Table 3.1: Phytochemicals isolated from fruits and vegetables for breast cancer chemoprevention.

Fruits/Vegetables	Active ingredient
Cruciferous vegetables like broccoli, cabbage, brussel sprouts, etc.	Sulforaphane, PEITC, indole-3-carbinol
Parsley	Flavones
Apples, onions, green leafy vegetables	Quercetin
Garlic	Diallyl sulfate
Tomato	Lycopene
Capsicum	Capsaicin
Soy foods	Genistein
Berries	Anthocyanins
Citrus fruits	Limonene
Pomegranates	Ellagic acid
Grapes	Resveratol

cell proliferation, acting as antioxidants, increasing the activity of protective detoxifying enzymes, and altering the estrogen levels.

Some of the phytochemicals along with their dietary sources that play a role in breast cancer chemoprevention are listed in Table 3.1.

Various preclinical and clinical trials have been carried out to establish the role of dietary phytochemicals (present in fruits and vegetables) in breast cancer.

IN VITRO STUDIES

Several studies have been carried out in various breast cancer cell lines to determine the chemopreventive mechanisms and effects of dietary phytochemicals in breast cancer. A study conducted by Lee *et al.*[28] showed that the flavone luteolin suppresses MDA-MB-231 ER-negative breast cancer cell growth, deriving its anticancer activity from the inhibitory effects on EGFR-mediated cell survival. Seo *et al.*[29] showed that the flavone apigenin inhibited the proliferation of MCF-7 vec and MCF-7 HER2 breast cancer cells by targeting the p53-dependant pathway, thus indicating that apigenin could be used as a potential candidate to prevent or treat HER2 overexpressing breast cancer. Ying *et al.*[30] showed that the flavonoid quercetin inhibits cell growth and induces apoptosis in MCF-7 human breast cancer cells by the downregulation of Bcl-2 protein expression and upregulation of Bax expression. It has been reported by Jin *et al.*[31] that the isoflavone daidzein induces breast cancer cell apoptosis through the mitochondrial caspase-dependent apoptotic pathway. Another flavonoid kaempferol was shown to inhibit cell proliferation in human breast carcinoma MDA-MB-453 cells by induction of cell cycle arrest at G2/M phase which leads to apoptosis via the p53-mediated pathway.[32] Sulforaphane has been shown to inhibit cell growth, activate apoptosis, inhibit HDAC activity, and decrease the expression of key proteins involved in breast cancer proliferation in human breast cancer cells according to a study conducted in 2007.[33] It was revealed that benzyl isothiocyanate (BITC) (a component of cruciferous vegetables) suppresses growth of cultured human breast cancer cells (MDA-MB-231 and MCF-7) by causing G2/M phase cell cycle arrest and induction of apoptosis. The BITC-mediated cell cycle arrest was due to decrease in protein levels involved in regulation of G2/M transition, such as cyclin B1, cyclin-dependent kinase 1, and cell division cycle. The BITC-induced apoptosis was due to induction of pro-apoptotic proteins Bax (MCF-7) and Bak (MDA-MB-231 and MCF-7) and downregulation of antiapoptotic proteins Bcl-2 and Bcl-x_L (MDA-MB-231).[34] Another study concluded that phenethyl isothiocyanate (PEITC) inhibited the expression of heat shock proteins (HSPs) (particularly HSP 90) and HSF1 in breast cancer cell lines (breast adenocarcinoma MCF-7 and highly metastatic breast cancer cell MDA-MB-231) by downregulating cell-cycle regulatory proteins like cyclin B1, CDK1, Cdc25C, and PLK-1, and upregulating p21 irrespective of p53 status. These effects were accompanied by cell-cycle arrest at G2/M phase and apoptosis by activation of caspases 3 and 9.[35]

The chemopreventive activity of blueberries was studied by Yee *et al.*[22] in triple-negative breast cancer cell lines. It was revealed that the phytochemicals present in blueberries decreased proliferation of HCC38, HCC1937, and MDA-MB-231 cells. Blueberry phytochemicals inhibited the growth and metastatic potential of MDA-MB-231 cells via modulation of the PI3K/Akt/NF-κB pathway. A study conducted on cranberries showed that the phytochemicals present in these fruits suppresses the proliferation of human breast cancer MCF-7 cells by inducing cell cycle arrest at G1 phase and induction of apoptosis.[23] Limonoids present in citrus fruits have shown to exhibit anti-aromatase activity and cytotoxicity on breast cancer cells by caspase 7-dependant pathways.[24] Phytochemicals present in pomegranate extracts (ellagic acid, punicic acid, ursolic acid, luteolin, and several anthocyanin pigments) have shown to induce anti-proliferative effects and inhibit metastatic processes in breast cancer cell lines.[36]

A study was conducted by Chang *et al.*[19] to study the effect of capsaicin on human breast cancer cell lines MCF-7 and BT-20. The results showed decreased cell viability in these cell lines by induction of apoptosis and arresting the cell cycle at S phase. Capsaicin was found to significantly decrease mitochondria membrane potential, induce the cleavage of PARP-1, and decrease procaspase-7 expression in both cells. Chiu *et al.*[37] showed that chlorophyllin deactivates ERK to inhibit the proliferation of human breast carcinoma MCF-7 cells. A study was carried out to determine the effects of six phenolic acids (caffeic acid, ferrulic acid, sinapic acid, syringic acid, protocatechuic acid, and 3,4-dihydroxyphenylacetic acid) on human breast cancer T47D cell line. The results indicated inhibition of growth of these cells, indicating a protective effect on hormone-dependent breast tumors.[38] In a study conducted by Zhang *et al.*,[39] it was observed that the triterpenoids in apples showed anti-proliferative activities against human breast cancer cell lines MCF-7 and MDA-MB-231.

IN VIVO STUDIES

Several *in vivo* studies have been carried out to confirm the role of dietary phytochemicals in breast cancer. Takashi *et al.*[40] showed that the monoterpene perillyl alcohol suppresses tumor cell growth and metastasis in a nude mouse model. The cell cycle progression was preceded by a decrease in cyclins D1 and E, along with an increase in p21 and a decrease in proliferating cell nuclear antigen level. However, there was no change in levels of p53 and cyclin A. Another study confirmed that supplementation of nude mice (inoculated with MDA-MB-231 cells) with the flavones luteolin significantly reduced the tumor burden. The results showed that luteolin suppresses ^{3}H thymidine incorporation indicating growth inhibition, and this was accompanied by cell cycle arrest at the G2/M and S stages and apoptotic activity. Further analyses revealed that luteolin caused cell cycle arrest and apoptotic activity by decreasing Akt, PLK1, cyclin B1, cyclin A, CDC2, CDK2, and Bcl-x_L expression and increasing p21 and Bax expression.[28] A study conducted in SV40-immortalized mouse embryonic fibroblasts (derived from Bax and Bak double-knock-out mice) revealed that BITC treatment causes arrest of growth and induction of apoptosis by a complex signaling pathway involving formation of reactive oxygen species and various caspases (caspases 3, 8, and 9).[34] Another PEITC has been reported to inhibit the growth of mammary cancers in a breast cancer mouse model. This inhibition was associated with reduced cellular proliferation and neoangiogenesis, increased apoptosis, and altered expression of several proteins, including decreased ATP synthase in the tumor and increased plasma levels of transthyretin and not because of suppression of human epidermal growth factor receptor-2 expression.[41] The inhibition of triple-negative breast tumor growth by blueberries was studied using MDA-MB-231 xenograft model, thus revealing that blueberries have inhibitory effect on growth and metastatic potential of these cells by decreasing the activation of Akt and p65 NF-κB signaling proteins.[22] It has been revealed in a study that resveratrol in diet significantly reduced the incidence and multiplicity of DMBA-induced mammary tumors, thus extending the latency period, in mice by decreasing COX-2 and matrix metalloproteinase-9 expression and suppression of NF-κB activation. 7,12-dimethylbenz(a)anthracene (DMBA)-induced mammary cancer in rats was prevented by dietary resveratrol by reducing cell proliferation, increasing mammary epithelial cell apoptosis and causing maturation of the mammary gland. Resveratrol combined with soy isoflavone genistein showed better effects in extending tumor latency in rats as compared to resveratrol alone.[26] It was revealed by another study that supplementation of HER2/neu-overexpressing transgenic mice with resveratrol delayed spontaneous mammary tumor development and reduced metastasizing capacity by downregulating the expression of HER2/neu and induction of apoptosis in tumor cells.[42] Ellagic acid present in berries was reported to significantly reduce the breast cancer burden on rats according to a study conducted in 2010 by Aiyer *et al.*[43] The induction of breast cancer was associated with increase in a number of metabolic enzymes including cytochrome P450, 17β-HSD, and catechol-O-methyl-transferase. The flavonoid quercetin has been reported to show apoptotic activities in breast tumors *in vivo*.[44] A study was conducted by Kanematsu *et al.*[45] in 2011 to determine the effect of sulforaphane, an isothiocyanate, in breast cancer. Treatment of female athymic BALB/c mice, orthotopically (right thoracic mammary fat pad) transplanted with KPL-1 cells, showed reduced axillary lymph node metastasis by suppressing proliferation of cells and induction of apoptosis. A progestin-dependent mammary cancer model was developed by treating Sprague–Dawley rats with DMBA. These rats were then exposed to the flavonoid apigenin, commonly found in parsley. Apigenin was found to significantly delay the development of, and decrease the incidence and multiplicity of DMBA-induced mammary tumors in this animal model, thus suggesting a chemopreventive role of apigenin in breast cancers that develop in response to progestins.[46] Studies showed that the triterpenoids in apples could substantially reduce the occurrence and growth of mammary tumor in a rat model.[39]

CLINICAL TRIALS AND EPIDEMIOLOGICAL STUDIES

Numerous clinical trials and epidemiological studies have been carried out to investigate the association between consumption of dietary phytochemicals and breast cancer. Studies conducted on 3,055 patients and 3,956 control subjects showed that women who have higher circulating levels of carotenoids are at reduced risk of breast cancer.[15] A large population-based study was carried out in women staying in the states of Massachusetts, New Hampshire, and Wisconsin to examine the association between carotenoids and breast cancer risk. The study comprised 5,707 women with invasive breast cancer and 6,389 population controls. It was revealed that high consumption of carotenoids may lessen the risks of premenopausal breast cancer but not postmenopausal breast cancer.[47] A case control study comprising 678 breast cancer patients and 3,390 controls was conducted to elucidate the association between soy food intake and risk of breast cancer based on receptor status. It was found that phytochemicals present in soy foods significantly reduced the chances of breast cancer.[48] Another study revealed that regular consumption of soy foods may play a role in reducing the risks of ER- and PR-positive breast cancer.[49]

Case control studies conducted on women revealed that higher consumption of cruciferous vegetables led to a lower risk of breast cancer. A study conducted on 2,569 Italian women suffering from breast cancer showed that the risks of developing the disease was significantly reduced by increasing consumption of flavones like apigenin and luteolin in their diet.[50] Another study was conducted by Zhang *et al.* in 2009 in Guangdong, China. The study comprised 438 breast cancer patients and an equal number of controls matched by age and area of residence (rural/urban). It was reported that higher intake of fruits and vegetables in Chinese women led to decreased risks of breast cancer.[51]

Another study was conducted to determine the relation between dietary consumption of resveratrol and breast cancer risk. The study was conducted between 1993 and 2003 in the Swiss canton of Vaud on 369 breast cancer cases and 602 matched controls. A reduction of breast cancer risk was observed in women consuming resveratrol from grapes.[52] Epidemiological studies have reported an inverse correlation between dietary intake of cruciferous vegetables and the risks of developing breast cancer.[34] Retinoids have also been studied in clinical trials as chemopreventive agents as they have been proven to show anticancer properties. It was reported that fenretinide, the most-studied retinoid in breast cancer clinical trials, has demonstrated the potential to reduce second breast malignancies in premenopausal women (according to a phase III breast cancer prevention trial).[53]

Nevertheless, one of the major difficulties of the clinical usage of phytochemicals lies in poor bioavailability due to incomplete absorption and rapid first-pass metabolism. Therefore, intense further research needs to be carried out in this field.

PHYTOCHEMICAL–DRUG INTERACTIONS

Dietary factors in fruits and vegetables may enhance the efficacy of cancer therapeutics by altering cell proliferation and survival pathways. Phytochemicals rich in antioxidants have shown their efficacy in tumor response to chemotherapy by improving the overall survival of the patients. Some of these phytochemicals like quercetin can work synergistically with doxorubicin in multi-drug resistant (MDR) human breast cancer cells. Furthermore, quercetin has been found to enhance the cytotoxic efficacy of cyclophosphamide and doxorubicin and at the same time decrease the resistance to certain chemotherapeutic drugs like gemcitabine, topotecan, vincristine, tamoxifen, and paclitaxel.[54,55] Another isoflavonoid diadzein confers protection against mammary carcinogenesis in combination with tamoxifen. Genestein in combination with tamoxifen synergistically inhibits growth in ER-negative human breast carcinoma cells MDA-MB-435.[56]

Flavonoids can increase the bioavailability of drugs by inhibiting ATP transporters-mediated drug efflux *in vitro*.[55] A report showed that an indole derivative 3,3′-diindolylmethane (DIM), when used in combination with Herceptin to treat breast cancers, having high levels of HER2/neu, DIM enhanced the effectiveness of Herceptin by inducing apoptosis.[57] The synergistic association of phytochemicals with chemotherapeutic drugs might result in lowering drug doses and consequential reduction of drug induced toxicity. The results of the ongoing clinical trials might thus provide a platform for planning and executing future clinical trials to assess the efficacy of phytochemicals.[58]

CONCLUSION

With rapid improvements in screening, early detection, and treatment modalities, breast cancer is the most common cancer among women. Some of the causative factors of breast cancer include age, family history, and hormonal factors are beyond the scope of modification. Therefore, other preventive measures may pave a way to control breast cancer. It has been seen from various preclinical (*in vitro* and *in vivo*) studies and clinical trials that dietary phytochemicals are associated with chemoprevention in breast cancer. A promising role of dietary products from fruits and vegetables for prevention and treatment of cancer is gaining popularity. A chemopreventive strategy could protect DNA from further damage. Active ingredients in diet are efficient in inhibiting or reversing the process of initiation, promotion, and progression. They also maintain a balance between phase I and phase II enzyme levels. Fruits and vegetables contain diverse mixtures of phytonutrients and can act as antioxidants, aiding protection against free radicals. Thus, they may confer protection against cancer. Chemoprevention by phytochemicals is cheap, readily consumable, acceptable to the society, and safe. Breast cancer, which poses a critical problem among women, can be controlled by means of daily intake of fruits and vegetables. This would be cost-effective and a novel way of cancer control. Therefore, it would be a great endeavor to promote awareness among society to consume fruits and vegetables; at the same time, this will be an excellent cancer chemopreventive strategy for breast cancer. In addition, strengthening of cellular defense mechanism or restoration of stress–response signaling by administrating dietary phytonutrients from fruits and vegetables provides an important strategy for cancer chemoprevention. It is a challenge to the scientific community to make the best out of these phytochemicals in different populations who are at risk.

REFERENCES

1. Ferlay, J., H.R. Shin, F. Bray, D. Forman, C. Mathers, and D.M. Parkin, Estimates of worldwide burden of cancer in 2008: GLOBOCAN 2008, *Int J Cancer* **127**(12): 2893–2917 (2010).
2. Agarwal, G. and P. Ramakant, Breast cancer care in India: The current scenario and the challenges for the future, *Breast Care (Basel)* **3**(1): 21–27 (2008).
3. Agarwal, G., P. Ramakant, E.R. Forgach, J.C. Rendón, J.M. Chaparro, C.S. Basurto, and M. Margaritoni, Breast cancer care in developing countries, *World J Surg* **33**(10): 2069–2076 (2009).
4. Ali, R., I. Barnes, S.W. Kan, and V. Beral, Cancer incidence in British Indians and British whites in Leicester, 2001–2006, *Br J Cancer* **103**(1): 143–148 (2010).
5. Coleman, M.P., M. Quaresma, F. Berrino, J.M. Lutz, R. De Angelis, R. Capocaccia, P. Baili, B. Rachet, G. Gatta, T. Hakulinen, A. Micheli, M. Sant, H.K. Weir, J.M. Elwood, H. Tsukuma, S. Koifman, G.A.E. Silva, S. Francisci, M. Santaquilani, A. Verdecchia, H.H. Storm, and J.L. Young, CONCORD Working Group., Cancer survival in five continents: A worldwide population-based study (CONCORD), *Lancet Oncol* **9**(8): 730–756 (2008).
6. Doll, R. and R. Peto, The causes of cancer: Quantitative estimates of avoidable risks of cancer in the United States today, *J Natl Cancer Inst* **66**(6): 1191–1308 (1981).
7. Cho, E., W.Y. Chen, D.J. Hunter, M.J. Stampfer, G.A. Colditz, S.E. Hankinson, and W.C. Willett, Red meat intake and risk of breast cancer among premenopausal women, *Arch Intern Med* **166**(20): 2253–2259 (2006).

8. Romieu, I., E. Lazcano-Ponce, L.M. Sanchez-Zamorano, W. Willett, and M. Hernandez-Avila, Carbohydrates and the risk of breast cancer among Mexican women, *Cancer Epidemiol Biomarkers Prev* **13**(8): 1283–1289 (2004).
9. Ju, Y.H., K.E. Carlson, J. Sun, D. Pathak, B.S. Katzenellenbogen, J.A. Katzenellenbogen, and W.G. Helferich, Estrogenic effects of extracts from cabbage, fermented cabbage, and acidified brussels sprouts on growth and gene expression of estrogen-dependent human breast cancer (MCF-7) cells, *J Agric Food Chem* **48**(10): 4628–4634 (2000).
10. Bonovas, S., A. Tsantes, T. Drosos, and N.M. Sitaras, Cancer chemoprevention: A summary of the current evidence, *Anticancer Res* **28**(3B): 1857–1866 (2008).
11. Surh, Y.J., Cancer chemoprevention with dietary phytochemicals, *Nat Rev Cancer* **3**(10): 768–780 (2003).
12. Gopalakrishnan, A. and A. Kong, Anticarcinogenesis by dietary phytochemicals: Cytoprotection by Nrf2 in normal cells and cytotoxicity by modulation of transcription factors NF-kappa B and AP-1 in abnormal cancer cells, *Food Chem Toxicol* **46**(4): 1257–1270 (2008).
13. Hayes, J.D., M.O. Kelleher, and I.M. Eggleston, The cancer chemopreventive actions of phytochemicals derived from glucosinolates, *Eur J Nutr* **47** (Suppl. 2): 73–88 (2008).
14. Juge, N., R.F. Mithen, and M. Traka, Molecular basis for chemoprevention by sulforaphane: A comprehensive review, *Cell Mol Life Sci* **64**(9): 1105–1127 (2007).
15. Eliassen, A.H., S.J. Hendrickson, L.A. Brinton, J.E. Buring, H. Campos, Q. Dai, J.F. Dorgan, A.A. Franke, Y.T. Gao, M.T. Goodman, G. Hallmans, K.J. Helzlsouer, J. Hoffman-Bolton, K. Hultén, H.D. Sesso, A.L. Sowell, R.M. Tamimi, P. Toniolo, L.R. Wilkens, A. Winkvist, A. Zeleniuch-Jacquotte, W. Zheng, and S.E. Hankinson, Circulating carotenoids and risk of breast cancer: Pooled analysis of eight prospective studies, *J Natl Cancer Inst* **104**(24): 1905–1916 (2012).
16. Bianchini, F. and H. Vainio, Allium vegetables and organosulfur compounds: Do they help prevent cancer? *Environ Health Perspect* **109**(9): 893–902 (2001).
17. Miean, K.H. and S. Mohamed, Flavonoid (myricetin, quercetin, kaempferol, luteolin, and apigenin) content of edible tropical plants, *J Agric Food Chem* **49**: 3106–3112 (2001).
18. Teodoro, A.J., F.L. Oliveira, N.B. Martins, A. Maia Gde, R.B. Martucci, and R. Borojevic, Effect of lycopene on cell viability and cell cycle progression in human cancer cell lines, *Cancer Cell Int* **12**(1): 36–44 (2012).

19. Chou, C.C., Y.C. Wu, Y.F. Wang, M.J. Chou, S.J. Kuo, and D.R. Chen, Capsaicin-induced apoptosis in human breast cancer MCF-7 cells through caspase-independent pathway, *Oncol Rep* **21**(3): 665–671 (2009).
20. Pilšáková, L., I. Riečanský, and F. Jagla, The physiological actions of isoflavone phytoestrogens, *Physiol Res* **59**(5): 651–664 (2010).
21. Kang, J., T.M. Badger, M.J. Ronis, and X. Wu, Non-isoflavone phytochemicals in soy and their health effects, *J Agric Food Chem* **58**(14): 8119–8133 (2010).
22. Adams, L.S., S. Phung, N. Yee, N.P. Seeram, L. Li, and S. Chen, Blueberry phytochemicals inhibit growth and metastatic potential of MDA-MB-231 breast cancer cells through modulation of the phosphatidylinositol 3-kinase pathway, *Cancer Res* **70**(9): 3594–3605 (2010).
23. Neto, C.C., Cranberry and its phytochemicals: A review of *in vitro* anticancer studies, *J Nutr* **137**(1 Suppl.): 186S–193S (2007).
24. Kim, J., G.K. Jayaprakasha, and B.S. Patil, Limonoids and their anti-proliferative and anti-aromatase properties in human breast cancer cells, *Food Funct* **4**(2): 258–265 (2013).
25. Adhami, V.M., N. Khan, and H. Mukhtar, Cancer chemoprevention by pomegranate: Laboratory and clinical evidence, *Nutr Cancer* **61**(6): 811–815 (2009).
26. Bishayee, A., Cancer prevention and treatment with resveratrol: From rodent studies to clinical trials, *Cancer Prev Res (Phila)* **2**(5): 409–418 (2009).
27. Boyer, J. and R.H. Liu, Apple phytochemicals and their health benefits, *Nutr J* **3**: 5–20 (2004).
28. Lee, E.J., S.Y. Oh, and M.K. Sung, Luteolin exerts anti-tumor activity through the suppression of epidermal growth factor receptor-mediated pathway in MDA-MB-231 ER-negative breast cancer cells, *Food Chem Toxicol* **50**(11): 4136–4143 (2012).
29. Seo, H.S., H.S. Choi, S.R. Kim, Y.K. Choi, S.M. Woo, I. Shin, J.K. Woo, S.Y. Park, Y.C. Shin, and S.G. Ko, Apigenin induces apoptosis via extrinsic pathway, inducing p53 and inhibiting STAT3 and NFκB signaling in HER2-overexpressing breast cancer cells, *Mol Cell Biochem* **366**(1–2): 319–334 (2012).
30. Scambia, G., F.O. Ranelletti, P. Benedetti Panici, M. Piantelli, G. Bonanno, R. De Vincenzo, G. Ferrandina, L. Pierelli, A. Capelli, and S. Mancuso, Quercetin inhibits the growth of a multidrug-resistant estrogen-receptor-negative MCF-7 human breast-cancer cell line expressing type II estrogen-binding sites, *Cancer Chemother Pharmacol* **28**(4): 255–258 (1991).
31. Jin, S., Q.Y. Zhang, X.M. Kang, J.X. Wang, and W.H. Zhao, Daidzein induces MCF-7 breast cancer cell apoptosis via the mitochondrial pathway, *Ann Oncol* **21**(2): 263–268 (2010).

32. Choi, E.J. and W. Ahn, Kaempferol induced the apoptosis via cell cycle arrest in human breast cancer MDA-MB-453 cells, *Nutr Res Pract* **2**(4): 322–325 (2008).
33. Pledgie-Tracy, A., M.D. Sobolewski, and N.E. Davidson, Sulforaphane induces cell type-specific apoptosis in human breast cancer cell lines, *Mol Cancer Ther* **6**(3): 1013–1021 (2007).
34. Xiao, D., V. Vogel, and S.V. Singh, Benzyl isothiocyanate-induced apoptosis in human breast cancer cells is initiated by reactive oxygen species and regulated by Bax and Bak, *Mol Cancer Ther* **5**(11): 2931–2945 (2006).
35. Sarkar, R., S. Mukherjee, and M. Roy, Targeting heat shock proteins by phenethyl isothiocyanate results in cell-cycle arrest and apoptosis of human breast cancer cells, *Nutr Cancer* **65**(3): 480–493 (2013).
36. Rocha, A., L. Wang, M. Penichet, and M.M. Green, Pomegranate juice and specific components inhibit cell and molecular processes critical for metastasis of breast cancer, *Breast Cancer Res Treat* **136**(3): 647–658 (2012).
37. Chiu, L.C., C.K. Kong, and V. Ooi, The chlorophyllin-induced cell cycle arrest and apoptosis in human breast cancer MCF-7 cells is associated with ERK deactivation and Cyclin D1 depletion, *Int J Mol Med* **16**(4): 735–740 (2005).
38. Marilena, K., I.A. Vassilia, N. George, P.N. Artemissia, N. Anastassia, H. Anastassia, B. Efstathia, K. Elena, B. George, B. Dimitrios, G. Achille, and C. Elias, Antiproliferative and apoptotic effects of selective phenolic acids on T47D human breast cancer cells: Potential mechanisms of action, *Breast Cancer Res* **6**: 63–67 (2003).
39. He, X., Y. Wang, H. Hu, and Z. Zhang, *In vitro* and *in vivo* antimammary tumor activities and mechanisms of the apple total triterpenoids, *J Agric Food Chem* **60**(37): 9430–9436 (2012).
40. Yuri, T., N. Danbara, M. Tsujita-Kyutoku, Y. Kiyozuka, H. Senzaki, N. Shikata, H. Kanzaki, and A. Tsubura, Perillyl alcohol inhibits human breast cancer cell growth *in vitro* and *in vivo*, *Breast Cancer Res Treat* **84**(3): 251–260 (2004).
41. Singh, S.V., S.H. Kim, A. Sehrawat, J.A. Arlotti, E.R. Hahm, K. Sakao, J.H. Beumer, R.C. Jankowitz, C.K. Kumar, J. Lee, A.A. Powolny, and R. Dhir, Biomarkers of phenethyl isothiocyanate-mediated mammary cancer chemoprevention in a clinically relevant mouse model, *J Natl Cancer Inst* **104**(16): 1228–1239 (2012).
42. Athar, M., J.H. Back, X. Tang, K.H. Kim, L. Kopelovich, D.R. Bickers, and A. Kim, Resveratrol: A review of preclinical studies for human cancer prevention, *Toxicol Appl Pharmacol* **224**(3): 274–283 (2007).
43. Aiyer, H.S. and R.C. Gupta, Berries and ellagic acid prevent estrogen-induced mammary tumorigenesis by modulating enzymes of estrogen metabolism, *Cancer Prev Res (Phila)* **3**(6): 727–737 (2010).

44. Dechsupa, S., J. Vergote, G. Leger, A. Martineau, S. Berangeo, R. Kosanlavit, J.L. Moretti, and S. Mankhetkorn, Quercetin, Siamois 1 and Siamois 2 induce apoptosis in human breast cancer MDA-MB-435 cells xenograft *in vivo*, *Cancer Biol Ther* **6**(1): 56–61 (2007).
45. Kanematsu, S., K. Yoshizawa, N. Uehara, H. Miki, T. Sasaki, M. Kuro, Y.C. Lai, A. Kimura, T. Yuri, and A. Tsubura, Sulforaphane inhibits the growth of KPL-1 human breast cancer cells *in vitro* and suppresses the growth and metastasis of orthotopically transplanted KPL-1 cells in female athymic mice, *Oncol Rep* **26**(3): 603–608 (2011).
46. Mafuvadze, B., I. Benakanakere, F.R. López Pérez, C. Besch-Williford, M.R. Ellersieck, and S.M. Hyder, Apigenin prevents development of medroxyprogesterone acetate-accelerated 7,12-dimethylbenz(a)anthracene-induced mammary tumors in Sprague-Dawley rats, *Cancer Prev Res (Phila)* **4**(8): 1316–1324 (2011).
47. Mignone, L.I., E. Giovannucci, P.A. Newcomb, L. Titus-Ernstoff, A. Trentham-Dietz, J.M. Hampton, W.C. Willett, and K.M. Egan, Dietary carotenoids and the risk of invasive breast cancer, *Int J Cancer* **124**(12): 2929–2937 (2009).
48. Suzuki, T., K. Matsuo, N. Tsunoda, K. Hirose, A. Hiraki, T. Kawase, T. Yamashita, H. Iwata, H. Tanaka, and K. Tajima, Effect of soybean on breast cancer according to receptor status: A case-control study in Japan, *Int J Cancer* **123**(7): 1674–1680 (2008).
49. Dai, Q., X.O. Shu, F. Jin, J.D. Potter, L.H. Kushi, J. Teas, Y.T. Gao, and W. Zheng, Population-based case-control study of soyfood intake and breast cancer risk in Shanghai, *Br J Cancer* **85**(3): 372–378 (2001).
50. Bosetti, C., L. Spertini, M. Parpinel, P. Gnagnarella, P. Lagiou, E. Negri, S. Franceschi, M. Montella, J. Peterson, J. Dwyer, A. Giacosa, and C. La Vecchia, Flavonoids and breast cancer risk in Italy, *Cancer Epidemiol Biomarkers Prev* **14**(4): 805–808 (2005).
51. Zhang, C.X., S.C. Ho, Y.M. Chen, J.H. Fu, S.Z. Cheng, and F.Y.Lin, Greater vegetable and fruit intake is associated with a lower risk of breast cancer among Chinese women, *Int J Cancer* **125**(1): 181–188 (2009).
52. Levi, F., C. Pasche, F. Lucchini, R. Ghidoni, M. Ferraroni, and C. La Vecchia, Resveratrol and breast cancer risk, *Eur J Cancer Prev* **14**(2): 139–142 (2005).
53. Zanardi, S., D. Serrano, A. Argusti, M. Barile, M. Puntoni, and A. Decensi, Clinical trials with retinoids for breast cancer chemoprevention, *Endocr Relat Cancer* **13**(1): 51–68 (2006).
54. Li, S.Z., K. Li, J.H. Zhang, and Z. Dong, The effect of quercetin on doxorubicin cytotoxicity in human breast cancer cells, *Anticancer Agents Med Chem* **13**(2): 352–355 (2013).

55. Bansal, T., M. Jaggi, R.K. Khar, and S. Talegaonkar, Emerging significance of flavonoids as P-glycoprotein inhibitors in cancer chemotherapy, *J Pharm Pharm Sci* **12**(1): 46–78 (2009).
56. Constantinou, A.I., B.E. White, D. Tonetti, Y. Yang, W. Liang, W. Li, and R.B. van Breemen, The soy isoflavone daidzein improves the capacity of tamoxifen to prevent mammary tumours, *Eur J Cancer* **41**(4): 647–654 (2005).
57. Ahmad, A., S. Ali, A. Ahmed, A.S. Ali, A. Raz, W.A. Sakr, and K.M. Rahman, 3,3′-diindolylmethane enhances the effectiveness of Herceptin against HER-2/neu-expressing breast cancer cells, *PLoS One* **8**(1): e54657 (2013).
58. Russo, M., C. Spagnuolo, I. Tedesco, and G.L. Russo, Phytochemicals in cancer prevention and therapy: Truth or dare? *Toxins (Basel)* **2**(4): 517–551 (2010).

4

Anti-Proliferative and Pro-Apoptotic Effects of Bioactive Constituents Derived from Fruits and Vegetables Against Colorectal Cancer

*Sakshi Sikka and Gautam Sethi**

INTRODUCTION

Colorectal cancer is defined as any malignant neoplasm arising from the inner lining of the colonic epithelium. It is the third most common cancer and the third leading cause of cancer related deaths for both men and women in the United States.[1] The five-year survival rate of colon cancer after diagnosis at an early and localized stage is 90%; however, when distant metastasis has occurred, the five-year survival rate drops to 10%.[1] The occurrence of colon cancer is mainly associated with the incidence of aberrant crypt foci (ACF), an earliest neoplastic lesion, which are clusters of mucosal cells with an enlarged and thicker layer of epithelia than the surrounding normal crypts that progress into polyps followed by adenomas and adenocarcinomas. These sequences of events are considered to be

*Corresponding author: Gautam Sethi, Ph.D., Assistant Professor, Department of Pharmacology, Yong Loo Lin School of Medicine and Cancer Science Institute of Singapore, National University of Singapore, Singapore 117597. Tel: (+65) 6516-3267, Fax: (+65) 6873-7690, Email: phcgs@nus.edu.sg.

a consequence of the accumulation of multiple genetic alterations in colonic epithelium.[2] The occurrence of colon cancer is strongly related to age, with 90% of the cases arising in people who are 50 years or older. It has been estimated that about 70–90% of colon cancer death can be linked to diet.[3] It is clearly established that only 5–10% of all cancer cases can be attributed to genetic defects, whereas the remaining 90–95% have their roots in the environment and lifestyle.[4] Furthermore, it is estimated that 75–85% of all chronic illnesses and diseases are linked to lifestyle and cannot be explained by differences in genetic makeup.[5] The lifestyle factors include cigarette smoking, diet (fried foods, red meat, etc.), alcohol, sun exposure, environmental pollutants, infections, stress, obesity,[6] and physical inactivity.[7] The evidence indicates that of all cancer-related deaths, as many as 30–35% are linked to diet. Therefore, cancer prevention requires increased ingestion of fruits and vegetables, moderate intake of alcohol, caloric restriction, exercise, avoidance of direct exposure to sunlight, minimal meat consumption and use of whole grains.[8] There is a positive association between fat and red meat and an inverse association between dietary fiber, fruits, and vegetable intake with the development of colorectal adenomas.[9,10] Recently, there is considerable interest in using dietary prevention and chemoprevention to decrease colorectal cancer mortality.[11,12] A number of important signalling molecules including pro-apoptotic proteins (e.g., caspases, PARP), protein kinases (e.g., Akt, IKK, PKC, p38, JNK, MAPK), cell-cycle proteins (e.g., cyclins, cyclin-dependent kinases), cell-adhesion molecules (ICAM, VCAM, ELAM) and metastatic proteins (COX-2, 5-LOX, MMP-9, VEGF) have been found to be inhibited by dietary agents.[3] While fruits and vegetables are recommended for prevention of cancer and other diseases, their active ingredients and mechanisms of actions are less well understood. Extensive research has identified various molecular targets that can potentially be used not only for the prevention of cancer but also for its treatment.[13,14] However, lack of desirable therapeutic effects with targeted therapies resulting from bypass mechanisms has forced researchers to employ either combination therapy or agents that interfere with multiple cell signalling pathways. In this chapter, we present evidence that numerous agents derived from fruits and vegetables can interfere with several cell signalling pathways in colorectal cancer.[15]

The active components of dietary fruits and vegetables that have exhibited significant anticancer effects include genistein, resveratrol, diallylsulfide, S-allylcysteine, allicin, lycopene, capsaicin, diosgenin, 6-gingerol, ellagic acid, ursolic acid, silymarin, anethol, catechins, eugenol, isoeugenol, dithiolthiones, isothiocyanates, indole-3-carbinol, isoflavones, saponins, phytosterols, inositol hexaphosphate, vitamin C, D-limonene, lutein, folic acid, β-carotene, selenium, vitamin E, flavonoids and dietary fiber.[15,16] These dietary agents are able to suppress the inflammatory processes that lead to transformation, hyperproliferation and initiation of carcinogenesis, angiogenesis and metastasis.[17,18]

MAJOR ONCOGENIC PATHWAYS TARGETED BY DIETARY AGENTS IN COLORECTAL CANCER

Tumorigenesis is a multi-step process that can be activated by various environmental carcinogens (such as cigarette smoke, industrial emissions, gasoline vapours), inflammatory agents (such as tumor necrosis factor (TNF) and H_2O_2) and tumor promoters (such as phorbol esters and okadaic acid).[19] A wide variety of molecular targets activated by distinct stimuli including transcription factors (e.g., NF-κB, AP-1, STAT3, HIF-1α, Nrf2, Wnt/β-catenin pathway), anti-apoptotic proteins (e.g., Bcl-2, Bcl-x_L, survivin, Mcl-1), pro-apoptotic proteins (e.g., caspases, PARP), protein kinases (e.g., Akt, EGFR, HER2, JNK,MAPK), cell cycle proteins (e.g., cyclins, cyclin-dependent kinases), cell-adhesion molecules (ICAM, VCAM, ELAM), pro-inflammatory enzymes (COX-2, 5-LOX) and regulators of angiogenesis (VEGF, FGF)[20,21] have been implicated in the initiation and progression of colorectal cancer. A few of these important signalling cascades that can be modulated by dietary agents are discussed in brief below.

NF-κB Pathway

It is now well established that NF-κB is constitutively activated in colon cancer and helps in the transition of benign carcinomas towards a metastatic phenotype.[22] The activation of NF-κB also leads to resistance of colon cancer cells to chemotherapy.[23] NF-κB is activated by free radicals, inflammatory stimuli, cytokines, carcinogens, tumor promoters, endotoxins, γ-radiation, ultraviolet (UV) light and X-rays. Under resting conditions, the NF-κB dimers reside in the cytoplasm. Upon activation, it is translocated to the nucleus, where it induces the expression of more than 200 genes that have been shown to suppress apoptosis and induce cellular transformation, proliferation, invasion, metastasis, chemo-resistance, radio-resistance and inflammation.[24,25] Several target genes that are activated are critical to the establishment of the early and late stages of aggressive cancers, including expression of cyclin D1, apoptosis suppressor proteins such as Bcl-2 and Bcl-X_L, and those required for metastasis and angiogenesis, such as matrix metalloproteinases (MMP) and vascular endothelial growth factor (VEGF).[26,27] Dietary agents can suppress the TNF-induced activation of IKK that leads to the inhibition of TNF-dependent phosphorylation and degradation of IκBα and translocation of the p65 subunit.[28] They can thus abrogate NF-κB activation and block the expression of various gene products regulated by this transcription factor (Fig. 4.1). For example, cyclin D1 expression is regulated by NF-κB, and the suppression of NF-κB activation leads to a downregulation of cyclin D1. This can lead to a decrease in the formation of cyclinD1/Cdk4 holoenzyme complex, resulting in the suppression of

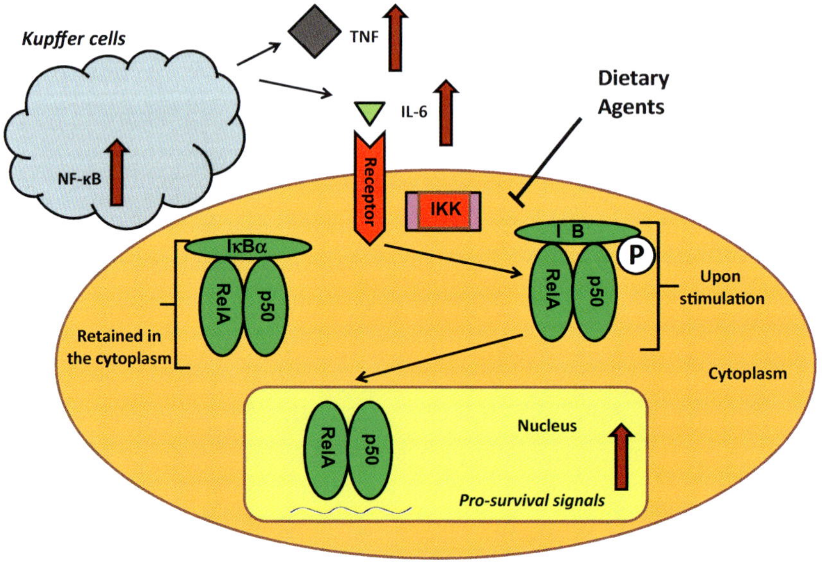

Figure 4.1: Modulation of NF-κB signalling pathway by dietary agents.

proliferation and induction of apoptosis. In addition, dietary agents can induce G0/G1 and/or G2/M phase cell-cycle arrest, upregulate Cdk inhibitors such as p21/Cip1/waf1 and p27Kip1 and downregulate cyclin B1 and Cdc2. Overall, modulation of NF-κB activation by various dietary agents has been found to suppress tumor proliferation, metastasis and angiogenesis in various tumor cell lines and xenograft mice models.

Signal Transducer and Activator of Transcription (STAT3) Pathway

STAT3 is one of the members of a family of STAT transcription factors.[29] The binding of growth factors (e.g., EGF and PDGF) or cytokines (e.g., IL-6) to their receptors results in the activation of their receptor tyrosine kinase or of receptor-associated tyrosine kinases that subsequently phosphorylate the cytoplasmic part of the receptor and provide docking sites for monomeric STAT3. Once recruited, STAT3 is phosphorylated on a specific tyrosine-705 residue, allowing its dimerisation and translocation to the nucleus.[30] Rebouissou *et al.*[31] showed that STAT3 is linked to inflammation-associated tumorigenesis. In addition, elevated STAT3 activity has been detected in a wide variety of cancers.[30] Moreover, the role of STAT3 is implicated in intestinal inflammation and in colon cancer.[32] Consistent with its role in various cancers, STAT3 regulates various genes involved in different aspects of cancer progression such as c-myc, cyclin D3, cyclin A, cdc25a, p21, cyclin D1, Pim-1 and Pim-2.[33] Genes regulated by STAT3 that are involved in survival include proteins belonging to the family of Bcl-2 and IAPs, namely, Bcl-2, Bcl-x_L, Mcl-1 and survivin. STAT3-mediated angiogenesis is regulated by VEGF and it can also control the expression of various MMP family members such as MMP2 and MMP9 that play an important role in tumor invasion and metastasis. Thus, various dietary agents also exert their anticancer effects through the suppression of STAT3 and its regulated oncogenic gene products in colorectal cancer (Fig. 4.2).

Wnt/β-catenin Pathway

An abnormal activation of the Wnt/β-catenin pathway has also been implicated in the development of human colon cancer, and therefore can be considered as a hallmark for this malignancy.[34] The nuclear accumulation

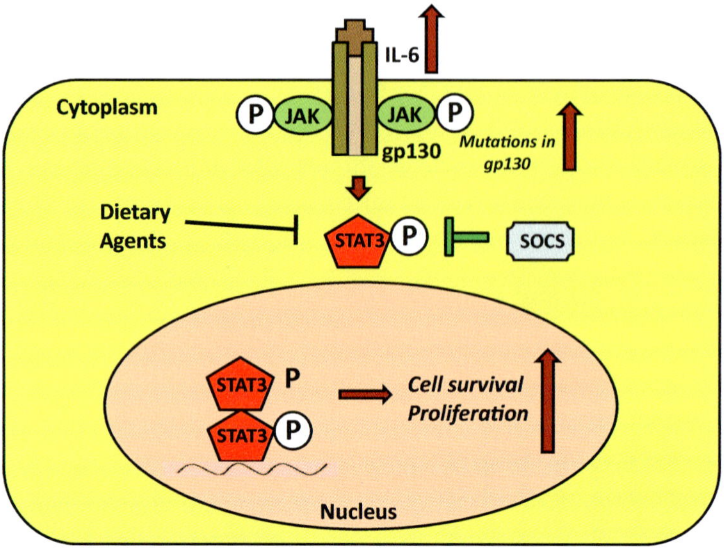

Figure 4.2: Effect of dietary agents on deregulated JAK2/STAT3 signalling pathway in colorectal cancer.

of β-catenin, a hallmark of activated Wnt signalling, has been clearly observed in cancer cells.[35] Seventy percent of colorectal cancers have been shown to bear mutations in APC, such that it fails to degrade β-catenin.[36] Hence, Wnt/β-catenin pathway plays a pivotal role in both the colorectal cancer initiation and progression.

REPORTED ANTICANCER EFFECTS OF DIETARY AGENTS AGAINST COLORECTAL CANCER

In this section, we discuss briefly the important constituents of fruits and vegetables that have shown significant potential in both the prevention and the treatment of colorectal cancer through the modulation of multiple signal transduction cascades.

Epigallocatechin-3-Gallate

Green tea polyphenols such as epigallocatechin-3-gallate (EGCG) and the flavins from black tea inhibits COX-dependent arachidonic acid metabolism in microsomes from tumors and normal colon mucosa, indicating that tea polyphenols can affect arachidonic acid metabolism in human colon mucosa and colon tumors, perhaps altering the risk for colon cancer in humans.[37,38] EGCG, a major component in green tea polyphenols, has been reported to suppress colonic tumorigenesis in animal models and epidemiological studies.[39] These dietary agents can be used either in their natural form for the prevention and perhaps in their pure form for the therapy, where large doses may be needed.[40] EGCG treatment of human colorectal carcinoma HT-29 cells resulted in classical features of apoptosis including nuclear condensation, DNA fragmentation, caspase activation, disruption of mitochondrial membrane potential and cytochrome c release, which all appeared to be mediated by the c-Jun N-terminal kinase (JNK) pathway.[39] EGCG can inhibit the growth and activation of EGFR and human EGFR-2 signalling pathways in human colon cancer cells.[41] Sah *et al.* found that EGCG can inhibit the EGFR signalling pathway, most likely through the direct inhibition of ERK1/2 and Akt kinases.[42] In Asian countries with relatively lower incidence of colon cancer, such as China, Japan and Korea, one of the prominent lifestyle habits is the daily consumption of green tea beverages by a large population.[43] A single cup of green tea can contain up to 200 mg of EGCG.[44] As EGCG is retained in the gastrointestinal tract after oral administration, this pharmacokinetics property gives it the potential to function as a chemopreventive agent against colon cancer. Moreover, treatment of EGCG has been shown to inhibit HT-29 colon cancer cell growth and activate caspases 3 and 9 accompanied by mitochondrial transmembrane potential transition and cytochrome c release. Activation of MAPKs was detected as early signalling event elicited by EGCG. Inhibition of the JNK pathway showed the involvement of JNK in EGCG-induced cytochrome c release and cell death.[45,46] It has been reported that EGCG inhibits azoxymethane (AOM)-induced colon tumorigenesis in the rat[47] and also drinking green tea blocks the formation of 1,2-dimethylhydrazine-induced colonic aberrant crypt foci, which is a typical precursor lesion of chemical-initiated colon cancer.[48] In HT-29 cells, treatment with EGCG can increase protein levels of E-cadherin by 27% to 58%, induce the translocation of β-catenin from the nucleus to the cytoplasm as well as the plasma membrane, and decrease c-Myc and cyclin D1. Zhang *et al.*[49] observed that EGCG decreased cyclin D1 protein stability and triggered ubiquitin-dependent proteasomal degradation in colorectal cancer cells. EGCG also increases

ERK-, IKK-, and PI3K-dependent p21 promoter activity, which in turn increases p21 mRNA and protein expression, leading to growth suppression in these cells.

Moreover, the combination of anticancer drugs with green tea catechin synergistically induces apoptosis in human cancer cells, inhibits tumor formation in mice, and enhances inhibition of tumor growth in xenograft mouse models. The effects of combining EGCG and anticancer drugs have been studied, focusing on inhibition of cell growth and induction of apoptosis. In one experiment, Min mice were fed CE-2 diet with 0.03% sulindac and took water containing 0.1% green tea extract for 10 weeks. All mice ingested about 5 mg sulindac and 10 mg of green tea extract per day. At 16 weeks of age, the average number of tumors per mouse in the control group (without sulindac and green tea extract), sulindac alone, green tea extract alone and the combination (sulindac and green tea extract) were 72.3 ± 28.3, 49.0 ± 12.7, 56.7 ± 3.5 and 32.0 ± 18.7, respectively, which shows a decrease of 55.7% of the average number of tumors per mouse in the combination group. Histologically, the control group produced 10.8% adenocarcinomas, whereas the groups treated with the combination, sulindac alone and green tea extract alone, induced only adenomas.[50] Moreover, mice treated with the combination showed an increase in body weight, as did those treated with sulindac alone and green tea extract alone, indicating that the treatment with the combination did not have any toxic effects.[50]

Resveratrol

Resveratrol (3,5,4′-trihydroxystilbene), a phytoalexin found in grapes, has shown to have cancer chemopreventive activity.[51,52] However, the mechanism of the anticarcinogenic activity is not well understood. Wolter *et al.* showed the downregulation of the cyclin D1/Cdk4 complex by resveratrol in colon cancer cell lines.[53] Colonic epithelial cells undergo a sequential process of proliferation, differentiation, apoptosis and exfoliation as they migrate along the crypt–villus axis, which is deregulated in carcinogenesis.[54] This process is largely regulated by periodical activation and inactivation of a highly conserved family of cyclin-dependent kinases (Cdk).[55] Cdk activity is modulated by the cyclins, which bind to and activate the Cdk.[56] They are regulated primarily by their expression levels.

Also, resveratrol was demonstrated to induce G2 arrest through the inhibition of Cdk7 and Cdc2 kinases in colon carcinoma HT-29 cells.[51] Moreover, resveratrol inhibited the proliferation of HT-29 colon cancer cells and resulted in their accumulation in the G_2 phase of the cell cycle. Western blot analysis and kinase assays demonstrated that the perturbation of G_2 phase progression by resveratrol was accompanied by the inactivation of $p34^{CDC2}$ protein kinase, and an increase in the tyrosine-phosphorylated (inactive) form of $p34^{CDC2}$. Kinase assays revealed that the reduction of $p34^{CDC2}$ activity by resveratrol was mediated through the inhibition of Cdk7 kinase activity, while Cdc25A phosphatase activity was not affected. In addition, resveratrol-treated cells were shown to have a low level of Cdk7 kinase-Thr^{161}-phosphorylated $p34^{CDC2}$. These results demonstrated that resveratrol induced cell cycle arrest at the G_2 phase through the inhibition of Cdk7 kinase activity, suggesting that its antitumor activity might occur through the disruption of cell division at the G_2/M phase.[51] Studies demonstrated that levels of cyclin D1 and Cdk4 proteins were decreased, as revealed by immunoblotting. In addition, resveratrol enhanced the expression of cyclin E and cyclin A. However, the protein levels of cdk2, cdk6 and proliferating cell nuclear antigen (PCNA) were unaffected. These findings suggest that resveratrol exerts chemopreventive effects on colonic cancer cells by inhibition of the cell cycle.[57]

The absorption rate of resveratrol in the perfused small intestine of the rat was estimated to be only 20.5%,[58] therefore the fact that the intestinal epithelium might be confronted with much higher concentrations than cells in other tissues implies that resveratrol could have an important role in the prevention of colon cancer by blocking hyperproliferation of the epithelium and by promoting apoptosis.[58] Limited data in humans have revealed that resveratrol is pharmacologically quite safe. Delmas *et al.* analyzed the molecular mechanisms of resveratrol-induced apoptosis in colon cancer cells, with special attention to the role of the death receptor Fas pathway.[59,60] They showed that resveratrol activates various caspases and triggers apoptosis in SW480 human colon cancer cells. Caspase activation was associated with accumulation of the pro-apoptotic proteins Bax and Bak, which underwent conformational changes and relocalization to the mitochondria. The concentrations of resveratrol, which can be achieved in human tissues after p.o. administration, have not yet been defined. The purpose of the study conducted by Patel *et al.*[61] was to measure concentrations of resveratrol and its metabolites in the colorectal tissue of 20 patients who consumed eight daily doses of resveratrol at 0.5 g or 1.0 g before surgical resection. The results showed that consumption of resveratrol reduced tumor cell proliferation by 5% without any side effects and the levels of resveratrol and its metabolites (resveratrol-3-O-glucuronide, resveratrol-4′-O-glucuronide, resveratrol-3-O-sulphate, resveratrol-4′-O-sulphate, resveratrol sulphate glucuronide and resveratrol disulphate) were consistently higher in tissues originating in the right side of the colon compared with the left.[61] Increasing lines of evidence suggest that microRNAs play important roles in all stages of cancer, from initiation to tumor promotion and progression, influencing cell proliferation, differentiation, apoptosis, angiogenesis and metastasis. Recent studies have shown that several "signature" miRNAs for colon cancer such as miR-21, miR-196a, miR-25, miR-17 and miR-92a-2 are significantly downregulated by resveratrol in experimental conditions.[62] Therefore, it can be concluded that resveratrol has high potential in the prevention of colorectal cancer.

Diosgenin

Research during the past decade has shown that diosgenin suppresses proliferation and induces apoptosis in a wide variety of cancer cells lines. Anti-proliferative effects of diosgenin are mediated through cell cycle arrest, disruption of Ca^{2+} homeostasis, activation of p53, release of apoptosis-inducing factor and modulation of caspase 3 activity.[63] Diosgenin has also been reported to inhibit AOM-induced aberrant colon crypt foci formation, inhibit intestinal inflammation and modulate the activity of LOX and COX-2.[64] Miyoshi *et al.*[65] investigated the effects of *sanyaku*, a traditional Chinese medicine and its major steroidal saponin constituent, diosgenin, on AOM-induced colon carcinogenesis. Colon cancer was induced by a single intraperitoneal injection of AOM followed by administration of 1.5% dextran sodium sulphate (DSS) in drinking water for seven days. The treatment with commercial diosgenin or *sanyaku* (which contained diosgenin at 63.8 ± 1.2 mg/kg dry weight) in the diet (at 20, 100, or 500 mg/kg) for 17 weeks significantly decreased colonic mucosal ulcers, dysplastic crypts and number of colon tumors compared with the control

(AOM/DSS-treated) mice, which was in accordance with the significant reduction of AOM/DSS-mediated increases in expression of inflammatory cytokines such as IL-1β and serum triglyceride. These studies suggest that the Chinese medicine *sanyaku* and the tubers of various yams containing diosgenin could be beneficial to prevent colon carcinogenesis in humans. Lepage *et al.*[66] investigated the effect of diosgenin on TNF-related apoptosis-inducing ligand (TRAIL)-induced apoptosis in HT-29 cells. It was shown that diosgenin sensitises HT-29 cells to TRAIL-induced apoptosis by p38 MAPK pathway activation and subsequent DR5 overexpression. Furthermore, diosgenin alone, TRAIL alone, or combination treatment increased COX-2 expression, and the use of a COX-2 inhibitor further increased apoptosis induction.

Eugenol

Eugenol, a natural compound available in honey and various plants extracts including cloves and *Magnoliae flos*, is exploited for various medicinal applications.[67] *Eugenia caryophyllata* Thunberg (Clove), a tropical tree originating in the Moluccas, is abundantly cultivated in Tanzania, Indonesia, Sri Lanka and the Malagasy Republic.[68,69] Studies indicated that eugenol can inhibit the proliferation of HT-29 cells and suppress the serum-stimulated mRNA expression of COX-2, but not COX-1.[70,71] Furthermore, Jaganathan *et al.*[67] analyzed the anticancer mechanism of eugenol against colon cancer cells. The treatment with eugenol inhibited proliferation and induced apoptosis in colon cancer cells by activating reactive oxygen species, polyadenosine diphosphate-ribose polymerase (PARP), p53 and caspase 3. These studies suggest that eugenol has the ability to act as an anticancer agent against colon cancer.

Silibinin

Silibinin from milk thistle suppresses the intestinal carcinogenesis in ApcMin mice as well as 1,2-dimethylhydrazine-induced colon cancer in male Wistar rats through the inhibition of the Wnt/β-catenin signalling pathwa.[72] Kaur *et al.*[73] assessed the anticancer efficacy of silibinin against advanced colorectal cancer LoVo cells both *in vitro* and *in vivo*. The results showed that silibinin treatment strongly inhibited the growth of LoVo cells and induced apoptotic death, which was associated with cell cycle arrest at G1 phase and G2/M phase (at higher concentration) and increased levels of cleaved caspases (3 and 9) and cleaved PARP. Moreover, silibinin decreased the level of cyclins (D1, D3, A and B1) and Cdks (1, 2, 4 and 6) and increased the level of Cdk inhibitors (p21 and p27). Furthermore, oral administration of silibinin for six weeks (at 100 and 200 mg/kg/d for five days/week) significantly inhibited the growth of LoVo xenograft in nude mice without any apparent toxicity. Together, these results suggest the potential efficacy of silibinin against advanced human colorectal cancer. Kauntz *et al.*[74] investigated the potential of silibinin as a chemopreventive agent in AOM-induced colon carcinogenesis. One week after AOM injection (post-initiation), animals were treated with silibinin (intragastric; 300 mg/kg/day) until their sacrifice (after seven weeks of treatment). Silibinin-treated animals exhibited a twofold reduction in the number of AOM-induced hyperproliferative crypts and aberrant crypt foci in the colon compared to AOM-injected control animals. Moreover, the colonic tissue analysis showed that silibinin-induced apoptosis in the colon mucosal cells, downregulated anti-apoptotic protein Bcl-2 and upregulated pro-apoptotic protein Bax.

In another study, Ravichandran *et al.*[75] investigated *in vivo* the efficacy of silibinin against AOM-induced colon tumorigenesis in A/J mice. Silibinin feeding showed a dose-dependent decrease in AOM-induced colon tumorigenesis with stronger efficacy in the pre-treatment versus post-treatment regimen. Analysis of tissue samples showed that silibinin inhibited cell proliferation, decreased PCNA, cyclin D1, inducible nitric oxide synthase, COX-2, and VEGF and increased Cip1/p21 levels suggesting its anti-inflammatory and antiangiogenic potential. Overall, these results support the translational potential of silibinin in colorectal cancer chemoprevention. However, its effects on cancer stem-like cells (CSLCs) remain unclear. A study was conducted to examine its effect on the development of CSLCs and disclose the underlying signalling.[76] The colorectal cancer spheroid culture system was used for enriching CSLCs. The effects of silibinin on CSLCs were evaluated by counting sphere numbers and calculating the percentage of CD133+ cells by flow cytometry and immunofluorescence both in the absence and presence of different concentrations of silibinin. The results showed silibinin reduced the sphere formation, decreased the CD133+ percentage cells and suppressed the activation of the AKT/mTOR pathway in spheroid culture through inhibiting the activity of protein phosphatase 2Ac subunit (PP2Ac). In a xenograft tumor model, treatment with silibinin also inhibited tumor formation rate and tumor growth.[76] These results showed that silibinin might have high potential for developing new strategies in modulating CSLCs in cancer therapy.

Capasaicin

Capsaicin (N-vanillyl-8-methyl-alpha-nonenamide), a spicy component of hot pepper, is a homovanillic acid derivative that preferentially induces certain cancer cells to undergo apoptosis and has a putative role in cancer chemoprevention.[77,78] Treatment with capsaicin induced apoptotic cell death in a dose-dependent manner in HT-29 human colon cancer cells.[79] Thus, capsaicin may have a beneficial effect for the treatment of colon cancer. It was also found in a study that capsaicin suppressed the transcriptional activity of β-catenin/TCF. Capsaicin treatment resulted in a decrease of intracellular β-catenin levels and a reduction of transcripts from the β-catenin gene (*CTNNB1*) contributing to the anticancer activity of capasaicin.[79] In addition, it was demonstrated that capsaicin decreased the levels of anti-apoptotic proteins such as Bcl-2 and increased the levels of pro-apoptotic proteins such as Bax. Capsaicin induced apoptosis in Colo 205 cells through the activation of caspases 3, 8 and 9. *In vivo* studies in immunodeficient nu/nu mice bearing Colo 205 tumor xenografts showed that capsaicin effectively inhibited tumor growth. The potent *in vitro* and *in vivo* antitumor activities of capsaicin suggest that capsaicin can be developed for the treatment of human colon cancer.[78]

Furthermore, Liu *et al.*[80] made the unexpected discovery that treatment with low concentrations of capsaicin upregulates tNOX (tumor-associated NADH oxidase) expression in HCT-116 human colon carcinoma cells in association with enhanced cell proliferation and migration, as evidenced by downregulation of epithelial markers and upregulation of mesenchymal markers. They found that tNOX knockdown in HCT-116 cells by RNA interference reversed capsaicin-induced cell proliferation and migration *in vitro* and decreased tumor growth *in vivo*. Therefore, caution should be taken when using capsaicin as a chemopreventive agent.

Fisetin

Fisetin is a naturally occurring flavonoid commonly found in various vegetables and fruits such as onions, cucumbers, apples, persimmons and strawberries.[81,82] It was found that the treatment of COX2-overexpressing HT-29 human colon cancer cells with fisetin (30–120 μM) induced apoptosis, inhibited Wnt signalling activity through downregulation of β-catenin and T cell factor 4, decreased the expression of target genes such as cyclin D1 and MMP-7, inhibited the secretion of prostaglandin E2 and downregulated COX-2 protein expression without affecting COX-1. Fisetin treatment of cells also inhibited the activation of EGFR and NF-κB pathway.[81] Moreover, Lim *et al.*[84] observed DNA condensations, cleavage of PARP and cleavage of caspases 3, 7 and 9 induced in HCT-116 cells treated with fisetin. Fisetin also induced a reduction in the protein levels of anti-apoptotic Bcl-x_L and Bcl-2 and an increase in the levels of pro-apoptotic Bak and Bim; however, this compound did not affect Bax protein levels, but induced its mitochondrial translocation. Fisetin also enhanced mitochondrial membrane permeability, induced the release of cytochrome c and Smac/DIABLO and increased in the protein levels of p53, cleaved caspase 8, Fas ligand, death receptor 5 and TRAIL. These results suggest that fisetin induces apoptosis in HCT-116 cells via the activation of the death receptor- and mitochondrial-dependent pathways and subsequent activation of the caspase cascade.[83]

Fruits

Blackberries, black raspberries, blueberries, cranberries, red raspberries and strawberry extracts have been shown to inhibit the growth and stimulate apoptosis in HT-29 and HCT-116 cells.[84] Cranberry fruit is high in content of phenolic compounds including three classes of flavonoids (flavonols, anthocyanins and PACs), catechins or flavan-3-ols; a variety of phenolic acids, among which the major is p-hydroxycinnamic acid; and triterpenoids of the ursane type.[85] Quercetin is the major flavonol in cranberries and exists in several glycosidic forms, primarily

In various human colon carcinoma cell lines, apigenin treatment resulted in cell growth inhibition and G2/M cell cycle arrest, which was associated with inhibition of p34 (Cdc2) kinase, and with reduced accumulation of p34 (Cdc2) and cyclin B1 proteins.[99] An important effect of apigenin is its ability to increase the stability of the tumor suppressor *p53* gene in normal cells.[100] It is hypothesized that apigenin may play a significant role in cancer prevention by modifying the effects of the p53 protein. Exposure of p53 mutant cancer cells to apigenin resulted in inhibition of cell growth and alteration of the cell cycle as demonstrated in a study in which apigenin treatment resulted in growth inhibition and G2/M phase arrest in two p53 mutant cancer cell lines, HT-29 and MG63.[101] These effects were associated with a marked increase in the protein expression of p21/WAF1 in a dose- and time-dependent manner. These results suggest that there is a p53-independent pathway for apigenin in p53 mutant cell lines, which induces p21/WAF1 expression and growth inhibition.

In addition, Turktekin *et al.*[102] explored the cytotoxic and apoptotic effects of various doses of apigenin administered alone and together with 5-fluorouracil (5-FU) — a chemotherapeutic agent with high cytotoxicity — for different incubation periods, on morphologic, DNA, RNA, mRN, and protein levels on the p53 mutant HT-29 human colon adenocarcinoma cell line. Treatment with apigenin resulted in 24.92% apoptosis, whereas the combination (same dose of apigenin plus 5-FU for the same incubation period) resulted in 29.13% of apoptosis in HT-29 cells. This was accompanied by an increase in mRNA and protein expression levels of caspases 3 and 8 and a decrease in mRNA expression levels of mammalian target of rapamycin (mTOR) and cyclin D1.[102] These studies demonstrate the therapeutic potential of apigenin alone and in combination with chemotherapeutic agents in colon cancer.

Delphinidin

Delphinidin, the major anthocyanidin present in vegetables such as eggplants, tomatoes, carrots, purple sweet potatoes, red cabbages and red onions possesses strong antioxidant and anti-inflammatory properties.[103] Treatment with delphinidin in HCT-116 cells resulted in decrease in cell viability, induction of apoptosis, cleavage of PARP, activation of caspases 3, 8, and 9, increase in Bax with a concomitant decrease in Bcl-2 protein, and G2/M phase cell cycle arrest. Delphinidin treatment also led to activation of initiator caspases 8 and 9 and downstream effector caspase 3. In addition, treatment of HCT116 cells with delphinidin resulted in the inhibition of IKKα, phosphorylation and degradation of IκBα, phosphorylation of NF-κB/p65, its nuclear translocation, NF-κB/p65 DNA binding activity and transcriptional activation of NF-κB. Additonally, delphinidin increased the expression of tumor suppressor protein p53 and its downstream target p21 in HCT-116 cells.[103,104] Recent studies have also shown that this compound induces cytotoxicity in Caco-2, LoVo and drug-resistant LoVo/ADR colon cancer cells in experimental conditions.[105] Overall, these studies illustrate the anticancer potential of delphinidin against colon cancer and its mechanisms of action.

CONCLUSION

Colorectal cancer remains a leading cause of cancer mortality throughout the world with few therapeutic options to combat this disease. Natural compounds obtained from different sources such as fruits, vegetables, herbs and even fungi, open up a novel and exciting prospective on colorectal cancer prevention and treatment. However, there still remains a lot to be determined about these agents' molecular mechanisms, including their effects on genes that are overexpressed or mutated in carcinogenesis, and subsequent studies may increase our knowledge as to whether any of these antioxidants have the capability to prevent colorectal cancer. These future studies should focus on molecular aspects of the antioxidant agents. Animal and cell culture models in which oncogenes are overexpressed or tumor suppressor genes are silenced will provide important information about antioxidant actions. Thus, there is a great need for the development of novel and effective cancer therapies.

ABBREVIATIONS

5-LOX: 5-lipoxygenase; ACF: aberrant crypt foci; AOM: azoxymethane; AP-1: activator protein-1; APC: adenomatous polyposis coli; Bcl-2:

B-cell lymphoma 2; Bcl-x_L: B-cell lymphoma-extra large; Cdk: cyclin-dependent kinases; COX-2: cyclooxygenase-2; CSLC: cancer stem-like cell; DAS: diallylsulphide; DR5: death receptor; EGCG: epigallocatechingallate; EGF: epidermal growth factor; ELAM: endothelial leukocyte adhesion molecule 1; ERK1/2: extracellular signal-regulated kinases; FAP: familial adenomatous polyposis; H_2O_2: hydrogen peroxide; HIF-1α: hypoxia-inducible factor 1-alpha; IAP: inhibitor of apoptosis; IKK: IκB kinase; IL-6: interleukin-6; JNK: c-Jun N-terminal kinases; MAPK-ERK: mitogen-activated protein kinase-extracellular signal regulated kinase; Mcl-1: myeloid leukemia cell differentiation protein; MMP: matrix metalloproteinase; NF-κB: nuclear factor-kappa B; Nrf2: nuclear factor (erythroid-derived 2)-like 2; P PARP: poly(ADP-ribose) polymerase; PDGF: platelet-derived growth factor; PI3K: phosphoinositide 3-kinase; PKC: protein kinase C; STAT3: signal transducer and activator of transcription; TNF-α: tumor necrosis factor-alpha; TRAIL: TNF-related apoptosis-inducing ligand; VCAM: vascular cell adhesion protein 1; VEGF: vascular endothelial growth factor; XIAP: X-linked inhibitor of apoptosis protein.

ACKNOWLEDGMENT

This work was supported by a grant from the National Medical Research Council of Singapore (Grant R-184-000-201-275) to Dr. Gautam Sethi.

REFERENCES

1. Rajamanickam, S. and R. Agarwal, Natural products and colon cancer: Current status and future prospects, *Drug Dev Res* **69**(7): 460–471 (2008).
2. Humphries, A. and N.A. Wright, Colonic crypt organization and tumorigenesis, *Nat Rev Cancer* **8**(6): 415–424 (2008).
3. Ries, L.A., P.A. Wingo, D.S. Miller, H.L. Howe, H.K. Weir, H.M. Rosenberg, S.W. Vernon, K. Cronin, and B.K. Edwards, The annual report to the nation on the status of cancer, 1973–1997, with a special section on colorectal cancer, *Cancer* **88**(10): 2398–2424 (2000).
4. Anand, P., A.B. Kunnumakkara, C. Sundaram, K.B. Harikumar, S.T. Tharakan, O.S. Lai, B. Sung, and B.B. Aggarwal, Cancer is a preventable disease that requires major lifestyle changes, *Pharm Res* **25**(9): 2097–2116 (2008).

5. Wong, A.H., I.I. Gottesman, and A. Petronis, Phenotypic differences in genetically identical organisms: The epigenetic perspective, *Hum Mol Genet* **14**(1): R11–R18 (2005).
6. Lund, E.K., N.J. Belshaw, G.O. Elliott, and I.T. Johnson, Recent advances in understanding the role of diet and obesity in the development of colorectal cancer, *Proc Nutr Soc* **70**(2): 194–204 (2011).
7. Sung, B., S. Prasad, V.R. Yadav, A. Lavasanifar, and B.B. Aggarwal, Cancer and diet: How are they related?, *Free Radic Res* **45**(8): 864–879 (2011).
8. Gonzalez, C.A., Nutrition and cancer: The current epidemiological evidence, *Br J Nutr* **96**(1 Suppl.): S42–S45 (2006).
9. Mathew, A., U. Peters, N. Chatterjee, M. Kulldorff, and R. Sinha, Fat, fiber, fruits, vegetables, and risk of colorectal adenomas, *Int J Cancer* **108**(2): 287–292 (2004).
10. Marshall, J.R., Prevention of colorectal cancer: Diet, chemoprevention, and lifestyle, *Gastroenterol Clin North Am* **37**(1): 73–82 (2008).
11. Steele, V.E., R.C. Moon, R.A. Lubet, C.J. Grubbs, B.S. Reddy, M. Wargovich, D.L. McCormick, M.A. Pereira, J.A. Crowell, D. Bagheri, *et al.*, Preclinical efficacy evaluation of potential chemopreventive agents in animal carcinogenesis models: Methods and results from the NCI Chemoprevention Drug Development Program, *J Cell Biochem Suppl* **20**: 32–54 (1994).
12. Schatzkin, A. and G. Kelloff, Chemo- and dietary prevention of colorectal cancer, *Eur J Cancer* **31A**(7–8): 1198–1204 (1995).
13. Pratheeshkumar, P., C. Sreekala, Z. Zhang, A. Budhraja, S. Ding, Y.O. Son, X. Wang, A. Hitron, K. Hyun-Jung, L. Wang, J.C. Lee, and X. Shi, Cancer prevention with promising natural products: Mechanisms of action and molecular targets, *Anticancer Agents Med Chem* **12**(10): 1159–1184 (2012).
14. Lee, K.W., A.M. Bode, and Z. Dong, Molecular targets of phytochemicals for cancer prevention, *Nat Rev Cancer* **11**(3): 211–218 (2011).
15. Aggarwal, B.B. and S. Shishodia, Molecular targets of dietary agents for prevention and therapy of cancer, *Biochem Pharmacol* **71**(10): 1397–1421 (2006).
16. Siu, D., Natural products and their role in cancer therapy, *Med Oncol* **28**(3): 888–900 (2011).
17. Deorukhkar, A., S. Krishnan, G. Sethi, and B.B. Aggarwal, Back to basics: How natural products can provide the basis for new therapeutics, *Expert Opin Investig Drugs* **16**(11): 1753–1773 (2007).
18. Priyadarsini, R.V. and S. Nagini, Cancer chemoprevention by dietary phytochemicals: Promises and pitfalls, *Curr Pharm Biotechnol* **13**(1): 125–136 (2012).

19. Aggarwal, B.B., G. Sethi, V. Baladandayuthapani, S. Krishnan, and S. Shishodia, Targeting cell signaling pathways for drug discovery: An old lock needs a new key, *J Cell Biochem* **102**(3): 580–592 (2007).
20. Sethi, G., M.K. Shanmugam, L. Ramachandran, A.P. Kumar, and V. Tergaonkar, Multifaceted link between cancer and inflammation, *Biosci Rep* **32**(1): 1–15 (2012).
21. Tan, A.C., I. Konczak, D.M. Sze, and I. Ramzan, Molecular pathways for cancer chemoprevention by dietary phytochemicals, *Nutr Cancer* **63**(4): 495–505 (2011).
22. Vaiopoulos, A.G., K.K. Papachroni, and A.G. Papavassiliou, Colon carcinogenesis: Learning from NF-kappaB and AP-1, *Int J Biochem Cell Biol* **42**(7): 1061–1065 (2010).
23. Sakamoto, K. and S. Maeda, Targeting NF-kappaB for colorectal cancer, *Expert Opin Ther Targets* **14**(6): 593–601 (2010).
24. Li, F. and G. Sethi, Targeting transcription factor NF-kappaB to overcome chemoresistance and radioresistance in cancer therapy, *Biochim Biophys Acta* **1805**(2): 167–180 (2010).
25. Ahn, K.S., G. Sethi, and B.B. Aggarwal, Nuclear factor-kappaB: From clone to clinic, *Curr Mol Med* **7**(7): 619–637 (2007).
26. Sethi, G. and V. Tergaonkar, Potential pharmacological control of the NF-kappaB pathway, *Trends Pharmacol Sci* **30**(6): 313–321 (2009).
27. Sethi, G., B. Sung, and B.B. Aggarwal, Nuclear factor-kappaB activation: From bench to bedside, *Exp Biol Med (Maywood)* **233**(1): 21–31 (2008).
28. Sethi, G., B. Sung, and B.B. Aggarwal, TNF: A master switch for inflammation to cancer, *Front Biosci* **13**: 5094–5107 (2008).
29. Akira, S., Y. Nishio, M. Inoue, X.J. Wang, S. Wei, T. Matsusaka, K. Yoshida, T. Sudo, M. Naruto, and T. Kishimoto, Molecular cloning of APRF, a novel IFN-stimulated gene factor 3 p91-related transcription factor involved in the gp130-mediated signaling pathway, *Cell* **77**(1): 63–71 (1994).
30. Aggarwal, B.B., A.B. Kunnumakkara, K.B. Harikumar, S.R. Gupta, S.T. Tharakan, C. Koca, S. Dey, and B. Sung, Signal transducer and activator of transcription-3, inflammation, and cancer: How intimate is the relationship?, *Ann NY Acad Sci* **1171**: 59–76 (2009).
31. Rebouissou, S., M. Amessou, G. Couchy, K. Poussin, S. Imbeaud, C. Pilati, T. Izard, C. Balabaud, P. Bioulac-Sage, and J. Zucman-Rossi, Frequent in-frame somatic deletions activate gp130 in inflammatory hepatocellular tumours, *Nature* **457**(7226): 200–204 (2009).

32. Atreya, R. and M.F. Neurath, Signaling molecules: The pathogenic role of the IL-6/STAT-3 trans signaling pathway in intestinal inflammation and in colonic cancer, *Curr Drug Targets* **9**(5): 369–74 (2008).
33. Subramaniam, A., M.K. Shanmugam, E. Perumal, F. Li, A. Nachiyappan, X. Dai, S.N. Swamy, K.S. Ahn, A.P. Kumar, B.K. Tan, K.M. Hui, and G. Sethi, Potential role of signal transducer and activator of transcription (STAT)3 signaling pathway in inflammation, survival, proliferation and invasion of hepatocellular carcinoma, *Biochim Biophys Acta* **1835**(1): 46–60 (2012).
34. Tarapore, R.S., I.A. Siddiqui, and H. Mukhtar, Modulation of Wnt/beta-catenin signaling pathway by bioactive food components, *Carcinogenesis* **33**(3): 483–491 (2012).
35. Bienz, M. and H. Clevers, Armadillo/beta-catenin signals in the nucleus — proof beyond a reasonable doubt?, *Nat Cell Biol* **5**(3): 179–182 (2003).
36. Giles, R.H., J.H. van Es, and H. Clevers, Caught up in a Wnt storm: Wnt signaling in cancer, *Biochim Biophys Acta* **1653**(1): 1–24 (2003).
37. Hong, J., T.J. Smith, C.T. Ho, D.A. August, and C.S. Yang, Effects of purified green and black tea polyphenols on cyclooxygenase- and lipoxygenase-dependent metabolism of arachidonic acid in human colon mucosa and colon tumor tissues, *Biochem Pharmacol* **62**(9): 1175–1183 (2001).
38. Stoicov, C., R. Saffari, and J. Houghton, Green tea inhibits *Helicobacter* growth *in vivo* and *in vitro*, *Int J Antimicrob Agents* **33**(5): 473–478 (2009).
39. Chen, C., G. Shen, V. Hebbar, R. Hu, E.D. Owuor, and A.N. Kong, Epigallocatechin-3-gallate-induced stress signals in HT-29 human colon adenocarcinoma cells, *Carcinogenesis* **24**(8): 1369–1378 (2003).
40. Khan, N. and H. Mukhtar, Modulation of signaling pathways in prostate cancer by green tea polyphenols, *Biochem Pharmacol* **85**(5): 667–672 (2012).
41. Shimizu, M., A. Deguchi, J.T. Lim, H. Moriwaki, L. Kopelovich, and I.B. Weinstein, (−)-Epigallocatechin gallate and polyphenon E inhibit growth and activation of the epidermal growth factor receptor and human epidermal growth factor receptor-2 signaling pathways in human colon cancer cells, *Clin Cancer Res* **11**(7): 2735–2746 (2005).
42. Sah, J.F., S. Balasubramanian, R.L. Eckert, and E.A. Rorke, Epigallocatechin-3-gallate inhibits epidermal growth factor receptor signaling pathway. Evidence for direct inhibition of ERK1/2 and AKT kinases, *J Biol Chem* **279**(13): 12755–12762 (2004).
43. Tomata, Y., M. Kakizaki, N. Nakaya, T. Tsuboya, T. Sone, S. Kuriyama, A. Hozawa, and I. Tsuji, Green tea consumption and the risk of incident functional disability in elderly Japanese: The Ohsaki Cohort 2006 Study, *Am J Clin Nutr* **95**(3): 732–739 (2012).

44. Mukhtar, H. and N. Ahmad, Mechanism of cancer chemopreventive activity of green tea, *Proc Soc Exp Biol Med* **220**(4): 234–238 (1999).
45. Chen, L., M.J. Lee, H. Li, and C.S. Yang, Absorption, distribution, elimination of tea polyphenols in rats, *Drug Metab Dispos* **25**(9): 1045–1050 (1997).
46. Kim, S., M.J. Lee, J. Hong, C. Li, T.J. Smith, G.Y. Yang, D.N. Seril, and C.S. Yang, Plasma and tissue levels of tea catechins in rats and mice during chronic consumption of green tea polyphenols, *Nutr Cancer* **37**(1): 41–48 (2000).
47. Yamane, T., H. Nakatani, N. Kikuoka, H. Matsumoto, Y. Iwata, Y. Kitao, K. Oya, and T. Takahashi, Inhibitory effects and toxicity of green tea polyphenols for gastrointestinal carcinogenesis, *Cancer* **77**(8 Suppl.): 1662–1667 (1996).
48. Jia, X. and C. Han, Effects of green tea on colonic aberrant crypt foci and proliferative indexes in rats, *Nutr Cancer* **39**(2): 239–243 (2001).
49. Zhang, X., K.W. Min, J. Wimalasena, and S.J. Baek, Cyclin D1 degradation and p21 induction contribute to growth inhibition of colorectal cancer cells induced by epigallocatechin-3-gallate, *J Cancer Res Clin Oncol* **138**(12): 2051–2060 (2012).
50. Fujiki, H. and M. Suganuma, Green tea: An effective synergist with anticancer drugs for tertiary cancer prevention, *Cancer Lett* **324**(2): 119–125 (2012).
51. Liang, Y.C., S.H. Tsai, L. Chen, S.Y. Lin-Shiau, and J.K. Lin, Resveratrol-induced G2 arrest through the inhibition of CDK7 and p34 CDC2 kinases in colon carcinoma HT29 cells, *Biochem Pharmacol* **65**(7): 1053–1060 (2003).
52. Whitlock, N.C. and S.J. Baek, The anticancer effects of resveratrol: Modulation of transcription factors, *Nutr Cancer* **64**(4): 493–502 (2012).
53. Wolter, F., B. Akoglu, A. Clausnitzer, and J. Stein, Downregulation of the cyclin D1/Cdk4 complex occurs during resveratrol-induced cell cycle arrest in colon cancer cell lines, *J Nutr* **131**(8): 2197–2203 (2001).
54. Bishayee, A., Cancer prevention and treatment with resveratrol: From rodent studies to clinical trials, *Cancer Prev Res (Phila)* **2**(5): 409–418 (2009).
55. van den Heuvel, S. and E. Harlow, Distinct roles for cyclin-dependent kinases in cell cycle control, *Science* **262**(5142): 2050–2054 (1993).
56. Morgan, D.O., Principles of CDK regulation, *Nature* **374**(6518): 131–134 (1995).
57. Wolter, F., B. Akoglu, A. Clausnitzer, and J. Stein, Downregulation of the cyclin D1/Cdk4 complex occurs during resveratrol-induced cell cycle arrest in colon cancer cell lines, *J Nutr* **131**(8): 2197–2203 (2001).
58. Andlauer, W., J. Kolb, K. Siebert, and P. Fürst, Assessment of resveratrol bioavailability in the perfused small intestine of the rat, *Drugs Exp Clin Res* **26**(2): 47–55 (2000).

59. Aggarwal, B.B., A. Bhardwaj, R.S. Aggarwal, N.P. Seeram, S. Shishodia, and Y. Takada, Role of resveratrol in prevention and therapy of cancer: Preclinical and clinical studies, *Anticancer Res* **24**(5A): 2783–2840 (2004).
60. Delmas, D., C. Rébé, S. Lacour, R. Filomenko, A. Athias, P. Gambert, M. Cherkaoui-Malki, B. Jannin, L. Dubrez-Daloz, N. Latruffe, and E. Solary, Resveratrol-induced apoptosis is associated with Fas redistribution in the rafts and the formation of a death-inducing signaling complex in colon cancer cells, *J Biol Chem* **278**(42): 41482–41490 (2003).
61. Patel, K.R., V.A. Brown, D.J. Jones, R.G. Britton, D. Hemingway, A.S. Miller, K.P. West, T.D. Booth, M. Perloff, J.A. Crowell, D.E. Brenner, W.P. Steward, A.J. Gescher, and K. Brown, Clinical pharmacology of resveratrol and its metabolites in colorectal cancer patients, *Cancer Res* **70**(19): 7392–7399 (2010).
62. Parasramka, M.A., E. Ho, D.E. Williams, and R.H. Dashwood, MicroRNAs, diet, and cancer: New mechanistic insights on the epigenetic actions of phytochemicals, *Mol Carcinog* **51**(3): 213–230 (2012).
63. Sung, B., S. Prasad, V.R. Yadav, and B.B. Aggarwal, Cancer cell signaling pathways targeted by spice-derived nutraceuticals, *Nutr Cancer* **64**(2): 173–197 (2012).
64. Shishodia, S. and B.B. Aggarwal, Diosgenin inhibits osteoclastogenesis, invasion, and proliferation through the downregulation of Akt, I kappa B kinase activation and NF-kappa B-regulated gene expression, *Oncogene* **25**(10): 1463–1473 (2006).
65. Miyoshi, N., T. Nagasawa, R. Mabuchi, Y. Yasui, K .Wakabayashi, T. Tanaka, and H. Ohshima, Chemoprevention of azoxymethane/dextran sodium sulfate-induced mouse colon carcinogenesis by freeze-dried yam sanyaku and its constituent diosgenin, *Cancer Prev Res (Phila)* **4**(6): 924–934 (2011).
66. Lepage, C., D.Y. Léger, J. Bertrand, F. Martin, J.L. Beneytout, and B. Liagre, Diosgenin induces death receptor-5 through activation of p38 pathway and promotes TRAIL-induced apoptosis in colon cancer cells, *Cancer Lett* **301**(2): 193–202 (2011).
67. Jaganathan, S.K., A. Mazumdar, D. Mondhe, and M. Mandal, Apoptotic effect of eugenol in human colon cancer cell lines, *Cell Biol Int* **35**(6): 607–615 (2011).
68. Kim, S.S., O.J. Oh, H.Y. Min, E.J. Park, Y. Kim, H.J. Park, Y. Nam Han, and S.K. Lee, Eugenol suppresses cyclooxygenase-2 expression in lipopolysaccharide-stimulated mouse macrophage RAW264.7 cells, *Life Sci* **73**(3): 337–348 (2003).
69. Zheng, G.Q., P.M. Kenney, and L.K. Lam, Sesquiterpenes from clove (*Eugenia caryophyllata*) as potential anticarcinogenic agents, *J Nat Prod* **55**(7): 999–1003 (1992).

70. Lu, J., C.T. Ho, G. Ghai, and K.Y. Chen, Differential effects of theaflavin monogallates on cell growth, apoptosis, and Cox-2 gene expression in cancerous versus normal cells, *Cancer Res* **60**(22): 6465–6471 (2000).
71. Goel, A., C.R. Boland, and D.P. Chauhan, Specific inhibition of cyclooxygenase-2 (COX-2) expression by dietary curcumin in HT-29 human colon cancer cells, *Cancer Lett* **172**(2): 111–118 (2001).
72. Sangeetha, N., S. Aranganathan, J. Panneerselvam, P. Shanthi, G. Rama, and N. Nalini, Oral supplementation of silibinin prevents colon carcinogenesis in a long term preclinical model, *Eur J Pharmacol* **643**(1): 93–100 (2010).
73. Kaur, M., B. Velmurugan, A. Tyagi, G. Deep, S. Katiyar, C. Agarwal, and R. Agarwal, Silibinin suppresses growth and induces apoptotic death of human colorectal carcinoma LoVo cells in culture and tumor xenograft, *Mol Cancer Ther* **8**(8): 2366–2374 (2009).
74. Kauntz, H., S. Bousserouel, F. Gosse, J. Marescaux, and F. Raul, Silibinin, A natural flavonoid, modulates the early expression of chemoprevention biomarkers in a preclinical model of colon carcinogenesis, *Int J Oncol* **41**(3): 849–854 (2012).
75. Ravichandran, K., B. Velmurugan, M. Gu, R.P. Singh, and R. Agarwal, Inhibitory effect of silibinin against azoxymethane-induced colon tumorigenesis in A/J mice, *Clin Cancer Res* **16**(18): 4595–4606 (2010).
76. Wang, J.Y., C.C. Chang, C.C. Chiang, W.M. Chen, and S.C. Hung, Silibinin suppresses the maintenance of colorectal cancer stem-like cells by inhibiting PP2A/AKT/mTOR pathways, *J Cell Biochem* **113**(5): 1733–1744 (2012).
77. Kim, C.S., W.H. Park, J.Y. Park, J.H. Kang, M.O. Kim, T. Kawada, H. Yoo, I.S. Han, and R. Yu, Capsaicin, a spicy component of hot pepper, induces apoptosis by activation of the peroxisome proliferator-activated receptor gamma in HT-29 human colon cancer cells, *J Med Food* **7**(3): 267–273 (2004).
78. Lu, H.F., Y.L. Chen, J.S. Yang, Y.Y. Yang, J.Y. Liu, S.C. Hsu, K.C. Lai, and J.G. Chung, Antitumor activity of capsaicin on human colon cancer cells *in vitro* and colo 205 tumor xenografts *in vivo*, *J Agric Food Chem* **58**(24): 12999–13005 (2010).
79. Lee, S.H., R.L. Richardson, R.H. Dashwood, and S.J. Baek, Capsaicin represses transcriptional activity of beta-catenin in human colorectal cancer cells, *J Nutr Biochem* **23**(6): 646–655 (2012).
80. Liu, N.C., P.F. Hsieh, M.K. Hsieh, Z.M. Zeng, H.L. Cheng, J.W. Liao, and P.J. Chueh, Capsaicin-mediated tNOX (ENOX2) up-regulation enhances cell proliferation and migration *in vitro* and *in vivo*, *J Agric Food Chem* **60**(10): 2758–2765 (2012).
81. Suh, Y., F. Afaq, J.J. Johnson, and H. Mukhtar, A plant flavonoid fisetin induces apoptosis in colon cancer cells by inhibition of COX2 and Wnt/EGFR/NF-kappaB-signaling pathways, *Carcinogenesis* **30**(2): 300–307 (2009).

82. Khan, N., D.N. Syed, N. Ahmad and H. Mukhtar, Fisetin: A dietary antioxidant for health promotion, *Antioxid Redox Signal* **10**(9): 151–162 (2012).
83. Lim do, Y. and J.H. Park, Induction of p53 contributes to apoptosis of HCT-116 human colon cancer cells induced by the dietary compound fisetin, *Am J Physiol Gastrointest Liver Physiol* **296**(5): G1060–G1068 (2009).
84. Seeram, N.P., L.S. Adams, Y. Zhang, R. Lee, D. Sand, H.S. Scheuller, and D. Heber, Blackberry, black raspberry, blueberry, cranberry, red raspberry, and strawberry extracts inhibit growth and stimulate apoptosis of human cancer cells *in vitro*, *J Agric Food Chem* **54**(25): 9329–9339 (2006).
85. Neto, C.C., J.W. Amoroso, and A.M. Liberty, Anticancer activities of cranberry phytochemicals: An update, *Mol Nutr Food Res* **52**(1 Suppl.): S18–S27 (2008).
86. Gossé, F., S. Guyot, S. Roussi, A. Lobstein, B. Fischer, N. Seiler, and F. Raul, Chemopreventive properties of apple procyanidins on human colon cancer-derived metastatic SW620 cells and in a rat model of colon carcinogenesis, *Carcinogenesis* **26**(7): 1291–1295 (2005).
87. Kaur, M., R.P. Singh, M. Gu, R. Agarwal, and C. Agarwal, Grape seed extract inhibits *in vitro* and *in vivo* growth of human colorectal carcinoma cells, *Clin Cancer Res* **12**(20 Pt 1): 6194–6202 (2006).
88. Khan, S.A., Short communication: The role of pomegranate (punica granatum l.) in colon cancer, *Pak J Pharm Sci* **22**(3): 346–348 (2009).
89. Boateng, J., M. Verghese, L. Shackelford, L.T. Walker, J. Khatiwada, S. Ogutu, D.S. Williams, J. Jones, M. Guyton, D. Asiamah, F. Henderson, L. Grant, M. DeBruce, A. Johnson, S. Washington, and C.B. Chawan, Selected fruits reduce azoxymethane (AOM)-induced aberrant crypt foci (ACF) in Fisher 344 male rats, *Food Chem Toxicol* **45**(2): 725–732 (2007).
90. Adams, L.S., N.P. Seeram, B.B. Aggarwal, Y. Takada, D. Sand, and D. Heber, Pomegranate juice, total pomegranate ellagitannins, and punicalagin suppress inflammatory cell signaling in colon cancer cells, *J Agric Food Chem* **54**(3): 980–985 (2006).
91. Waly, M.I., A. Ali, N. Guizani, A.S. Al-Rawahi, S.A. Farooq, and M.S. Rahman, Pomegranate (Punica granatum) peel extract efficacy as a dietary antioxidant against azoxymethane-induced colon cancer in rat, *Asian Pac J Cancer Prev* **13**(18): 4051–4055 (2012).
92. Nagini, S., Cancer chemoprevention by garlic and its organosulfur compounds — panacea or promise?, *Anticancer Agents Med Chem* **8**(3): 313–321 (2008).
93. Sriram, N., S. Kalayarasan, P. Ashokkumar, A. Sureshkumar, and G. Sudhandiran, Diallyl sulfide induces apoptosis in Colo 320 DM human

colon cancer cells: Involvement of caspase-3, NF-κB, and ERK-2, *Mol Cell Biochem* **311**(1–2): 157–165 (2008).

94. Kang, J.S., T.M. Kim, T.J. Shim, E.I. Salim, B.S. Han, and D.J. Kim, Modifying effect of diallyl sulfide on colon carcinogenesis in C57BL/6J-ApcMin/(+) mice, *Asian Pac J Cancer Prev* **13**(4): 1115–1118 (2012).
95. Pham, H., M. Chen, H. Takahashi, J. King, H.A. Reber, O.J. Hines, S. Pandol, and G. Eibl, Apigenin inhibits NNK-induced focal adhesion kinase activation in pancreatic cancer cells, *Pancreas* **41**(8): 1306–1315 (2012).
96. Leonardi, T., J. Vanamala, S.S. Taddeo, L.A. Davidson, M.E. Murphy, B.S. Patil, N. Wang, R.J. Carroll, R.S. Chapkin, J.R. Lupton, and N.D. Turner, Apigenin and naringenin suppress colon carcinogenesis through the aberrant crypt stage in azoxymethane-treated rats, *Exp Biol Med (Maywood)* **235**(6): 710–717 (2010).
97. Pierini, R., J.M. Gee, N.J. Belshaw, and I.T. Johnson, Flavonoids and intestinal cancers, *Br J Nutr* **99** (E Suppl. 1): ES53–ES59 (2008).
98. Cai, H., S. Sale, R. Schnid, R.G. Britton, K. Brown, W.P. Steward, and A.J. Gescher, Flavones as colorectal cancer chemopreventive agents — phenol-o-methylation enhances efficacy, *Cancer Prev Res (Phila)* **2**(8): 743–750 (2009).
99. Wang, W., L. Heideman, C.S. Chung, J.C. Pelling, K.J. Koehler, and D.F. Birt, Cell-cycle arrest at G2/M and growth inhibition by apigenin in human colon carcinoma cell lines, *Mol Carcinog* **28**(2): 102–110 (2000).
100. Plaumann, B., M. Fritsche, H. Rimpler, G. Brandner, and R.D. Hess, Flavonoids activate wild-type p53, *Oncogene* **13**(8): 1605–1614 (1996).
101. Takagaki, N., Y. Sowa, T. Oki, R. Nakanishi, S. Yogosawa, and T. Sakai, Apigenin induces cell cycle arrest and p21/WAF1 expression in a p53-independent pathway, *Int J Oncol* **26**(1): 185–189 (2005).
102. Turktekin, M., E. Konac, H.I. Onen, E. Alp, A. Yilmaz, and S. Menevse, Evaluation of the effects of the flavonoid apigenin on apoptotic pathway gene expression on the colon cancer cell line (HT29), *J Med Food* **14**(10): 1107–1117 (2011).
103. Yun, J.M., F. Afaq, N. Khan, and H. Mukhtar, Delphinidin, an anthocyanidin in pigmented fruits and vegetables, induces apoptosis and cell cycle arrest in human colon cancer HCT116 cells, *Mol Carcinog* **48**(3): 260–270 (2009).
104. Thomasset, S., N. Teller, H. Cai, D. Marko, D.P. Berry, W.P. Steward, and A.J. Gescher, Do anthocyanins and anthocyanidins, cancer chemopreventive pigments in the diet, merit development as potential drugs?, *Cancer Chemother Pharmacol* **64**(1): 201–211 (2009).
105. Cvorovic, J., F. Tramer, M. Granzotto, L. Candussio, G. Decorti, and S. Passamonti, Oxidative stress-based cytotoxicity of delphinidin and cyanidin in colon cancer cells, *Arch Biochem Biophys* **501**(1): 151–157 (2010).

5

Anticancer Activities of Fruits and Vegetables Against Gynecological Cancers

*Sankar Jagadeeshan, Ajaikumar B. Kunnumakkara, Indu Ramachandran and S. Asha Nair**

GYNECOLOGICAL CANCER: AN OVERVIEW

Gynecological cancers are cancers originating in the female reproductive system, types of which include cervix, fallopian tube, endometrium/uterus, ovary, vagina, and vulva. Increasing lines of evidence suggest that the compounds present in fruits and vegetables have protective roles against these malignancies. The present chapter will give detailed information about different types of gynecologic disorders and the potential of fruits and vegetables in preventing these diseases.

Cervical Cancer

Cervical cancer is the second most common cancer in women after breast cancer. More than 85% of the global burden occurs in developing countries, where it accounts for 13% of all female cancers.[1] High-risk regions are Eastern and Western Africa (age standardized rate (ASR) greater than

*Corresponding author: S. Asha Nair, Cancer Research Program, Rajiv Gandhi Centre for Biotechnology, Poojapura, Thiruvananthapuram, India.

30 per 100,000), Southern Africa (ASR: 26.8 per 100,000), South-Central Asia (ASR: 24.6 per 100,000), South America, and Middle Africa (ASRs: 23.9 and 23.0 per 100,000, respectively). Rates are lowest in Western Asia, Northern America, and Australia/New Zealand (ASRs less than 6 per 100,000). Cervical cancer remains the most common cancer in women only in Eastern Africa, South-Central Asia and Melanesia. Overall, the mortality:incidence ratio is 52%, and cervical cancer is responsible for 275,000 deaths in 2008, about 88% of which occurred in developing countries: 53,000 in Africa, 31,700 in Latin America and the Caribbean, and 159,800 in Asia.[2]

Cervical cancer is strongly associated with human papillomavirus (HPV) infection. The role of HPV infection in the pathogenesis of cervical cancer was first demonstrated in the 1980s by zur Hausen.[3] For cervical cancer to develop, the following may occur: infection with HPV; persistence of HPV infections; development of precancerous lesions in cervical cells that have been persistently infected with HPV; and invasion of cervical cells (cancer). HPV is detected in over 90% of cervical cancers.[4] Of these, HPV-16 and HPV-18 are the most common, being associated with 75% of cases worldwide.[5] The HPV genome encodes proteins that facilitate the accumulation of mutations in the host genome, which possibly leads to activation of cellular oncogenes or inactivation of tumor suppressor genes. Inactivation of p53, either by interaction with the HPV16 E6 oncoprotein or by gene mutation in the absence of the virus, appears to be a key step in cervical carcinogenesis resulting in the initial event in a multi-step progression to malignancy.[5]

Ovarian Cancer

Cancer that forms in tissues of the ovary are defined as ovarian cancers. There are two major types of ovarian cancer based on their tissue of origin: ovarian epithelial carcinomas (originating in the cells on the surface of the ovary) and malignant germ cell tumors (originating in egg cells). Worldwide, carcinoma of the ovary is the sixth most common cancer in women accounting for 4% of all female cancer cases worldwide. Ovarian cancer is the fourth leading cause of cancer deaths in the United States and the most common cause of death from a gynecological malignancy.

Similar findings are reported from all well-developed countries of the northern hemisphere. Many theories exist regarding the etiologies of ovarian cancer. The development of a conclusive system is hampered by the heterogeneity of epithelial ovarian cancer and the rarity of other ovarian malignancies. The best-developed concept at this time is the ovulation model, which theorizes that the trauma to the ovarian epithelium at time of ovulation and subsequent contact with fluids containing high estrogen concentrations may increase proliferation and inclusion cyst formation. The regenerating epithelium may also be more susceptible to external factors such as infectious agents and chemicals. Most ovarian cancers are associated with only vague symptoms. Therefore, the disease is commonly diagnosed at an advanced stage; about 75% of women diagnosed with Stage III/IV disease.

The etiology of ovarian cancer is poorly understood.[6] More than 90% of ovarian malignancies are epithelial in origin and most of these are sporadic. In these cases, nulliparity and infertility are associated with an increased ovarian cancer risk, whereas the oral contraceptive pill, multiparity, and lactation are protective. Similarly, tubal ligation and hysterectomy appear to be associated with a reduced risk, although the reasons for this are not clear.

Genetic predisposition is the strongest risk factor but only affects 10% of patients with ovarian cancer. The most frequently seen mutation in 60–65% of cases involves the *BRCA1* and *BRCA2* genes. Other genes that are inactivated during ovarian cancer development include *TP53*, *PTEN*, *OPCML*, *p16* (*CDKN2A*), *Disabled-2* (*Dab2*), and the *Deleted in Colorectal Carcinoma* (*DCC*) gene.

Endometrial Cancer

Cancer of the endometrium is the most common gynecological malignancy in the United States and is exceeded in frequency only by breast, colon, and lung cancers. In the United Kingdom, it is the second most common gynecological malignancy. Endometrial cancer is predominantly a disease of postmenopausal women; the median age at diagnosis is 63. It is usually associated with a good prognosis, probably because it is often detected at an early stage; 80% of patients present with Stage I disease.

Most studies have found that several risk factors for endometrial cancer relate to reproduction; these include early age at menarche, late menopause, and nulliparity.[7] Unopposed estrogen replacement therapy is associated with an increased risk and use of oral contraceptives has a protective effect. Obesity, diabetes, and hypertension increase the risk of endometrial cancer whereas smoking, exercise, and low-fat diet reduce the risk. Approximately 10% of endometrial cancers have a hereditary basis as part of hereditary non-polyposis colorectal cancer (HNPCC).[7]

Vulval Cancer

Vulval carcinoma is an uncommon gynecological malignancy; it accounts for ~6% of all gynecological malignancies. In the United Kingdom, approximately 1,000 new cases are reported each year. Risk factors include chronic vulval disease, past history of genital warts or vulval carcinoma *in situ* (VIN), other genital carcinomas (usually cervical carcinoma in 15–20% of cases) and smoking. Squamous cell carcinomas account for 90% of the cases, whereas melanomas, adenocarcinomas, and basal cell carcinomas are much less common.

A number of epidemiological studies have linked vulval squamous cell carcinoma to some of the risk factors described for cervical carcinoma. A proportion of vulval squamous cell carcinoma has been associated with HPV infection. In one study, there was a significantly increased risk of vulval cancer following HPV-16 infection (odds ratio 5, 95% CI: 1.1–22.0).[5] The association between HPV infection and vulval carcinoma appears to be related to a small number of cases, especially in younger women with basaloid subtype and associated VIN. It has been surmised that the rise in incidence in biopsy proven VIN in younger women is secondary to the rise of anogenital HPV prevalence in this age group. Most vulval carcinomas, however, occur in older patients, peaking in the seventh and eighth decades of life. These are predominantly of the keratinizing subtype and associated with lichen sclerosis suggesting that vulval carcinoma has different etiologies.

Vaginal Cancer

Carcinoma of the vagina is predominantly a disease of elderly postmenopausal woman. It is an uncommon gynecological cancer accounting for

1.4% of all gynecological tumors in the United Kingdom. Owing to the rarity of the disease, the molecular events underlying the development of the vaginal tumors are less well understood than for other gynecological malignancies. Similarly, relatively little is known about the epidemiology and etiology of the disease.

Squamous cell carcinomas of the vagina are the most common primary vaginal tumor (85–90%), though most are believed to be extensions from the cervix and vulva. Approximately one-third of patients with vulval cancer have had a previous gynecological malignancy, mostly cervical carcinoma, making it difficult at times to ascertain whether a vaginal tumor represents a new primary or recurrence of a previous cervical cancer. Consequently, it has been suggested that some vaginal cancers have the same etiology as cervical cancer. In a study of 341 cases of primary vaginal carcinomas by Hellman *et al.*, there appeared to be two types of vaginal carcinoma with age-related etiology.[8] In one group, the cancer occurred in younger women with similar etiological factors to those found in cervical carcinoma including HPV infection, smoking, and lower socio-economic status. In the other more common group, however, patients were older, the disease occurred as unifocal lesions and the etiology appeared possibly to be associated with hormonal factors and trauma to the vagina from pessaries and prolapse.

Primary Fallopian Tube Cancer

Primary carcinoma of the fallopian tube is reported to be the rarest of all gynecologic malignancies (<1%) with a yearly incidence of 3.6 per million women. As with vaginal cancer metastatic disease seems more common; however, in advanced stages, it is impossible to be differentiated from primary ovarian cancer. The mean age at presentation is 57 years old. The only risk factors that have been consistently identified are the *BRCA1* and *BRCA2* mutations, where a significant percentage of lesions develop in the distal aspect of the Fallopian tube.[9]

ANTICANCER COMPOUNDS PRESENT IN FRUITS AND VEGETABLES AND THEIR MECHANISMS OF ACTION

Researches over the past several years have shown that phytochemicals present in fruits and vegetables have high potential in the prevention and treatment of

Table 5.1: Anticancer activities of fruits and vegetables against gynecologic cancers: *in vitro, in vivo*, and clinical studies.

Compound	Cancer type	Type of study	References
Quercetin	Cervical and Ovarian	*In vitro, in vivo,* clinical trials	124, 125
Kaempferol	Ovarian	*In vitro*	15–17
Resveratol	Cervical	*In vitro*	51, 52–55, 126
Genistein	Cervical	*In vitro*	30, 37, 40, 45
Epigallocatechin-3-gallate	Ovarian	*In vitro*	63, 127
Gingerol	Ovarian	*In vitro*	73, 74
Anthocyanin	Ovarian and Cervical	*In vitro*	84, 93, 128
Sulforaphane	Ovarian	*In vitro*	129
Indole-3-carbinol	Ovarian, Cervical and Vulvar	*In vitro, in vivo,* clinical trials	99, 100
Carotenoids	Ovarian and Cervical	*In vitro*	105, 107
Hesperetin	Cervical	*In vitro*	113
Naringin	Cervical	*In vitro*	114
Glyceollin	Ovarian	*In vitro*	115
Frutalin	Cervical	*In vitro*	116
Garcinol	Cervical	*In vitro*	117

gynecologic malignancies (Table 5.1). Basic research has illuminated four potential mechanisms by which components in fruits and vegetables (Fig. 5.1) act to prevent cancer.[10] These are reflected in our understanding of the process of chemical carcinogenesis and factors that influence the different phases of the process. The process of "initiation" (earliest aspects of cancer induction) refers to the interactions between carcinogens and DNA that result in heritable mutations, and promotion and progression (later phases of carcinogenesis) refers to the clonal expansion of genetically altered cells and their invasion and metastatic spread to other organs.[10] In cancer prevention, two concepts of this carcinogenic process are important, interception of DNA-reactive elements and activation and detoxification of potential carcinogens. In later stages, food components inhibit the proliferation of genetically altered cells and disrupt the biology of the tumor that suppress further growth and metastasis.[10]

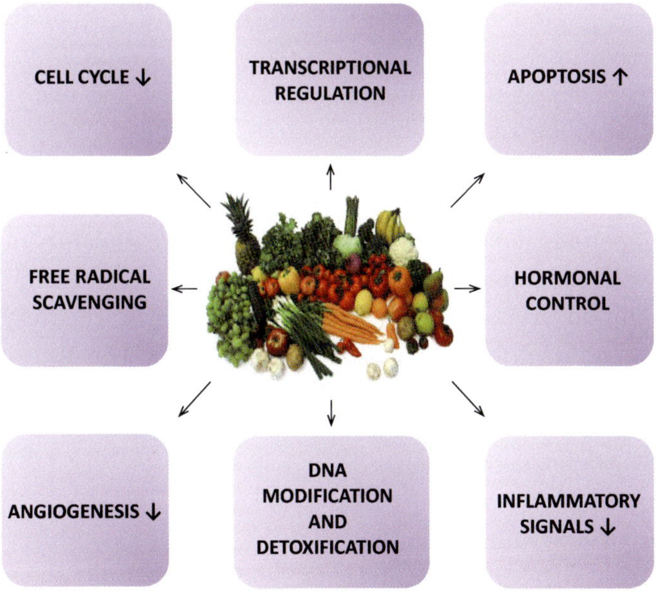

Figure 5.1: Mechanisms of action of anticancer activities of fruits and vegetables against gynecologic cancers.

Phytochemicals that are high in antioxidant potential are efficient interceptors of DNA-reactive elements. Being deficient in electrons, most mutagens/carcinogens are attracted to electron-rich sources in the cell. In terms of cancer development, DNA, RNA, and proteins have the highest nucleophilic potential to interact with an electrophile. Formation of stable bonds between the mutagenic agent and portions of nucleoprotein leads to adduct formation. Adduction of DNA is considered to be the sometimes repairable event that starts the carcinogenic process. Among the chemicals in fruits and vegetables, several have outstanding potential as antioxidants. Strong evidence exists that one class in particular, the plant phenolics, can prevent DNA adduction, presumably by presenting alternative targets for attack by carcinogens.

Another mechanism by which plant components can prevent cancer in the early phases of carcinogenesis is through modulation of carcinogen metabolism. A wealth of research has focused on chemicals in crucifers and *Allium sp.* vegetables that modify carcinogenesis by this mechanism.

Isothiocyanates, found in cabbage (*Brassica oleracea L. Capitata* Group), broccoli (*Brassica oleracea L. Botrytis* Group), and cauliflower (*Brassica oleracea L. Botrytis* Group), organosulfur compounds like diallyl disulfide from the members of the *Allium* genus, including garlic (*A. sativum L.*), onions (*A. cepa L.*), shallots (*A. cepa L.*), and chives (*A. schoenoprasum L.*), inhibit cervical cancer cells.[11] Extensive research in the metabolism of these compounds indicates that they are efficient modulators of carcinogen activation and detoxification.

In addition, fruits and vegetables can also impact carcinogenesis by modifying the behavior of cancer cells. Cancer cells may require abnormal stimulation of certain genes such as oncogenes, allowing them to escape factors that regulate cell growth.[10] Phytochemicals present in fruits and vegetables modulate the cellular process like the cell cycle; DNA replication interacts at the molecular level with kinases; and key receptors that initiates signaling pathways leading to apoptosis. The most recent development in the search for anticarcinogenic substances in fruits and vegetables involves the identification of anti-inflammatory compounds that influence the generation of prostaglandins. Prostaglandins are mediators of pain, inflammation, and swelling produced from arachidonic acid by the enzyme cyclooxygenase (COX).

Flavonoids and Gynecologic Cancers

Flavonoids are naturally occurring polyphenolic compounds that constitute the most abundant class of dietary natural products and are present in fruits, vegetables, and medicinal plants. They are classified into flavonols, flavanones, flavones, anthocyanidins, leucoanthocyanidins, and catechins. Extensive investigations of their bioactivity in the past 30 years have demonstrated their potential in the prevention of cancer. These compounds inhibit tumor formation and proliferation of cancer cells through various biological mechanisms.[12] Particularly, their effects on procarcinogen-activating enzymes (cytochrome P450 CYP1 family; CYP1A1 and CYP1B1), have been studied in detail. These enzymes are overexpressed in tumors and metabolize procarcinogens to epoxide intermediates, which are further activated to diol epoxides by the enzyme epoxide hydrolase.[12] The most common chemical, extensively studied for its carcinogenicity, is benzo[a]pyrene (B[a]P). Formation of B[a]P-7,8-diol-9,10-epoxides (bay region epoxides) causes accelerated DNA mutations due to their high reactivity, and any compound that blocks the formation of reactive intermediates, can potentially prevent the initiation of carcinogenesis.[12] The ability of flavonoids to inhibit CYP1 enzymatic activity is well established and it is known that flavonoids can act as substrates for CYP1 enzymes and can cause inhibition of tumor cell growth by the formation of more pharmacologically active conversion products.[12]

Kaempferol

Kaempferol is a relatively non-toxic, inexpensive natural flavonoid that is widely distributed in fruits and vegetables, and prospective studies revealed that over decades, consumption of kaempferol dramatically and significantly reduced the risk of ovarian cancer in American female nurses.[13] Moreover, studies have also demonstrated that kaempferol inhibits the expression of vascular epithelial growth factor (VEGF), induces Akt phosphorylation, and regulates the expression of *p53*, *Bad*, *Bax*, and *Bcl-*x_L genes leading to apoptosis in ovarian cancer cells.[13] Recent studies have shown that this compound reverses multi-drug resistance in human cervical carcinoma KB-V1 cells.[14–17] These studies thus suggest that kaempferol is a promising agent for the prevention and treatment of gynecologic cancer.

Phytoestrogens

Phytoestrogens are naturally occurring polycyclic phenols found in certain plants that may, when ingested and metabolized, have weak estrogenic effects due to the fact that they are structurally and functionally similar to 17β-estradiol, and therefore bind to estradiol receptors (mainly to estradiol β2 receptors).[18] The most important groups of phytoestrogens are isoflavones (formononetin, resveratrol, biochanin A, daidzein, genistein, quercetin, O-desmethylangolensin-ODMA, equol, etc.). Daidzein and genistein represent phytoestrogens that are most commonly used as food supplements and also the most thoroughly investigated.[19,20] They are the main isoflavones extracted from soy, the plant popular in human food. Isoflavones are well known not only as antioxidants, but also as chemo-preventive and anti-inflammatory agents that can modulate apoptosis.[21,22] They could be involved in regulation of the immune response and in that way reduce prevalence of chronic health disorders of their regular consumers. Phytoestrogens upregulate the expression of antioxidant enzymes via the estrogen receptor and mitogen activated protein kinase (MAPK) activation, which in turn activate the NF-κB signaling pathway, resulting in the upregulation of the expression of longevity-related genes.[21,22] Consequently, women who are treated with phytoestrogens in menopause have a benefit, apart from estrogenic, from the antioxidative effects of administered substances. Numerous anti-proliferative properties are suggested for phytoestrogens contrary to estrogen effects. This is due to diverse activities of the estrogen receptors and the higher affinity of phytoestrogens for ER-β than ER-α.[20] The effects of phytoestrogens on cell growth and proliferation may be explained by their ability to alter the expression of a number of proteins that control cell cycle and induce cell cycle arrest and apoptosis. Thus, isoflavones and other phenolic compounds decrease the increased level of markers of oxidative stress and boost DNA resistance to oxidative damage and consequently, menopausal women who are receiving phytoestrogens have multiple benefits.[16] Recently, Bandera *et al.*[23] conducted a population-based case-control study to determine the protective effect of phytoestrogens against ovarian cancer and found that there is an inverse association between phytoestrogen uptake and ovarian cancer risk.[24] Moreover, out of six population-based studies conducted in the last decade, five have suggested an inverse association between phytoestrogen uptake and ovarian cancer risk.[24–29] A meta-analysis including the four studies that evaluated the intake of soy also reported reduced risk of ovarian cancer.[24–29] These studies suggest that phytoestrogens have high potential in preventing ovarian cancer.

Genistein

Genistein is a soy-derived isoflavone that has shown protective effects against endocrine-related gynecological cancers.[30,31] This molecule has been shown to inhibit cell proliferation, and induce apoptosis in endometrial cancer, cervical cancer, and ovarian cancer cells by modulating different signaling pathways,[30–40] prevent the invasive potential of cervical cancer cells by downregulating matrix metalloproteinase (MMP)-9 and tissue inhibitors of MMP (TIMP)-1 expression,[41] and inhibit VEGF expression in ovarian cancer (OVCAR-3) cells.[37] Phenoxodiol (2H-1-benzopyran-7-0,1, 3-[4-hydroxyphenyl], PXD), a synthetic analog of genistein, also demonstrated a potent antitumor effect against ovarian cancer and inhibited tumor angiogenesis.[42] Genestein has been shown to enhance the apoptotic effect of cisplatin and TNF-related apoptosis-inducing ligand (TRAIL) in cervical cancer cells and endometrial cancer cells respectively, and sensitizes cervical cancer cells to radiotherapy.[35,43] In addition, genistein treatment also induces autophagic cell death in ovarian cancer cells, which may contribute to its potential to overcome chemoresistance developed from an altered apoptotic signaling pathway.[44] In both platinum-sensitive and platinum-resistant ovarian cancer cells, genistein abrogated NF-κB DNA binding activity and downregulated anti-apoptotic genes.[45]

Many studies have investigated the anticancer activities of genistein in animals against various gynecologic malignancies. Ghaemi *et al.*[46] investigated the potential immunomodulatory effects of genistein against the TC-1 cervical cancer cell line and found that administration of genistein significantly increased lymphocyte proliferation, lactase dehydrogenase (LDH) release, and interferon gamma (IFN-γ) production which contributed to the inhibition of tumor growth. The effects of isoflavones (genistein and daidzein) on 17β-estradiol endometrial carcinogenesis in mice has also been investigated, which shows that both the compounds significantly inhibited incidences of endometrial adenocarcinoma and atypical endometrial hyperplasia in mice by suppressing expression of estrogen-induced estrogen-related genes c-fos and c-jun, and internal cytokines IL-1α and TNF-α through a cytokine and estrogen receptor-mediated pathway.[47] These compounds has also been shown to inhibit 7,12-dimethylbenz[a]anthracene-induced mutagenicity and uterine dysplasia in ovariectomized rats.[48] In addition, this molecule has also been shown to inhibit human ovarian carcinoma cells lines SKOV3 and HO-8910PM induced tumor xenograft in nude mice by regulating the cell cycle and apoptotic genes, and by inhibiting the expression of epidermal growth factor receptor (EGFR) and its downstream nuclear transcription factors c-jun and c-fos at the mRNA and protein levels.[49,50] Collectively, these studies demonstrate that genestein and its derivatives inhibit various gynecological malignancies by modulating different signaling pathways.

Resveratrol

Resveratrol (3,4′,5-trihydroxy-trans-stilbene, $C_{14}H_{12}O_3$) is a natural phytoalexin synthesized in more than 70 plant species in response to injury, UV radiation, and insect or fungal attack. Because of its high concentration in grape skin, a significant amount of resveratrol is present in wines, especially red wines, and it is considered to be responsible for the beneficial effects of red wines against coronary heart disease.[51] Resveratrol is gaining tremendous importance as it possesses cancer preventive as well as anticancer activities in various biological systems. Resveratrol has also been shown to possess *in vitro* cytotoxic effects against a wide variety of human tumor cells, including ovary and cervix carcinoma cells.[52] Resveratrol displays pleiotropic effects and has a multitude of biochemical and molecular actions including inhibition of free radical formation and activities of COX, inducible nitric oxide synthase (iNOS), CYP450, and protein kinase C (PKC), and directly binds to estrogen receptors (ER) and the F1 component of mitochondrial ATP synthase.[53] It inhibits cell proliferation and DNA synthesis by downregulating ribonucleotide reductase, DNA polymerase, and ornithine decarboxylase activities, and induces apoptosis in various malignant cells through upregulation of CD95L expression, caspase activation, stabilization of p53, and inhibition of NF-κB activity.[52,53]

Several pathways are intertwined and influence additional mechanisms involved in cellular invasion and metastasis, such as the regulation of growth factors and matrix metalloproteins.[54] These multiple overlapping mechanisms contribute to the overall impact of resveratrol's effects against precancerous or cancer cells. Resveratrol possesses tremendous potential for ovarian cancer chemoprevention and treatment due to the aforementioned biochemical and molecular effects as well as its minimal toxicity. Moreover, specific inhibitors of COX-2 have been found to have chemopreventive action in a number of epithelial cancers.[55] Recently, it has been hypothesized that by inhibiting COX-2, the loss of the basement membrane of the ovarian surface epithelium may be reduced, and consequently the neoplastic transformation of the ovarian surface epithelial cells may be minimized.[53,56]

The oncogenesis of ovarian cancer appears to favor the development and subsequent expansion of cell clones that are resistant to apoptotic triggers. An important clinical prospect is to identify lead compounds that circumvent the resistance mechanisms that limit the success of conventional drugs.[53] Studies have shown that resveratrol induces death in ovarian cancer cells by autophagocytosis (a mechanism distinct from apoptosis), suggesting that it may provide leverage to treat ovarian cancer that is chemoresistant on the basis of ineffective apoptosis.[53,57] Increasing lines of evidence suggest that alterations in the angiogenic characteristics of ovarian surface epithelium play an important role in the etiology of ovarian cancer and resveratrol reduces human ovarian cancer progression and angiogenesis through suppression of hypoxia-inducible factor 1α (HIF-1α) and VEGF,[58,59] In addition, recent studies have shown that this compound inhibits proliferation, invasion and metastases, and induces apoptosis in cervical and endometrial cancer cells.[60–62]

Epigallocatechin-3-gallate

Epigallocatechin-3-gallate (EGCG), a polyphenol constituent of green tea, has shown anti-proliferative and pro-apoptotic effects on several cancer cells by inducing cell cycle arrest, apoptosis, stabilizing p53, and inhibiting NF-κB activity.[63] Studies have shown that EGCG inhibits proliferation, induces apoptosis, and sensitizes different ovarian cancer cells to chemotherapeutic agents such as cisplatin, oxaliplatin, etc.[64–66] This polyphenol has also been shown to inhibit proliferation, invasion, and metastasis, and induces apoptosis in different cervical cancer cells in experimental conditions.[67–68] Recent studies have shown that EGCG chemosensitizes the cervical cancer cells to cisplatin-induced growth inhibition and apoptosis.[69] The anticancer effect of EGCG on endometrial and vulval cancers have also been investigated, which demonstrate that this compound induces apoptosis in human endometrial adenocarcinoma cells via reactive oxygen species (ROS) generation and p38 MAPK activation and inhibits EGFR and the ErbB2 receptor phosphorylation in human vulva carcinoma cell line (A431).[70,71] Therefore, these studies demonstrate that EGCG has great potential in the prevention and treatment of gynecological malignancies.

[6]-gingerol and [6]-shogaol

Ginger (*Zingiber officinale Roscoe, Zingiberaceae*) has been used widely as a spicy or flavoring agent, and as a medicinal herb in traditional medicine. It has been used in Oriental medicine for the treatment of ameliorate symptoms such as nausea, gastrointestinal discomforts, headache, and cold.[72,73] The pungent phenolic constituents derived from ginger are believed to possess many interesting pharmacological and physiological activities and these include [6]-gingerol, [8]-gingerol, and [6]-shogaol.[72] [6]-gingerol was reported to exhibit antioxidant and anti-inflammatory properties and to have antimutagenic potentials.[73] Chakraborty *et al.*[74] showed that [6]-gingerol significantly downregulated NF-κB, AKT and Bcl2 and induced the expression of TNFα, Bax, and cytochrome c in HeLa cells, which suggest that [6]-gingerol has potential to bind with DNA and induce cell death by autophagy and caspase 3-mediated apoptosis. Recent studies have also shown that this compound induces apoptosis in cervical and ovarian cells by modulating the expression of different proteins.[75,76]

[6]-shogaol [(E)-1-(4-hydroxy-3-methoxyphenyl)-dec-4-en-3-one], a major biologically active compound of ginger, was reported to exhibit anticancer efficacy against different cancers by modulating different pathways such as extracellular signal-regulate kinase 1/2, c-Jun N-terminal kinase 1/2, p38 mitogen-activated protein kinase, phosphatidylinositol 3-kinase/Akt, and cell cycle checkpoint proteins Cdk1, cyclin B, and Cdc25C.[72,73] Liu and his colleagues[75] demonstrated that 6-shogaol induced apoptosis and G2/M phase arrest in human cervical cancer (HeLa) cells and that endoplasmic reticulum stress and mitochondrial pathway were involved in [6]-shogaol-mediated apoptosis. Proteomic analysis showed that treatment with [6]-shogaol results in the differential expression of a total of 287 proteins in HeLa cells and 14-3-3 signaling is the predominant canonical pathway involved in networks which may be significantly associated with the process of apoptosis and G2/M cell cycle arrest induced by [6]-shogaol.[76]

Anthocyanin

Anthocyanins are natural colorants which have triggered a growing interest due to their extensive range of colors, and innocuous and beneficial health effects.[77] There are several reports focused on the effect of anthocyanins in cancer treatments[78,79] and their biological activity.[80] The anthocyanidins and anthocyanins have shown a higher antioxidant activity than vitamins C and E.[81] In addition to their antioxidant activity, they also have cancer chemopreventive potential. These compounds exert their antitumor and anticancer activities through two main mechanisms: redox status modification and modulation of basic cellular functions of cancer cells such as cell cycle, apoptosis, inflammation, angiogenesis, invasion, and metastasis. These compounds have also been reported to modulate different cell signaling pathways such as extracellular regulated kinase (ERK), c-Jun N terminal kinase (JNK), MAPK, NF-κB, activator protein1 (AP1) pathway, etc. In addition, these molecules are known to inhibit VEGF, VEGF receptor, (VEGFR2), platelet-derived growth factor (PDGF), PDGF receptor (PDGFR), and HIF-1α, and prevent the growth and proliferation of various ovarian cancer cell lines. For example, proanthocyanidin from cranberry inhibits cancer cell viability, angiogenesis, and cell cycle progression (through G2/M phase), increase ROS generation, and induce apoptosis in chemotherapy-resistant SKOV-3 cells.[82] Moreover, many studies have shown that anthocyanidins isolated from different fruits inhibit proliferation of cervical cancer, ovarian cancer and vulval cancer cell lines in experimental conditions.[83–87]

Sulforaphane

Cruciferous vegetables, particularly broccoli, have a high content of glucosinolates, and their hydrolysis results in the generation of metabolites responsible for the anticarcinogenic activity.[88,89] One such bioactive compound is sulforaphane, which is derived from the breakdown of glucoraphanin; it is a potent inducer of phase II detoxification enzymes.[90] Many studies have demonstrated the anticancer potential of sulforaphane against different gynecological malignancies in experimental conditions. Studies have shown that this compound inhibits the proliferation of different cervical cancer (HeLa and C33A) and ovarian cancers (SKOV3,

OVCAR3, EOC, A2780, PA1, etc.) cell lines by modulating different signaling pathways.[91–94]

Indole-3-carbinol

Indole-3-carbinol (I3C), a natural compound present in cruciferous vegetables, has been shown to possess chemopreventive and therapeutic properties against different gynecologic malignancies in preclinical and clinical settings.[95,96] This molecule exerts its anticancer properties through various mechanisms such as induction of apoptosis, G1 cell cycle arrest, activation of the endoplasmic reticulum, reversal of multi-drug resistance, etc.[97] Many studies have shown that this compound inhibits proliferation of different cervical cancer, endometrial cancer, ovarian cancer, and vulval cancer cells in laboratory conditions, inhibit PTEN loss in cervical cancer, and suppress endometrial cancer development in rats.[98,99] Studies have also demonstrated the ability of this compound to prevent vulvar intraepithelial neoplasia and cervical cancer.[100] Moreover, 3,3′-diindolylmethane (DIM), an active metabolite of I3C, has been shown to inhibit proliferation of cancer cells by causing G_2/M cell cycle arrest; it possesses chemopreventive and therapeutic properties against various cancers.[100,101] DIM is nontoxic to normal cells and administration of this compound has been shown to improve cervical cancer in 50% of patients.[102,103]

Carotenoids

Carotenoids, found in nearly all brightly colored fruits and vegetables or seafood, have strong cancer-fighting properties.[104] Their anticancer effect comes from their antioxidant properties. Antioxidants protect cells from free radicals, which are substances that work to destroy cell membranes and DNA. In addition, studies have demonstrated that carotenoids enhance both specific and non-specific immune functions and tumor immunity by various mechanisms such as (1) quenching excessive reactive species formed by various immunoactive cells, (2) quenching immunosuppressive peroxides and maintaining membrane fluidity, (3) helping to maintain membrane receptors essential for immune functions, and (4) acting in the release of immunomodulatory lipid molecules such as prostaglandins and leukotrienes.[105] These compounds are known to inhibit proliferation of different ovarian cervical cancer, endometrial cancer, and ovarian cancer cell lines by modulating the expression of different proteins. Moreover, many studies in humans have demonstrated the intake of carotenoids and reduced risk of gynecologic malignancies. Studies conducted in Korea showed that β-carotene, lycopene, zeaxanthin, lutein, retinol, etc. play a role in reducing the risk of ovarian cancer.[104] Out of 10 case-control studies performed, five showed an inverse relation between dietary carotenoid and cervical neoplasia.[105] Studies have also suggested that carotenoids may help to prevent endometrial cancer.[106,107] A multicentric case-control study performed in Italy suggests that dietary carotenoid intake prevents endometrial cancer in Italian women.[108,109] These studies therefore demonstrate the potential of these carotenoids in the prevention of gynecologic malignancies.

Apart from these compounds, there are also several other compounds such as phloroglucinols, stilbenes, guttiferones, pycnogenol, and diterpenoid from wild fruits also showed considerable *in vitro* cytotoxicity against different gynecologic cancer cells whose mechanisms of action have yet to be elucidated and studied for therapeutic applications.[110–118]

CRUDE EXTRACTS FROM FRUITS AND VEGETABLES WITH ANTICANCER PROPERTIES AGAINST GYNECOLOGICAL CANCERS

In addition to the above-mentioned compounds, various crude extracts of fruits and vegetables have been shown to prevent gynecologic malignancies. Cacti have been used by Native Americans and Mexicans not only as common vegetation, but their products are also used as medicine for 1,000 years.[118] Cactus pear extract has been shown to inhibit proliferation and induce apoptosis in ovarian cancer cells through the production of ROS. The produced ROS activates several signaling pathways including JNK/SAPK and AKT to protect normal cells and initiate mitochondria-dependent apoptosis to inhibit the proliferation of OVC420 and SKOV3 ovarian cancer cell lines.[119] Another fruit which has been shown to prevent gynecological malignancies is *Momordica charantia* (MC). Various studies (*in vitro* as well as *in vivo*) have demonstrated the anticancer potential of this fruit against different types of cancers. Several studies have reported that bioactive compounds present in MC exert anticancer activity through the inhibition of cell cycle G2/M phase, inhibition of guanylate cyclase activity, activation of NK cells, induction of apoptosis,[120] and modulation of biotransformation and detoxification enzymes of the host.[121] Studies have shown that treatment of cervical cancer patients with MC significantly decreased multi-drug resistance protein 1 level from the basal value, while no such effect was seen in patients given only chemotherapy.[122,123] However, more studies are needed to validate these results in humans.

CONCLUSION

Gynecological malignancies such as cervical, endometrial, fallopian tube, ovarian, and vulval cancers are some of the most commonly occurring malignancies in women worldwide. Approximately, 90% of these malignancies arise from changes in lifestyle and are preventable if we adopt a healthy daily regime. Increasing lines of evidences suggest that a diet rich in fruits and vegetables can prevent most of these malignancies and dietary intake of these agents would help us to reduce the incidence of these cancers. Therefore, it is encouraged to eat more fruits and vegetables to prevent these malignancies.

REFERENCES

1. Ferlay, J., D.M Parkin, and E. Steliarova-Foucher, Estimates of cancer incidence and mortality in Europe in 2008, *Eur J Cancer* **46**(4): 765–781 (2010).
2. Ferlay, J., H.R. Shin, F. Bray, D. Forman, C. Mathers, and D.M. Parkin, Estimates of worldwide burden of cancer in 2008: GLOBOCAN 2008, *Int J Cancer,* **127**(12): 2893–2917 (2010).
3. zur Hausen, H., Papillomaviruses in human cancer, *Appl Pathol* **5**(1): 19–24 (1987).
4. Androutsopoulos, V.P., A. Papakyriakou, D. Vourloumis, A.M. Tsatsakis, and D.A. Spandidos, Dietary flavonoids in cancer therapy and prevention: Substrates and inhibitors of cytochrome P450 CYP1 enzymes, *Pharmacol Ther* **126**(1): 9–20 (2010).
5. Walboomers, J.M., M.V. Jacobs, M.M. Manos, F.X. Bosch, J.A. Kummer, K.V. Shah, P.J. Snijders, J. Peto, C.J. Meijer, and N. Muñoz, Human

papillomavirus is a necessary cause of invasive cervical cancer worldwide, *J Pathol* **189**(1): 12–19 (1999).
6. Tortolero-Luna, G. and M.F. Mitchell, The epidemiology of ovarian cancer, *J Cell Biochem* **59**(23): 200–207 (1995).
7. Purdie, D.M. and A.C. Green, Epidemiology of endometrial cancer, *Best Pract Res Clin Obstet Gynaecol* **15**(3): 341–354 (2001).
8. Hellman, K., C. Silfverswärd, B. Nilsson, A.C. Hellström, B. Frankendal, and F. Pettersson, Primary carcinoma of the vagina: Factors influencing the age at diagnosis. The Radiumhemmet series 1956–96, *Int J Gynecol Cancer* **14**(3): 491–501 (2004).
9. Aziz, S., G. Kuperstein, B. Rosen, D. Cole, R. Nedelcu, J. McLaughlin, and S.A. Narod, A genetic epidemiological study of carcinoma of the Fallopian tube, *Gyne Oncol* **80**(3): 341–345 (2001).
10. Wargovich, M.J., Anticancer properties of fruits and vegetables, *Hortscience OL* **35**(4): 573–575 (2000).
11. Yi, L. and Q. Su, Molecular mechanisms for the anti-cancer effects of diallyl disulfide, *Food Chem Toxicol* **57**: 362–370 (2013).
12. Androutsopoulos, V.P., A.M. Tsatsakis, and D.A. Spandidos, Cytochrome P450 CYP1A1: Wider roles in cancer progression and prevention, *BMC Cancer* **9**: 187 (2009).
13. Gates, M.A., S.S. Tworoger, J.L. Hecht, I.D. Vivo, B. Rosner, and S.E. Hankinson, A prospective study of dietary flavonoid intake and incidence of epithelial ovarian cancer, *Int J Cancer* **121**(10): 2225–2232 (2007).
14. Limtrakul, P., O. Khantamat, and K. Pintha, Inhibition of P-glycoprotein function and expression by kaempferol and quercetin, *J Chemother* **17**(1): 86–95 (2005).
15. Luo, H., G.O. Rankin, L. Liu, M.K. Daddysman, B.H. Jiang, and Y.C. Chen, Kaempferol inhibits angiogenesis and VEGF expression through both HIF dependent and independent pathways in human ovarian cancer cells, *Nutr Cancer* **61**(4): 554–563 (2009).
16. Luo, H., G.O. Rankin, Z. Li, L. Depriest, and Y.C. Chen, Kaempferol induces apoptosis in ovarian cancer cells through activating p53 in the intrinsic pathway, *Food Chem* **128**(2): 513–519 (2011).
17. Luo, H., M.K. Daddysman, G.O. Rankin, B.H. Jiang, and Y.C. Chen, Kaempferol enhances cisplatin's effect on ovarian cancer cells through promoting apoptosis caused by down regulation of cMyc, *Cancer Cell Int* **11**(10): 16 (2010).
18. Bedell, S., M. Nachtigall, and F. Naftolin, The pros and cons of plant estrogens for menopause, *J Steroid Biochem Mol Biol* [Epub ahead of print] (2012).

19. Terzic, M.M. and R.J. Dotlic, Phytoestrogens in gynecology — antioxidative role, *Oxid Antioxid Med Sci* **2**(1): 1–4 (2013).
20. Ondricek, A.J., A.K. Kashyap, S.I. Thamake, and J.K. Vishwanatha, A comparative study of phytoestrogen action in mitigating apoptosis induced by oxidative stress, *In Vivo* **26**(5): 765–775 (2012).
21. Rossi, M., C. Bosetti, E. Negri, P. Lagiou, and C. La Vecchia, Flavonoids, proanthocyanidins, and cancer risk: A network of case-control studies from Italy, *Nutr Cancer* **62**(7): 871–877 (2010).
22. Vina, J., J. Gambini, R. Lopez-Grueso, K.M. Abdelaziz, M. Jove, and C. Borras, Females live longer than males: Role of oxidative stress, *Curr Pharm Des* **17**(36): 3959–3965 (2011).
23. Bandera, E.V., M. King, U. Chandran, L.E. Paddock, L. Rodriguez-Rodriguez, and S.H. Olson, Phytoestrogen consumption from foods and supplements and epithelial ovarian cancer risk: A population-based case control study, *BMC Womens Health* **11**: 40 (2011).
24. Zhang, M., X. Xie, A.H. Lee, and C.W. Binns, Soy and isoflavone intake are associated with reduced risk of ovarian cancer in southeast China, *Nutr Cancer* **49**(2): 125–130 (2004).
25. Chang, E.T., V.S. Lee, A.J. Canchola, C.A. Clarke, D.M. Purdie, P. Reynolds, H. Anton Culver, L. Bernstein, D. Deapen, D. Peel, R. Pinder, R.K. Ross, D.O. Stram, D.W. West, W. Wright, A. Ziogas, and P.L. Horn-Ross, Diet and risk of ovarian cancer in the California Teachers Study cohort, *Am J Epidemiol* **165**(7): 802–813 (2007).
26. Sakauchi, F., M.M. Khan, M. Mori, T. Kubo, Y. Fujino, S. Suzuki, S. Tokudome, and A. Tamakoshi, Dietary habits and risk of ovarian cancer death in a large scale cohort study (JACC study) in Japan, *Nutr Cancer* **57**(2): 138–145 (2007).
27. McCann, S.E., J.L. Freudenheim, J.R. Marshall, and S. Graham, Risk of human ovarian cancer is related to dietary intake of selected nutrients, phytochemicals and food groups, *J Nutr* **133**(6): 1937–1942 (2003).
28. Hedelin, M., M. Lof, T.M. Andersson, H. Adlercreutz, and E. Weiderpass, Dietary phytoestrogens and the risk of ovarian cancer in the women's lifestyle and health cohort study, *Cancer Epidemiol Biomarkers Prev* **20**(2): 308–317 (2011).
29. Myung, S.K., W. Ju, H.J. Choi, and S.C. Kim, Soy intake and risk of endocrine related gynaecological cancer: A meta-analysis, *Br J Gynaecol* **116**(13): 1697–1705 (2009).
30. Ouyang, G., L. Yao, K. Ruan, G. Song, Y. Mao, and S. Bao, Genistein induces G2/M cell cycle arrest and apoptosis of human ovarian cancer cells via activation of DNA damage checkpoint pathways, *Cell Biol Int* **33**(12): 1237–1244 (2009).

31. Kim, M.K., K. Kim, J.Y. Han, J.M. Lim, and Y.S. Song, Modulation of inflammatory signaling pathways by phytochemicals in ovarian cancer, *Genes Nutr* **6**(2): 109–115 (2011).
32. Wang, S.Y., K.W. Yang, Y.T. Hsu, C.L. Chang, and Y.C. Yang, The differential inhibitory effects of genistein on the growth of cervical cancer cells *in vitro*, *Neoplasma* **48**(3): 227–233 (2001).
33. Kim, S.H., S.H. Kim, S.C. Lee, and Y.S. Song, Involvement of both extrinsic and intrinsic apoptotic pathways in apoptosis induced by genistein in human cervical cancer cells, *Ann NY Acad Sci* **1171**: 196–201 (2009).
34. Kim, S.H., S.H. Kim, Y.B. Kim, Y.T. Jeon, S.C. Lee, and Y.S. Song, Genistein inhibits cell growth by modulating various mitogen-activated protein kinases and AKT in cervical cancer cells, *Ann NY Acad Sci* **1171**: 495–500 (2009).
35. Sahin, K., M. Tuzcu, N. Basak, B. Caglayan, U. Kilic, F. Sahin, and O. Kucuk, Sensitization of cervical cancer cells to cisplatin by genistein: The role of NFκB and Akt/mTOR signaling pathways, *J Oncol* **2012**: 461562 (2012).
36. Sha, G.H. and S.Q. Lin, Genistein inhibits proliferation of human endometrial endothelial cell *in vitro*, *Chin Med Sci J* **23**(1): 49–53 (2008).
37. Gossner, G., M. Choi, L. Tan, S. Fogoros, K.A. Griffith, M. Kuenker, and J.R. Liu, Genistein-induced apoptosis and autophagocytosis in ovarian cancer cells, *Gynecol Oncol* **105**(1): 23–30 (2007).
38. Ouyang, G., L. Yao, K. Ruan, G. Song, Y. Mao, and S. Bao, Genistein induces G2/M cell cycle arrest and apoptosis of human ovarian cancer cells via activation of DNA damage checkpoint pathways, *Cell Biol Int* **33**(12): 1237–1244 (2009).
39. Hwang, K.A., N.H. Kang, B.R. Yi, H.R. Lee, M.A. Park, and K.C. Choi, Genistein, a soy phytoestrogen, prevents the growth of BG-1 ovarian cancer cells induced by 17β-estradiol or bisphenol A via the inhibition of cell cycle progression, *Int J Oncol* **42**(2): 733–740 (2013).
40. Choi, E.J., T. Kim, and M.S. Lee, Pro-apoptotic effect and cytotoxicity of genistein and genistin in human ovarian cancer sk-ov-3 cells, *Life sci* **80**(15): 1403–1408 (2007).
41. Hussain, A., G. Harish, S.A. Prabhu, J. Mohsin, M.A. Khan, T.A. Rizvi, and C. Sharma, Inhibitory effect of genistein on the invasive potential of human cervical cancer cells via modulation of matrix metalloproteinase-9 and tissue inhibitors of matrix metalloproteinase-1 expression, *Cancer Epidemiol* **36**(6): e387–e393 (2012).
42. Gamble, J.R., P. Xia, C.N. Hahn, J.J. Drew, C.J. Drogemuller, D. Brown, and M.A. Vadas, Phenoxodiol, an experimental anticancer drug, shows potent antiangiogenic properties in addition to its antitumour effects, *Int J Cancer* **118**(10): 2412–2420 (2006).

43. Parajuli, B., S.J. Shin, S.H. Kwon, S.D. Cha, H.G. Lee, I. Bae, and C.H. Cho, The synergistic apoptotic interaction of indole-3-carbinol and genistein with TRAIL on endometrial cancer cells, *J Korean Med Sci* **28**(4): 527–533 (2013).
44. Hwang, K.A., N.H. Kang, B.R. Yi, S.H. Hyun, E.B. Jeung, and K.C. Choi, Anticancer effect of genistein on BG-1 ovarian cancer growth induced by 17β-estradiol or bisphenol A via the suppression of the crosstalk between estrogen receptor and insulin-like growth factor 1 receptor signaling pathways, *Toxicol Appl Pharmacol* **272**(3): 637–646 (2013).
45. Solomon, L.A., S. Ali, S. Banerjee, A.R. Munkarah, R.T. Morris, and F.H. Sarkar, Sensitization of ovarian cancer cells to cisplatin by genistein: The role of NF-κB, *J Ovarian Res* **1**(1): 9 (2008).
46. Ghaemi, A., H. Soleimanjahi, S. Razeghi, A. Gorji, A. Tabaraei, A. Moradi, A. Alizadeh, and M.A. Vakili, Genistein induces a protective immunomodulatory effect in a mouse model of cervical cancer, *Iran J Immuno* **9**(2): 119–127 (2012).
47. Lian, Z., K. Niwa, K. Tagami, M. Hashimoto, J. Gao, Y. Yokoyama, H. Mori, and T. Tamaya, Preventive effects of isoflavones, genistein and daidzein, on estradiol-17 beta-related endometrial carcinogenesis in mice, *Jpn J Cancer Res* **92**(7): 726–734 (2001).
48. Aidoo, A., M.E. Bishop, S.D. Shelton, L.E. Lyn-Cook, T. Chen, and M. Manjanatha, Effects of daidzein, genistein, and 17beta-estradiol on 7,12-dimethylbenz[a]anthracene-induced mutagenicity and uterine dysplasia in ovariectomized rats, *Nutr Cancer* **53**(1): 82–90 (2005).
49. Wang, X., X.Y. Xin, and Y.H. Huang, Regulative effect of genistein on xenografted tumor of ovarian carcinoma cell on nude mice, *Zhongguo Zhong Yao Za Zhi* **31**(11): 901–904 (2006).
50. Li, Y., C. Mi, Y.Z. Wu, S.F. Yang, and Z.Q. Yang, The effects of genistein on epidermal growth factor receptor mediated signal transduction pathway in human ovarian carcinoma cells lines SKOV3 and its xenograft in nude mice, *Zhonghua Bing Li Xue Za Zhi* **33**(6): 546–549 (2004).
51. Shukla, Y. and R. Singh, Resveratrol and cellular mechanisms of cancer prevention, *Ann NY Acad Sci* **1215**: 1–8 (2011).
52. Stakleff, K.S., T. Sloan, D. Blanco, S. Marcanthony, T.D. Booth, and A. Bishayee, Resveratrol exerts differential effects *in vitro* and *in vivo* against ovarian cancer cells, *Asian Pac J Cancer Prev* **13**(4): 1333–1340 (2012).
53. Weng, C.J. and G.C. Yen, Chemopreventive effects of dietary phytochemicals against cancer invasion and metastasis: Phenolic acids, monophenol, polyphenol, and their derivatives, *Cancer Treat Rev* **38**(1): 76–87 (2012).

54. Smith, E.R., M.B. Daly, and X.X. Xu, A mechanism for COX-2 inhibitor anti-inflammatory activity in chemoprevention of epithelial cancers, *Cancer Epidem Biomarkers Prev* **13**(1): 144–145 (2004).
55. Opipari Jr, A.W., L. Tan, A.E. Boitano, D.R. Sorenson, A. Aurora, and J.R. Liu, Resveratrol-induced autophagocytosis in ovarian cancer cells, *Cancer Res* **64**(2): 696–703 (2004).
56. Schumacher, J.J., R.P. Dings, J. Cosin, I.V. Subramanian, N. Auersperg, and S. Ramakrishnan, Modulation of angiogenic phenotype alters tumorigenicity in rat ovarian epithelial cells, *Cancer Res* **67**(8): 3683–3690 (2007).
57. Cao, Z., J. Fang, C. Xia, X. Shi, and B.H. Jiang, Trans-3,4,5′-trihydroxystilbene inhibits hypoxia-inducible factor 1α and vascular endothelial growth factor expression in human ovarian cancer cells, *Clin Cancer Res* **10**(15): 5253–5263 (2004).
58. García-Zepeda, S.P., E. García-Villa, J. Díaz-Chávez, R. Hernández-Pando, and P. Gariglio, Resveratrol induces cell death in cervical cancer cells through apoptosis and autophagy, *Eur J Cancer Prev* **22**(6): 577–584 (2013).
59. Kim, Y.S., J.W. Sull, and H.J. Sung, Suppressing effect of resveratrol on the migration and invasion of human metastatic lung and cervical cancer cells, *Mol Biol Rep* **39**(9): 8709–8716 (2012).
60. Zoberi, I., C.M. Bradbury, H.A. Curry, K.S. Bisht, P.C. Goswami, J.L. Roti Roti, and D. Gius, Radiosensitizing and anti-proliferative effects of resveratrol in two human cervical tumor cell lines, *Cancer Lett* **175**(2): 165–173 (2002).
61. Bhat, K.P. and J.M. Pezzuto, Resveratrol exhibits cytostatic and antiestrogenic properties with human endometrial adenocarcinoma (Ishikawa) cells, *Cancer Res* **61**(16): 6137–6144 (2001).
62. Kaneuchi, M., M. Sasaki, Y. Tanaka, R. Yamamoto, N. Sakuragi, and R. Dahiya, Resveratrol suppresses growth of Ishikawa cells through down-regulation of EGF, *Int J Oncol* **23**(4): 1167–1172 (2003).
63. Rao, S.D. and K. Pagidas, Epigallocatechin-3-gallate, a natural polyphenol, inhibits cell proliferation and induces apoptosis in human ovarian cancer cells, *Anticancer Res* **30**(7): 2519–2523 (2010).
64. Mazumder, M.E., P. Beale, C. Chan, J.Q. Yu, and F. Huq., Epigallocatechin gallate acts synergistically in combination with cisplatin and designed trans-palladiums in ovarian cancer cells, *Anticancer Res* **32**(11): 4851–4860 (2012).
65. Yunos, N.M., P. Beale, J.Q. Yu, and F. Huq, Synergism from the combination of oxaliplatin with selected phytochemicals in human ovarian cancer cell lines, *Anticancer Res* **31**(12): 4283–4289 (2011).
66. Yokoyama, M., M. Noguchi, Y. Nakao, M. Ysunaga, F. Yamasaki, and T. Iwasaka, Antiproliferative effects of the major tea polyphenol, (−)-epigallocatechin

gallate and retinoic acid in cervical adenocarcinoma, *Gynecol Oncol* **108**(2): 326–331 (2008).
67. Yokoyama, M., M. Noguchi, Y. Nakao, A. Pater, and T. Iwasaka, The tea polyphenol, (–)-epigallocatechin gallate effects on growth, apoptosis, and telomerase activity in cervical cell lines, *Gynecol Oncol* **92**(1): 197–204 (2004).
68. Sharma, C., A. Nusri Qel, S. Begum, E. Javed, T.A. Rizvi, and A. Hussain, (–)-Epigallocatechin-3-gallate induces apoptosis and inhibits invasion and migration of human cervical cancer cells, *Asian Pac J Cancer Prev* **13**(9): 4815–4822 (2012).
69. Singh, M., K. Bhui, R. Singh, and Y. Shukla, Tea polyphenols enhance cisplatin chemosensitivity in cervical cancer cells via induction of apoptosis, *Life Sci* **93**(1): 7–16 (2013).
70. Manohar, M., I. Fatima, R. Saxena, V. Chandra, P.L. Sankhwar, and A. Dwivedi, (–)-Epigallocatechin-3-gallate induces apoptosis in human endometrial adenocarcinoma cells via ROS generation and p38 MAP kinase activation, *J Nutr Biochem* **24**(6): 940–947 (2013).
71. Fridrich, D., N. Teller, M. Esselen, G. Pahlke, and D. Marko, Comparison of delphinidin, quercetin and (–)-epigallocatechin-3-gallate as inhibitors of the EGFR and the ErbB2 receptor phosphorylation, *Mol Nutr Food Res* **52**(7): 815–822 (2008).
72. Dorai, T. and B.B. Aggarwal, Role of chemopreventive agents in cancer therapy, *Cancer Lett* **215**(2): 129–140 (2004).
73. Liu, Q., Y.B. Peng, L.W. Qi, X.L. Cheng, X.J. Xu, L.L. Liu, E.H. Liu, and P. Li, The Cytotoxicity mechanism of 6-shogaol-treated HeLa human cervical cancer cells revealed by label-free shotgun proteomics and bioinformatics analysis, *Evid Based Complement Alternat Med* 278652 (2012).
74. Chakraborty, D., K. Bishayee, S. Ghosh, R. Biswas, S.K. Mandal, and A.R. Khuda-Bukhsh, [6]-gingerol induces caspase 3 dependent apoptosis and autophagy in cancer cells: Drug-DNA interaction and expression of certain signal genes in HeLa cells, *Eur J Pharmacol* **694**(1–3): 20–29 (2012).
75. Rhode, J., S. Fogoros, S. Zick, H. Wahl, K.A. Griffith, J. Huang, and J.R. Liu, Ginger inhibits cell growth and modulates angiogenic factors in ovarian cancer cells, *BMC Complement Altern Med* **7**: 44 (2007).
76. Ruangnoo, S., A. Itharat, I. Sakpakdeejaroen, R. Rattarom, P. Tappayutpijam, and K.K. Pawa, *In vitro* cytotoxic activity of Benjakul herbal preparation and its active compounds against human lung, cervical and liver cancer cells, *J Med Assoc Thai* **95**(1 Suppl.): S127–S134 (2012).
77. Konczak, I. and W. Zhang, Anthocyanins-more than nature's colours, *J Biomed Biotechnol* **2004**(5): 239–240 (2004).

78. Lule, S.U. and W. Xia, Food phenolics, pros and cons: A review, *Food Rev Int* **21**(4): 367–388 (2005).
79. Nichenametla, S.N., T.G. Taruscio, D.L. Barney, and J.H. Exon, A review of the effects and mechanisms of polyphenolics in cancer, *Crit Rev Food Sci Nutr* **46**(2): 161–183 (2006).
80. Kong, J.M., L.S. Chia, N.K. Goh, T.F. Chia, and R. Brouillard, Analysis and biological activities of anthocyanins, *Phytochemistry* **64**(5): 923–933 (2003).
81. Chen, Z.Y., P.T. Chan, K.Y. Ho, K.P. Fung, and J. Wang, Antioxidant activity of natural flavonoids is governed by number and location of their aromatic hydroxyl groups, *Chem Phys Lipids* **79**(2): 157–163 (1996).
82. Kim, K.K., A.P. Singh, R.K. Singh, A. Demartino, L. Brard, N. Vorsa, T.S. Lange, and R.G. Moore, Anti-angiogenic activity of cranberry proanthocyanidins and cytotoxic properties in ovarian cancer cells, *Int J Oncol* **40**(1): 227–235 (2012).
83. Zeng, L., J. Gao, and R. Zhang, Study on anti-tumor effect of cyanidin-3-glucoside on ovarian cancer, *Zhongguo Zhong Yao Za Zhi* **37**(11): 1651–1654 (2012).
84. Rugină, D., Z. Sconţa, L. Leopold, A. Pintea, A. Bunea, and C. Socaciu, Antioxidant activities of chokeberry extracts and the cytotoxic action of their anthocyanin fraction on HeLa human cervical tumor cells, *J Med Food* **15**(8): 700–706 (2012).
85. Lu, J.N., W.S. Lee, J.W. Yun, M.J. Kim, H.J. Kim, D.C. Kim, J.H. Jeong, Y.H. Choi, G.S. Kim, C.H. Ryu, and S.C. Shin, Anthocyanins from vitis coignetiae pulliat inhibit cancer invasion and epithelial–mesenchymal transition, but these effects can be attenuated by tumor necrosis factor in human uterine cervical cancer HeLa cells, *Evid Based Complement Alternat Med* **2013**: 503043 (2013).
86. Marko, D., N. Puppel, Z. Tjaden, S. Jakobs, and G. Pahlke, The substitution pattern of anthocyanidins affects different cellular signaling cascades regulating cell proliferation, *Mol Nutr Food Res* **48**(4): 318–325 (2004).
87. Teller, N., W. Thiele, T.H. Marczylo, A.J. Gescher, U. Boettler, J. Sleeman, and D. Marko, Suppression of the kinase activity of receptor tyrosine kinases by anthocyanin-rich mixtures extracted from bilberries and grapes, *J Agric Food Chem* **57**(8): 3094–3101 (2008).
88. Chaudhuri, D., S. Orsulic, and B.T. Ashok, Antiproliferative activity of sulforaphane in Akt-overexpressing ovarian cancer cells, *Mol Cancer Ther* **6**(1): 334–345 (2007).
89. Wang, X., S. Govind, S.P. Sajankila, L. Mi, R. Roy, and F.L. Chung, Phenethyl isothiocyanate sensitizes human cervical cancer cells to apoptosis induced by cisplatin, *Mol Nutr Food Res* **55**(10): 1572–1581 (2011).

90. Park, S.Y., G.Y. Kim, S.J. Bae, Y.H. Yoo, and Y.H. Choi, Induction of apoptosis by isothiocyanate sulforaphane in human cervical carcinoma HeLa and hepatocarcinoma HepG2 cells through activation of caspase-3, *Oncol Rep* **18**(1): 181–187 (2007).
91. Chang, C.C., C.M. Hung, Y.R. Yang, M.J. Lee, and Y.C. Hsu, Sulforaphane induced cell cycle arrest in the G2/M phase via the blockade of cyclin B1/CDC2 in human ovarian cancer cells, *J Ovarian Res* **6**(1): 41 (2013).
92. Chen, H., C.N. Landen, Y. Li, R.D. Alvarez, and T.O. Tollefsbol, Enhancement of cisplatin-mediated apoptosis in ovarian cancer cells through potentiating G2/M arrest and p21 upregulation by vombinatorial rpigallocatechin gallate and sulforaphane, *J Oncol* **2013**: 872957 (2013).
93. Kim, K.K., A.P. Singh, R.K. Singh, A. Demartino, L. Brard, N. Vorsa, T.S. Lange, and R.G. Moore, Anti-angiogenic activity of cranberry proanthocyanidins and cytotoxic properties in ovarian cancer cells, *Int J Oncol* **40**(1): 227–235 (2012).
94. Chaudhuri, D., S. Orsulic, and B.T. Ashok, Antiproliferative activity of sulforaphane in Akt-overexpressing ovarian cancer cells, *Mol Cancer Ther* **6**(1): 334–345 (2007).
95. Weng, J.R., C.H. Tsai, S.K. Kulp, and C.S. Chen, Indole-3-carbinol as a chemopreventive and anti-cancer agent, *Cancer Lett* **262**(2): 153–163 (2008).
96. Taylor-Harding, B., H. Agadjanian, H. Nassanian, S. Kwon, X. Guo, C. Miller, B.Y. Karlan, S. Orsulic, and C.S. Walsh, Indole-3-carbinol synergistically sensitises ovarian cancer cells to bortezomib treatment, *Br J Cancer* **106**(2): 333–343 (2012).
97. Qi, M., A.E. Anderson, D.Z. Chen, S. Sun, and K.J. Auborn, Indole-3-carbinol prevents PTEN loss in cervical cancer *in vivo*, *Mol Med* **11**(1–12): 59–63 (2005).
98. Kojima, T., T. Tanaka, and H. Mori, Chemoprevention of spontaneous endometrial cancer in female Donryu rats by dietary indole-3-carbinol, *Cancer Res* **54**(6): 1446–1449 (1994).
99. Reed, G.A., K.S. Peterson, H.J. Smith, J.C. Gray, D.K. Sullivan, M.S. Mayo, J.A. Crowell, and A. Hurwitz, A phase I study of indole-3-carbinol in women: Tolerability and effects, *Cancer Epidemiol Biomarkers Prev* **14**(8): 1953–1960 (2005).
100. Naik, R., S. Nixon, A. Lopes, K. Godfrey, M.H. Hatem, and J.M. Monaghan, A randomized phase II trial of indole-3-carbinol in the treatment of vulvar intraepithelial neoplasia, *Int J Gynecol Cancer* **16**(2): 786–790 (2006).

101. Kandala, P.K. and S. K. Srivastava, Activation of checkpoint kinase 2 by 3,3′-diindolylmethane is required for causing G2/M cell cycle arrest in human ovarian cancer cells, *Mol Pharmacol* **78**(2): 297–309 (2010).
102. Rajoria, S., R. Suriano, Y.L. Wilson, S.P. Schantz, A. Moscatello, J. Geliebter, and R.K. Tiwari, 3,3-diindolylmethane inhibits migration and invasion of human cancer cells through combined suppression of ERK and AKT pathways, *Oncol Rep* **25**(2): 491–497 (2011).
103. Del Priore, G., D.K. Gudipudi, N. Montemarano, A.M. Restivo, J. Malanowska-Stega, and A.A. Arslan, Oral diindolylmethane (DIM): Pilot evaluation of a non-surgical treatment for cervical dysplasia, *Gynecol Oncol* **116**(3): 464–467 (2010).
104. Mou, X., S. Kesari, P.Y. Wen, and X. Huang, Crude drugs as anticancer agents, *Int J Clin Exp Med* **4**(1): 17–25 (2011).
105. Burri B.J., Beta-carotene and human health: A review of current research, *Nutr Res* **17**: 547–580 (1997).
106. Jeong, N.H., E.S. Song, J.M. Lee, K.B. Lee, M.K. Kim, J.E. Cheon, J.K. Lee, S.K. Son, J.P. Lee, J.H. Kim, S.Y. Hur, and Y.I. Kwon, Plasma carotenoids, retinol and tocopherol levels and the risk of ovarian cancer, *Acta Obstet Gynecol Scand* **88**(4): 457–462 (2009).
107. Potischman, N., and L.A. Brinton, Nutrition and cervical neoplasia, *Cancer Causes Control* **7**(1): 113–126 (1996).
108. Pelucchi, C., L. Dal Maso, M. Montella, M. Parpinel, E. Negri, R. Talamini, A. Giudice, S. Franceschi, and C. La Vecchia, Dietary intake of carotenoids and retinol and endometrial cancer risk in an Italian case-control study, *Cancer Causes Control* **19**(10): 1209–1215 (2008).
109. Bosetti, C., A. Altieri, and C. La Vecchia, Diet and environmental carcinogenesis in breast/gynaecological cancers, *Curr Opin Obstet Gynecol* **14**(1): 13–18 (2002).
110. Cao, S., P.J. Brodie, J.S. Miller, F. Ratovoson, C. Birkinshaw, S. Randrianasolo, E. Rakotobe, V.E. Rasamison, and D.G. Kingston, Guttiferones K and L, antiproliferative compounds of *Rheediacalcicola* from the Madagascar rain forest, *J Nat Prod* **70**(4): 686–688 (2007).
111. Yoder, B.J., S. Cao, A. Norris, J.S. Miller, F. Ratovoson, J. Razafitsalama, R. Andriantsiferana, V.E. Rasamison, and D.G. Kingston, Antiproliferative prenylated stilbenes and flavonoids from *Macarangaalnifolia* from the Madagascar rainforest, *J Nat Prod* **70**(3): 342–346 (2007).
112. Pan, E., L. Harinantenaina, P.J. Brodie, J.S. Miller, M.W. Callmander, S. Rakotonandrasana, E. Rakotobe, V.E. Rasamison, and D.G. Kingston, Four diphenylpropanes and a cycloheptadibenzofuran from *Busseasakalava* from the Madagascar dry forest, *J Nat Prod* **73**(11): 1792–1795 (2010).

113. Alshatwi, A.A., E. Ramesh, V.S. Periasamy, and P. Subash-Babu, The apoptotic effect of hesperetin on human cervical cancer cells is mediated through cell cycle arrest, death receptor, and mitochondrial pathways, *Fundam Clin Pharmacol* **27**(6): 581–592 (2012).
114. Ramesh, E. and A.A. Alshatwi, Naringin induces death receptor and mitochondria-mediated apoptosis in human cervical cancer (SiHa) cells, *Food Chem Toxicol* **51**: 97–105 (2013).
115. Ng, T.B., X.J. Ye, J.H. Wong, E.F. Fang, Y.S. Chan, W. Pan, X.Y. Ye, S.C. Sze, K.Y. Zhang, F. Liu, and H.X. Wang, Glyceollin, a soybean phytoalexin with medicinal properties, *Appl Microbiol Biotechnol* **90**(1): 59–68 (2011).
116. Oliveira, C., A. Nicolau, J.A. Teixeira, and L. Domingues, Cytotoxic effects of native and recombinant frutalin, a plant galactose-binding lectin, on HeLa cervical cancer cells, *J Biomed Biotechnol* **2011:** 568932 (2011).
117. Oike, T., H. Ogiwara, K. Torikai, T. Nakano, J. Yokota, and T. Kohno, Garcinol, a histone acetyltransferase inhibitor, radiosensitizes cancer cells by inhibiting non-homologous end joining, *Int J Radiat Oncol Biol Phys* **84**(3): 815–821 (2012).
118. Cornett, J.W., *How Indians Used Desert Plants*, Palm Springs, CA: Nature Trails Press (2000).
119. Feugang, J.M., F. Ye, D.Y. Zhang, Y. Yu, M. Zhong, S. Zhang, and C. Zou, Cactus pear extracts induce reactive oxygen species production and apoptosis in ovarian cancer cells, *Nutr Cancer* **62**(5): 692–699 (2010).
120. Jilka, C., B. Strifler, G.W. Fortner, E.F. Hays, and D.J. Takemoto, *In vivo* antitumor activity of the bitter melon (*Momordicacharantia*), *Cancer Res* **43**(11): 5151–5155 (1983).
121. Kusamran, W.R., A Ratanavila, and A. Tepsuwan, Effects of neem flowers, Thai and Chinese bitter gourd fruits and sweet basil leaves on hepatic monooxygenases and glutathione S-transferase activities, and *in vitro* metabolic activation of chemical carcinogens in rats, *Food Chem Toxicol* **36**(6): 475–484 (1998).
122. Pongnikorn, S., D. Fongmoon, W. Kasinrerk, and P.N. Limtrakul, Effect of bitter melon (*Momordicacharantia Linn*) on level and function of natural killer cells in cervical cancer patients with radiotherapy, *Journal of Medical Association of Thailand* **86**(1): 61–68 (2003).
123. Limtrakul, P., O. Khantamat, and K. Pintha, Inhibition of P-glycoprotein activity and reversal of cancer multidrug resistance by *Momordica charantia* extract, *Cancer Chemother Pharmacol* **54**(6): 525–530 (2004).
124. Bishayee, K., S. Ghosh, A. Mukherjee, R. Sadhukhan, J. Mondal, A.R. Khuda-Bukhsh, Quercetin induces cytochrome-c release and ROS accumulation to

promote apoptosis and arrest the cell cycle in G2/M, in cervical carcinoma: Signal cascade and drug-DNA interaction, *Cell Prolif* **46**(2): 153–163 (2013).
125. Ferry, D.R., A. Smith, J. Malkhandi, D.W. Fyfe, P.G. deTakats, D. Anderson, J. Baker, and D.J. Kerr, Phase I clinical trial of the flavonoid quercetin: Pharmacokinetics and evidence for *in vivo* tyrosine kinase inhibition, *Clin Cancer Res* **2**(4): 659–668 (1996).
126. Delmas, D., E. Solary and N. Latruffe, Resveratrol, a phytochemical inducer of multiple cell death pathways: Apoptosis, autophagy and mitotic catastrophe, *Curr Med Chem* **18**(8): 1100–1121 (2011).
127. Huh, S.W., S.M. Bae, Y.W. Kim, J.M. Lee, S.E. Namkoong, I.P. Lee, S.H. Kim, C.K. Kim, and W.S. Ahn, Anticancer effects of (−)-epigallocatechin-3-gallate on ovarian carcinoma cell lines, *Gynecol Oncol* **94**(3): 760–768 (2004).
128. Kamei, H., T. Kojima, M. Hasegawa, T. Koide, T. Umeda, T. Yukawa, and K. Terabe, Suppression of tumor cell growth by anthocyanins *in vitro*, *Cancer Investigation* **13**(6): 590–594 (1995).
129. Zhang, Y., T.W. Kensler, C.G. Cho, G.H. Posner, and P. Talalay, Anticarcinogenic activities of sulforaphane and structurally related synthetic norbornyl isothiocyanates, *Proc Natl Acad Sci USA* **91**(8): 3147–3150 (1994).

6

Cancer Chemopreventive and Therapeutic Properties of Fruits and Vegetables Against Head and Neck Malignancies

Jesil Mathew Aranjani, Ganesan Padmavathi,
Ajaikumar B. Kunnumakkara and Atulya Mathew

INTRODUCTION

Head and neck squamous-cell carcinoma (HNSCC), one of most common cancers in the world, is an epithelial malignancy that arises in the upper aerodigestive tract (UADT), including regions such as the paranasal sinuses, nasal cavity, oral cavity, pharynx, and larynx.[1–3] Cancers of the brain, eye, esophagus, and thyroid gland, as well as those of the scalp, skin, muscles, and bones of the head and neck, are not usually classified as head and neck cancers. In India, it is the most prevalent form of cancer (one-fourth of all the cancers in men and one-tenth of all the cancers in women). The incidence of oral cavity cancer is higher in Melanesia (a region in Australia), South and Central Asia, Western and Southern Europe, and Southern Africa than other parts of the world, whereas the incidence of laryngeal cancer is higher in Southern and Central Europe, South America, and Western Europe than other regions of the world.[4]

HNSCC has a multi-factorial etiology which involves genetic susceptibility and exogenous exposure to substances such as tobacco, alcohol, betel quid, and viral interventions (human papillomavirus). Head and neck cancer caused by the human papillomavirus has a better prognosis with only 50% from their cancer compared to other HNSCC patients.[5] Poor diet is another risk factor for the development of head and neck cancers. Studies have shown that a Mediterranean diet of fruits, vegetables, fish, and reduced red-meat minimizes the incidence of HNSCC.[6,7]

In spite of development in the diagnosis, surgery, and treatment of HNSCC, the five-year survival rate of patients diagnosed with head and neck cancer in the developed countries has improved only by 40% compared to that of the five-year survival rate of similar patients in 1970s.[8,9]

Stages of Development and Precancerous Forms

The advancement of HNSCC includes a series of genetic insults. In general, approximately 5–20% of the dysplatic leukoplakia and erythroplakia (premalignant lesions) will grow into carcinoma *in situ* and develop as an invasive cancer. Another characteristic feature observed in patients with HNSCC is the field cancerization. There can be genetic aberrations in the normal-looking mucosa of the upper aerodigestive tract caused by constant exposure to various inducers such as tobacco smoke, betal quid chewing, and alcohol consumption. These silent lesions can develop as multiple malignant cells of various stages in the lifespan of HNSCC patients. Early stages of cancerogenesis is characterized by various physiological alterations such as increased proliferation, reduction of apoptosis followed by angiogenesis, and lyphangiogenesis that leads to regional nodal metastasis followed by distant metastasis.

It has been established that HNSCC arises from field cancerization, i.e., the exposure of an entire area of tissues to repeated carcinogenic insult that initiates a multi-stage pathogenesis process. Molecular alterations in epithelial cells may cause phenotypic histologic changes that may lead to malignant transformation from the benign to premalignant and invasive states. The term 'field cancerization' was coined by Slaughter *et al.*[10] while studying oral cancer, and since then, this terminology has been used to indicate the following:

1. Oral cancer developing in multifocal areas of a precancerous change.
2. Abnormal tissues surrounding the tumor.

3. Oral cancer which consists of multiple independent lesions that may coalesce.
4. The persistence of abnormal tissue even after surgery (a second primary tumor or local recurrences).

Multiple events occurring in the differentiation of the normal cells to a "field" initiates with a stem cell that acquires genetic alterations and forms a "patch," which is a clonal unit of altered daughter cells. Such a patch can be commonly identified by mutations in the *TP53* gene. In the next stage, the cells of the patch experiences additional genetic alterations. By virtue of its growth advantages, a proliferating field gradually displaces the normal mucosa. This is a logical and critical step in epithelial carcinogenesis is responsible for the conversion of a patch into an expanding field. Finally, the clonal divergence results into the development of one or more tumors within a contiguous field of preneoplastic cells.[11]

The second primary cancers are a leading cause of death of patients diagnosed with early stage head and neck cancer. Even after receiving a curative therapy for the early diagnosed head and neck cancer, there is almost a 20% recurrence rate in the first year, and an incidence of 5% of second primary cancers are noticed in subsequent years. The rate of second primary cancer will not get reduced with time as of recurrence, and at present, there is no efficient chemotherapeutic agent which constantly reduces the rate of second primary cancer. Reducing the incidence of second primary cancer is a key factor in the prognosis of the disease. The upper aerodigestive tract is the major area affected with the second primaries of lung cancer, esophageal cancer, pharyngeal, laryngeal, and oral cancers.[12] Thus, a precautionary approach before the advance of invasive cancer or progress of second primary tumors is highly desirable.

Cancers of the nasal cavity and paranasal sinuses are rare and constitute only three percent of those arising in the head and neck carcinoma. These tumors are more prevalent in males than females. They are difficult to treat and have been associated with a poor prognosis. As the location of tumor is in very close proximity to many vital anatomical structures, the complete surgical removal of such tumors are extremely difficult and sometimes an impossible goal. The majority of these tumors are squamous cell carcinoma, although a wide variety of other malignancies including sarcoma, adenoid cystic carcinoma, lymphoma, melanoma, and olfactory neuroblastoma may occur at this site.

According to the National Institutes of Health (NIH), in the United States, more than 10,000 men and about 3,000 women are diagnosed with laryngeal cancer every year. Like many other forms of head and neck cancers, the risk factors increasing incidence of laryngeal cancer include aging, smoking, heavy consumption of alcohol, poor diet, long-standing acid reflux from the stomach, and long-term exposure to pollutants, fumes, and certain chemicals. There is accumulating evidence from several population-based and laboratory studies to support an inverse relationship between regular consumption of fruits and vegetables and the risk of specific cancers. Head and neck cancer risk is one among them. These studies resulted in dietary guidelines to help people reduce the cancer risk.

ANTICANCER PROPERTIES OF FRUITS AND VEGETABLES AGAINST HEAD AND NECK CANCER AND THEIR MECHANISMS OF ACTION

Cancer is a disorder associated with lifestyles and thus many cancer incidences can be prevented by introducing lifestyle interventions. From the literature, it is evident that nearly 25% of the cancer cases are preventable by improving the consumption of fruits and vegetables among the population. According to the meta-analysis of epidemiology data published by the World Cancer Research Fund (WCRF) and American Institute of Cancer Research (AICR) on the potential of fruit and vegetable consumption to protect against cancer, there is probable evidence that eating fruits and vegetables conveyed protection against mouth, pharynx, larynx, esophageal, lung, and stomach cancers. This protection may be granted by micronutrients associated with fruits and vegetables such as foliates, carotenoids, β-carotene, lycopene and vitamin C. In addition studies have shown that a Mediterranean diet of fruits, vegetables, fish, and red-meat reduces the incidence of HNSCC.[6,7]

An epidemiological study on European populations has shown only a marginal benefit of the consumption of fruits and vegetables in preventing the esophageal, laryngeal, lung, and stomach cancer.[13] Boffetta *et al.*[14] reported a very small but significant inverse association between intake of

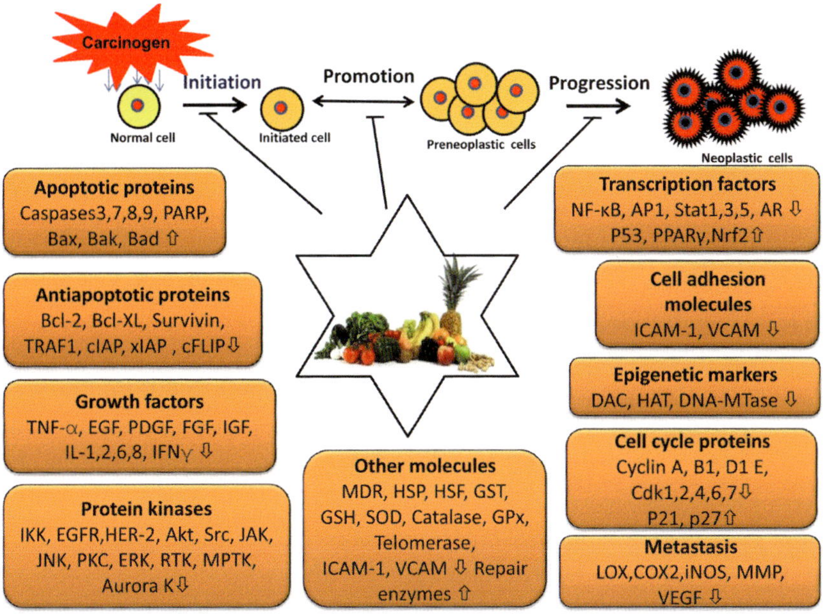

Figure 6.1: Effects of fruits and vegetables on initiation, promotion, and progression of head and neck cancers and their mechanisms of action.

total fruits and vegetables and non-specific cancer risk. There are few more epidemiologic studies indicating that the association of diet and alcohol on oral, pharyngeal, and laryngeal cancer is evident.[15,16] An attempt to review the available literature on anticancer potential of fruits and vegetables are made in this chapter. Figure 6.1 describes the important mechanisms of action of fruits and vegetables by which they inhibit the initiation, promotion, and progression of head and neck cancer.

Avocado

Avocado (*Persea americana*), also known as butter fruit, is a tree of Mexican origin. It belongs to the family Lauraceae. It has a very high content of monounsaturated fat and potassium. Widely consumed across the world as food, it has an amazing property of lowering LDL cholesterol and triglycerides, while promoting HDL cholesterol in the body.[17] The lipophilic extract of this fruit was reported to prevent various cancers principally due to the presence of highly functionalized alkanols or "aliphatic acetogenins." These agents are primarily found in the unusual idioblast oil cells of avocado fruit. Apart from these, other active molecules like terpenoid glycosides, various furan ring-containing derivatives, flavonoids, and a coumarin are also present in this plant. Ding *et al.* tested the various extracts of *P. americana* for growth inhibition against a normal (TE 1177), premalignant (SCC83-01-82), and malignant (SCC83-01-82CA) human oral cell lines. Among the extracts tested, the chloroform soluble fraction was found to have a good selective growth inhibition of both premalignant and malignant human oral epithelial cells.[18] Further studies using chromatographic techniques revealed that the active components are largely distributed in less polar subfractions and belongs to the aliphatic acetogenins. Two such active acetogenins were isolated and found to be (2S,4S)-2,4-dihydroxyheptadec-16-enyl acetate and (2S,4S)-2,4-dihydroxyheptadec-16-ynyl acetate. Both the molecules inhibited phosphorylation of EGFR (Tyr1173), c-RAF (Ser338), and ERK1/2 (Thr202/Tyr204) in the EGFR/RAS/RAF/MEK/ERK1/2 cancer pathway. The second molecule (2S,4S)-2,4-dihydroxyheptadec-16-ynyl acetate), but not the first one, prevented EGF-induced activation of the EGFR (Tyr1173). When combined, they act synergistically and inhibited phosphorylation of c-RAF (Ser338) and ERK1/2 (Thr202/Tyr204) and proliferation of human oral cancer cells. Therefore, it can be concluded that the potential anticancer activity of avocados is due to a combination of specific aliphatic acetogenins that target two key components of the EGFR/RAS/RAF/MEK/ERK1/2 cancer pathway.[19]

Raspberry

Black raspberry or *Rabus occidentalis* is a shrub of North American origin. The fruit has a diameter of 13–15 mm and a high content of anthocyanins and ellagic acid, which contributes to its antioxidant potential and nutraceutical value. Studies on the mechanism of chemoprevention revealed that this fruit exerts its anticancer activity through the modulation of multiple pathways.

Mallery *et al.* studied the effect of topical application of a bioadhesive black raspberry gel in human pre-malignant oral lesions. This study examined the effects of freeze-dried black raspberry gel (10% w/w) on oral intraepithelial neoplasia (IEN) histopathology, gene expression profiles, intraepithelial COX-2 and iNOS proteins, and microvascular densities. This study showed that freeze-dried black raspberries exhibited antioxidant properties and also induced keratinocyte apoptosis and terminal differentiation. Topical application of berry gel suppressed genes associated with RNA processing, growth factor recycling, and inhibition of apoptosis. Although the majority of patients showed that post-treatment of berry gel decreases epithelial iNOS and COX-2 proteins, only inhibition of COX-2 was statistically significant, indicating that berry gel application modulated oral IEN gene expression profiles, ultimately reducing epithelial COX-2 protein. It was also shown that in a subset of patients, application of berry gel reduced vascular densities in the superficial connective tissues and induced genes associated with keratinocyte terminal differentiation.[20,21]

Tomato

Tomato or *Solanum lycopersicum* is an edible red fruit-bearing plant originating in America. Its berries are consumed as a vegetable across the world. The anticancer properties of this plant are well studied, which are principally attributed to the presence of a bright-red carotenoid pigment lycopene, present in the fruits. Lycopene is a powerful antioxidant. In a case-control study on the relationship between tomatoes, tomato products, lycopene, and cancers of upper respiratory tract conducted in Uruguay, it was found that tomato intake was associated with a reduction in risk of 0.30 (95% confidence interval (CI), 0.18–0.51), whereas tomato sauce-rich foods displayed a protective effect of 0.57 (95% CI, 0.33–0.96 for the highest quartile of intake). The food group composed of raw tomato and tomato-rich foods showed a strong inverse association with upper aerodigestive tract cancer. It is also found that the joint effect of lycopene and total phytosterols was associated with a significant reduction in cancer risk.[22]

A review on the epidemiologic literature regarding intake of tomatoes and tomato-based products and blood lycopene levels in relation to the risk of various cancers was performed by Giovannucci *et al.*[23] Among 72 studies identified, 57 reported inverse associations between tomato intake or blood lycopene level and the risk of cancer at a defined anatomic site; 35 of these inverse associations were statistically significant. No study indicated that higher tomato consumption or blood lycopene level significantly increased the risk of cancer at any of the investigated sites. Data were suggestive of a benefit for cancers of the pancreas, colon and rectum, esophagus, oral cavity, breast, and cervix.

The chemopreventive effects of lycopene in a chemical-induced oral carcinogenesis rat model were investigated by El-Rouby.[24] Lycopene could decrease cell proliferation in 4-nitroquinoline-1-oxide (4-NQO)-induced tongue squamous cell carcinoma. Immunohistochemical studies have shown a reduced expression of proliferating cell nuclear antigen (PCNA) associated with lycopene treatment. Immunoexpression of E-cadherin and β-catenin was improved in lycopene treated groups. The results were indicative of anti-invasive effects of lycopene.

Lycopene can also selectively inhibit cancer cell (KB-1 cell line) proliferation, inducing a dose-dependent downregulation of PCNA associated with upregulation of connexin 43 (Cx-43) expression.[25] Studies using human and animal cells have identified that the expression of connexin-43 is upregulated by lycopene, and this allows direct intercellular gap junctional communication (GJC). GJC is deficient in many human tumors and its restoration or upregulation is associated with decreased proliferation.[26] Other potential anticancer mechanisms of lycopene include stimulation of xenobiotic metabolism,[27] inhibition of cholesterogenesis,[28] modulation of cyclooxygenase pathways,[29] and inhibition of inflammation.[30] In addition to lycopene, tomatoes contain numerous other potentially beneficial compounds which also contributes to the anticancer properties of this fruit.

Pomegranate

Pomegranate (*Punica granatum*) is a native of Persia. In olden days, physicians of Greece prescribed the juice for treating inflammation. The fruit is highly nutritious and rich in vitamin C. It is a good source of pantothenic acid and natural phenols such as ellagitannins, punicalagin, and flavonoids. It also contains a good proportion of nutritional oils, fibers, and potassium. Pomegranate juice was found to be anti-proliferative on human oral cancer cell lines.[31] The presence of a high quantity of antioxidant chemicals such as catechin, phenolics, and flavonoids (e.g., anthocyanins) are responsible for the significant anticancer potential of this plant. There are three major anthocyanidins found in this plant: delphinidin, cyanidin, and pelargonidin. Another important antioxidant present in pomegranates with promising anticancer activity is ellagitannins. These polyphenols are hydrolyzed to the anticancer compounds ellagic acid and urolithin. Apart from the above, the fruit extract also contains compounds such as pelargonidin, pseudopelletierine, isopelletierine, methyl isopelletierine, genistein, genistin, diadzein, diadzein, estrone, and gallic acid.

Indian Gooseberry (Amla, *Phyllanthus emblica, Emblica officinalis*)

Phyllanthus emblica Linn, commonly known as Indian gooseberry or amla, is a medicinal tree belonging to the family Phyllanthaceae. It is one of the most important medicinal plants in the Ayurvedic system of medicine. Various parts of this plant are used to treat a wide range of diseases, but the most important is the fruit. A number of phyto-constituents of amla, such as gallic acid, ellagic acid, pyrogallol, some norsesquiterpenoids, corilagin, geraniin, elaeocarpusin, and prodelphinidins B1 and B2, possess anticancer properties.[32] Ellagic acid formed from ellagitannins were found to be an important polyphenol with significant anticancer potential against HNSCC. It performs its anti-proliferative action by various mechanisms such as the activation of expression of tumor suppressor genes *p53/p21* and downregulation of insulin like growth factor (IGF II).[33] Ellagic acid prevents carcinogen induced tumorigenesis by activating detoxifying enzymes and inhibiting formation of mutagens by cytochrome P450 enzymes. The extract of amla is reported to possess beneficial radioprotective properties and are able to reduce the deleterious effects of radiation in head and neck cancer patients undergoing radiotherapy.[34,35] Triphala, the Ayurvedic rejuvenating formulation containing amla (emblica), bibhitaki (*Terminalia bellirica*), and haritaki (*Terminalia chebula*) fruits, is one of the most commonly used formulation in Ayurveda. Studies have shown that triphala possesses excellent radioprotective and chemotherapeutic properties.[36–39] The fruit also contains chebulinic acid, chebulagic acid, emblicanin A, emblicanin B, punigluconin, pedunculagin, citric acid, ellagotannin, trigallayl glucose, pectin, 1-O-galloyl-β D-glucose, 3,6-di-O-galloyl-D-glucose, corilagin, 1,6-di-O-galloyl-β-D-glucose, 3-ethyl gallic acid, and isostrictinin.[40–43]

Persimmon

Persimmon is the edible fruit of a number of species of *Diospyros* (family: Ebenaceae). It is most widely known as kaki and is native to China. The fruit has high content of sugar and tannins which makes the immature fruit astringent and bitter. Fractionated extracts of persimmon (*Diospyros kaki*) peels were studied for cytotoxic activity, multi-drug resistance (MDR) reversal activity, anti-human immunodeficiency virus (HIV) activity, and anti-*Helicobacter pylori* (*H. pylori*) activity by various groups. Acetone fraction of the fruits was shown to have significant cytotoxic effect against human oral squamous cell carcinoma (HSC-2) and human submandibular gland tumor (HSC) cells.[44]

Persimmons are rich in proanthocyanidins, which are condensed tannins. According to Lee *et al.*, proanthocyanidins from persimmon peel has a potential to act against oxidative damage in the nucleus of normal human lung diploid fibroblasts, and they modulate oxidative DNA damage under hydrogen peroxide induced cellular senescence.[45] Cryptoxanthin is a natural carotenoid pigment found in persimmons, petals, and flowers of plants in the genus *Physalis*, orange rind, papaya, and apples. Cryptoxanthin is found to be chemopreventive against oral cancer.[46] In a nested case-control study, Nomura *et al.* found that α-carotene, β-carotene, β-cryptoxanthin, total carotenoids, and γ-tocopherol levels were significantly lower in the upper aerodigestive tract cancer patients than in their controls.[47]

Garlic

Allium sativum is an integral part of Indian diet. It is commonly known as garlic and has well known pharmacological properties. The anticancer activity of this bulb is well known.[40–50] From a population-based case-control study of human laryngeal cancers conducted in China, Zheng reported a protective effect of garlic on laryngeal cancer[51] and similar effects with *Allium* vegetables on nasal tumors.[52] Only very few case control studies have reported the relationship between cancers of the head and neck and consumption of garlic. In a case control study conducted in Northeast China, Hu *et al.* reported a weak inverse relationship between garlic consumption and risk of cancers of head and neck.[53]

The different phytoconstituents of garlic possessing anticancer activity are found to be alliin, allicin, alliinase, S-allyl cysteine (SAC), diallyl disulfide (DADS), diallyl trisulfide (DATS), and methylallyltrisufide.[54,55] Allin is converted to allicin by an enzyme called allinase when garlic is crushed, chopped, or chewed. Allicin is then converted to a number of other compounds such as DAS, DADS, and ajoene.[56] Garlic is believed to confer a better protection against cancers caused by nitrosamines which is found in preserved meat products. Organosulfur compounds such as DADS and ajoene have the ability induce cell cycle arrest in cancer cell lines,[57] while DADS and DAS induce apoptosis in cancer cell lines.[58] Allicin is reported to inhibit proliferation of nasopharyngeal carcinoma (KB cells) *in vitro* with an IC_{50} value of 2.2 ± 0.2 μg/mL. Even though there are reports indicating *in vitro* anticancer activity of garlic and phytochemicals present in the garlic, the case-control studies and meta-analyses are not showing a promising inverse relation between garlic consumption and head and neck cancers.[59] Even though garlic promising in several other cancers, its involvement in chemoprevention of head and neck cancers needs to be analyzed in different populations.

Grape

Grapes (*Vitis vinifera*) and wine have been part of human civilization since thousands of years ago. The chemoprotective role of resveratrol (3,5,4′-trihydroxy-*trans*-stilbene), a natural phenol found in the seeds of grapes, is well documented. This compound was found to inhibit the proliferation of many head and neck cancer cell lines in experimental conditions.[60] *In vitro* studies showed that resveratrol induces dose-dependent growth suppression, cell-cycle arrest in the S phase, and caspase-dependent apoptosis in human nasopharyngeal carcinoma (NPC) cell lines NPC-TW076 and NPC-TW039. Moreover, it has also been shown that resveratrol enhanced chemotheraptic drug-induced apoptosis in human nasopharyngeal carcinoma cells.[61] In another study, Huang *et al.* showed that this compound significantly decreased cell viability of NPC cell lines in a dose- and time-dependent manner by decreasing mitochondrial transmembrane potential, releasing cytochrome c, enhancing expression of Fas ligand (FasL), suppressing glucose-regulated protein 78 kDa (GRP78), upregulating pro-apoptotic Bax, and downregulating of anti-apoptotic Bcl-2 protein.[62] This compound is also known to inhibit hypoxia-inducible factor-1alpha (HIF-1α) and VEGF, which are overexpressed in many human tumors and their metastases, and are closely associated with a more aggressive tumor phenotype.[63] Recent studies showed that this compound prevented 7,12-dimethylbenz[a]anthracene (DMBA)-induced oral carcinogenesis in hamster cheek pouch and significantly inhibited the growth of NPC tumor xenografts in nude mice.[64,65] Recent studies also showed that resveratrol triggers impairment of tumor-initiating stem-like property, reversed epithelial–mesenchymal transdifferentiation, and reduced self-renewal property and stemness genes signatures (*Oct4*, *Nanog*, and *Nestin*) expression in sphere-forming head and neck cancer-derived tumor-initiating cells (HNC-TICs).[66]

Lupeol is a triterpene found in grapes and many other fruits and vegetables, and was shown to selectively induce substantial HNSCC cell death, but exhibit only a minimal effect on a normal tongue fibroblast cell line *in vitro*. The major mechanism of the cytotoxic action of lupeol in HNSCC was found to be the downregulation of NF-κB. It also inhibited HNSCC cell invasion by reversal of the NF-κB-dependent epithelial-to-mesenchymal transition. Lupeol exerted a synergistic effect with cisplatin, resulting in the chemosensitization of HNSCC cell lines with high NF-κB activity *in vitro*. In *in vivo* studies, using an orthotopic metastatic nude mouse model of oral tongue squamous cell carcinoma, lupeol dramatically decreased tumor volume and suppressed local metastasis, which was more efficient than cisplatin alone. Lupeol also exerted a significant synergistic cytotoxic effect when combined with low-dose cisplatin without side effects.[67] Moreover, it has also been shown that grape seed extract selectively inhibits the growth and cell cycle arrest and induced apoptotic death in human HNSCC, by activating the DNA damage checkpoint cascade, including ataxia telangiectasia mutated/ataxia telangiectasia-Rad3-related–checkpoint kinase 1/2-Cdc25C as well as caspases 8, 9, and 3.[68]

Cruciferous Vegetables

Cruciferous vegetables include vegetables of the family Brassicaceae (Cruciferae). Examples include cabbage, broccoli, cauliflower, Brussels sprouts, kale, horse radish, arugula, radishes, rutabaga, turnips, watercress, wasabi, bok choy, etc. They have effected a lot of attention from cancer researchers due to their rich source of nutrients such as carotenoids, vitamins C, E, and K, foliates, and minerals. They are also a rich source of fiber.

The sulfur-containing molecules known as glucosinolates present in these vegetables are responsible for their pungent aroma and bitter flavor.[69] During different stages of food preparation, chewing and digestion induces metabolism of glucosinolates (Fig. 6.2) into biologically active compounds such as thiocyanates, isothiocyanates, and indoles.[70,71] Indole-3-carbinol (I3C) and sulforaphane are the most-studied molecules for their anticancer properties.

I3C is reported to induce apoptosis in many human cancer cell lines. Xu *et al.* demonstrated the apoptotic effects of I3C in nasopharyngeal cancer cells (CNE-2), which was associated with a significant reduction in

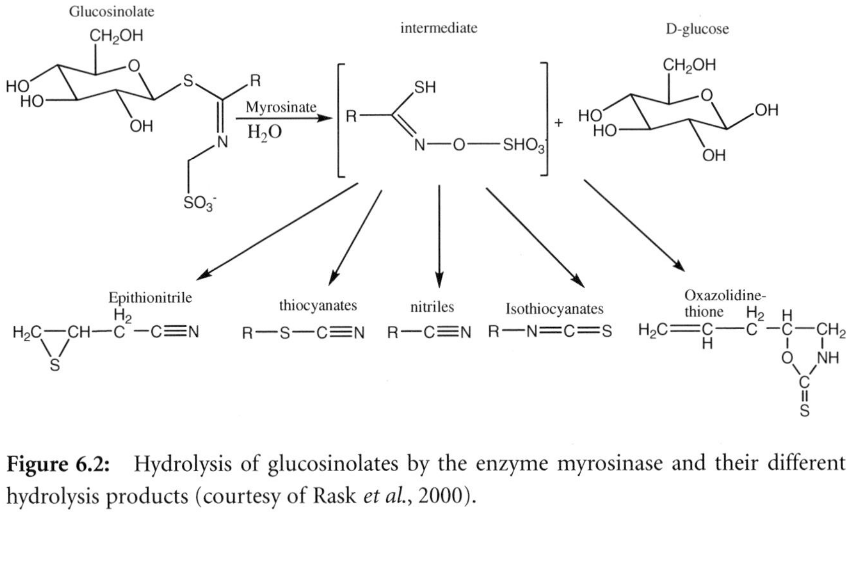

Figure 6.2: Hydrolysis of glucosinolates by the enzyme myrosinase and their different hydrolysis products (courtesy of Rask *et al.*, 2000).

mitochondrial potential and mitochondrial membrane dysfunction.[72] The data suggested that I3C-induced apoptosis induction may be associated with the signaling activation of the mitogen-activated protein kinase (MAPK) and Fas/FasL pathways. This study recommended I3C as a preventive and therapeutic agent against nasopharyngeal cancer. In another study conducted in China, researchers at Nanfang Medical University reported similar effect of I3C. They further reported the antioxidant activity of I3C along with its ability to reduce the levels of malonaldehyde and apoptotic effects both *in vitro* and *in vivo*.[73]

There have been several mechanisms of action reported for the anticancer activities of I3C. It suppresses NF-κB activation induced by various agents, which is correlated with suppression of IKK and IκBα phosphorylation, ubiquitination, and degradation, and with nuclear translocation and acetylation. I3C also down regulates the transcription of NF-κB-regulated reporter gene and expression of gene products involved in cell proliferation (e.g., cyclin D1 and COX-2), prevention of apoptosis (e.g., survivin, IAP1, IAP2, XIAP, Bcl-2, Bfl-1/A1, TRAF1, and FLIP), and invasion (MMP-9), thus enhancing apoptosis induced by cytokines and chemotherapeutic agents.[74] It is found that I3C downregulates cyclin D1 expression, which mediates G1/S transition.[74] I3C also downregulates the expression of iNOS and Bcl-2, which could also be due to the downregulation of NF-κB.[74]

Sulforaphane is the most-characterized isothiocyanate present in cruciferous vegetables. It has several pharmacological benefits such as anti-inflammatory,[75] anticancer,[76] and antioxidant activity.[77] Having low toxicity, the compound is safe to animals, making it as an excellent choice of a chemopreventive agent. It has the ability to also induce apoptosis in cancer cells.[78,79] It can also prevent the development of benign tumors to malignant tumors and interrupt metastasis. The effects of sulforaphane on tongue cancer proliferation and its mechanisms were studied by Yao *et al.*[80] Overexpression of HIF-1 expression is associated with tumorigenesis and angiogenesis. It regulates the expression of many genes including VEGF, iNOS, and lactate dehydrogenase A. Yao *et al.* investigated the effects of sulforaphane on the expression of HIF-1α, which was overexpressed in human tongue squamous cell carcinoma. Sulforaphane inhibited hypoxia-induced expression of HIF-1α via inhibiting synthesis of HIF-1α.

Sulforaphane was also found to inhibit hypoxia-induced HIF-1α expression through the activation of the JNK and ERK signaling pathways, but not the AKT pathway. Inhibition of HIF-1α by sulforaphane resulted in the decreased expression of VEGF. This clearly demonstrates the antiangiogenetic and chemopreventive action of sulforaphane against tongue cancers *in vitro.*

Soybean

This is a legume of East Asian origin. It is an edible bean rich in proteins, which account for nearly 60% of its dry seeds. The lipid portion of soybean (soybean oil) consists mainly of phytosterols such as campesterol (20–23%), β-sitosterol (53–56%), and stigmasterol (17–21%), accounting for 2.5% of the lipid fraction. Its anticancer property is mainly due to the presence of isoflavones like genistein and daidzein.[81] It also contains glycitein, an O-methylated isoflavone. Genistein can induce cell growth inhibition by arresting the cells at S/G2-M phases. It also induces apoptosis in HN4 squamous cell carcinoma of the head and neck cell line. These changes are achieved by the downregulation of cyclin B1 and Cdk1 and also by upregulation of Cdk inhibitor p21WAF1.[82] This could possibly be the reason for apoptosis and cell cycle arrest. Genistein and daidzein are able to inhibit DNA topoisomerases as well.[83]

In a case-control study conducted in China, the relationship between nasopharyngeal carcinoma and consumption of fruits and vegetables were analyzed by Lyu *et al.* A negative relationship was found between consumption of fruits and vegetables and risk on nasopharyngeal carcinoma.[84] A cohort study was conducted in the United States from 1995/96 to 2000 among 490,802 participants to investigate the relationship between diet and head and neck cancer. An inverse relationship was reported between total food and vegetable intake and head and neck cancer risk. In models mutually adjusted for fruits and vegetables intake, the association was stronger for vegetables (hazard ratio 0.65; CI 0.5–0.850) than fruits (hazard ratio 0.87; CI 0.68–1.11). Among various botanical groups, significant associations were found in leguminosae (dried beans, string beans, and peas), rosaceae (apples, peach, nectarines, plums, pears, and strawberries), solanaceae (peppers and tomatoes), and umbeliferrae (carrots). Therefore, it is clear that consumption of fruits and vegetables decreases the risk of head and neck cancer.

CONCLUSION

The recent past made substantial progress in exploring the biochemical events and modifications leading to the multi-stage process of carcinogenesis. This has improved our understanding on the possible targets of dietary phytochemicals that can significantly regulate carcinogenesis. The attempt to define cellular and molecular targets of chemopreventive phyotochemicals is still incomplete. One of the major pathways is the family of proline-directed serine/threonine kinases — the MAPKs. Some phytochemicals "switch on" or "turn off" the specific signaling molecule(s), depending on the nature of the signaling cascade they target, preventing abnormal cell proliferation and growth. Cell-signaling kinases other than MAPKs, such as protein kinase C (PKC) and phosphatidylinositol 3-kinase (PI3K), are also important targets of certain chemopreventive phytochemicals. These upstream kinases activate a distinct set of transcription factors, including NF-κB and activator protein 1 (AP1).

Chemoprevention by fruits and vegetables can be considered as an inexpensive, applicable, and acceptable approach. It is rather affordable and very safe compared to any synthetic chemopreventive agent. Several nutrients and non-nutritive phytochemicals are being evaluated in intervention trials for their potential as anticancer agents. Case-control and cohort studies indicate an inverse relationship between the consumption of fruits and vegetables and risk of head and neck cancer. Therefore, it is clear that a diet rich in fruits and vegetables can reduce the incidence of such a cancer.

REFERENCES

1. Jemal, A., F. Bray, M.M. Center, J. Ferlay, E. Ward, and D. Forman, Global cancer statistics, *CA Cancer J Clin* **61**(2): 69–90 (2011).
2. Hunter, K.D., E.K. Parkinson, and P.R. Harrison, Profiling early head and neck cancer, *Nat Rev Cancer* **5**(2): 127–135 (2005).
3. Wu, K.H.J., The management of head and neck cancer, *Surgery (Oxford)* **27**(12): 540–545 (2009).

4. Argiris, A., M.V. Karamouzis, D. Raben, and R.L. Ferris, Head and neck cancer, *Lancet* **371**(9625): 1695–1709 (2008).
5. Fakhryand, C. and M.L. Gillison, Clinical implications of human papillomavirus in head and neck cancers, *J Clin Oncol* **24**(17): 2606–2611 (2006).
6. Bosetti, C., S. Gallus, A. Trichopoulou, R. Talamini, S. Franceschi, E. Negri, and C. La Vecchia, Influence of the Mediterranean diet on the risk of cancers of the upper aerodigestive tract, *Cancer Epidem Biomar* **12**(10): 1091–1094 (2003).
7. Gallus, S., C. Bosetti, and C.L. Vecchia, Mediterranean diet and cancer risk, *Eur J Cancer Prev* **13**(5): 447 (2004).
8. Laramore, G., C. Scott, M. Al-Sarraf, R. Haselow, T. Ervin, R. Wheeler, J. Jacobs, D. Schuller, R. Gahbauer, and J. Schwade, Adjuvant chemotherapy for resectable squamous cell carcinomas of the head and neck: Report of Intergroup Study 0034, *Int J Radiat Oncol* **23**(4): 705–713 (1992).
9. Argirisand, A. and C. Eng, Epidemiology, staging, and screening of head and neck cancer, *Cancer Treat Res* **114**: 15–60 (2003).
10. Slaughter, D.P., H.W. Southwick, and W. Smejkal, Field cancerization in oral stratified squamous epithelium: Clinical implications of multicentric origin, *Cancer* **6**(5): 963–968 (1953).
11. Braakhuis, B.J., M.P. Tabor, J.A. Kummer, C.R. Leemans, and R.H. Brakenhoff, A genetic explanation of Slaughter's concept of field cancerization: Evidence and clinical implications, *Cancer Res* **63**(8): 1727–1730 (2003).
12. Cartmel, B., D. Bowen, D. Ross, E. Johnson, and S.T. Mayne, A randomized trial of an intervention to increase fruit and vegetable intake in curatively treated patients with early-stage head and neck cancer, *Cancer Epidem Biomar* **14**(12): 2848–2854 (2005).
13. Soerjomataram, I., D. Oomen, V. Lemmens, A. Oenema, V. Benetou, A. Trichopoulou, J.W. Coebergh, J. Barendregt, and E. de Vries, Increased consumption of fruit and vegetables and future cancer incidence in selected European countries, *Eur J Cancer* **46**(14): 2563 (2010).
14. Boffetta, P., E. Couto, J. Wichmann, P. Ferrari, D. Trichopoulos, H.B. Bueno-de-Mesquita, F.J.B. van Duijnhoven, F.L. Büchner, T. Key, and H. Boeing, Fruit and vegetable intake and overall cancer risk in the European Prospective Investigation into Cancer and Nutrition (EPIC), *J Natl Cancer Inst* **102**(8): 529–537 (2010).
15. Longnecker, M.P. and S.M. Enger, Epidemiologic data on alcoholic beverage consumption and risk of cancer, *Clin Chim Acta* **246**(1-2): 121–141 (1996).
16. Ziegler, R.G., Alcohol nutrient interactions in cancer etiology, *Cancer* **58**(8 Suppl.): 1942–1948 (2006).

17. Colquhoun, D., D. Moores, S.M. Somerset, and J.A. Humphries, Comparison of the effects on lipoproteins and apolipoproteins of a diet high in monounsaturated fatty acids, enriched with avocado, and a high-carbohydrate diet, *Am J Clin Nutr* **56**(4): 671–677 (1992).
18. Ding, H., Y.W. Chin, A.D. Kinghorn, and S.M. D'Ambrosio, Chemopreventive characteristics of avocado fruit, *Semin Cancer Biol* **17**(5): 386–394 (2007).
19. D'Ambrosio, S.M., C. Han, L. Pan, A.D. Kinghorn, and H. Ding, Aliphatic acetogenin constituents of avocado fruits inhibit human oral cancer cell proliferation by targeting the EGFR/RAS/RAF/MEK/ERK1/2 pathway, *Biochem Biophys Res Commun* **409**(3): 465–469 (2011).
20. Mallery, S.R., J.C. Zwick, P. Pei, M. Tong, P.E. Larsen, B.S. Shumway, B. Lu, H.W. Fields, R.J. Mumper, and G.D. Stoner, Topical application of a bioadhesive black raspberry gel modulates gene expression and reduces cyclooxygenase 2 protein in human premalignant oral lesions, *Cancer Res* **68**(12): 4945–4957 (2008).
21. Mallery, S.R., G.D. Stoner, P.E. Larsen, H.W. Fields, K.A. Rodrigo, S.J. Schwartz, Q. Tian, J. Dai, and R.J. Mumper, Formulation and *in-vitro* and *in-vivo* evaluation of a mucoadhesive gel containing freeze dried black raspberries: Implications for oral cancer chemoprevention, *Pharm Res* **24**(4): 728–737 (2007).
22. De Stefani, E., F. Oreggia, P. Boffetta, H. Deneo-Pellegrini, A. Ronco, and M. Mendilaharsu, Tomatoes, tomato-rich foods, lycopene and cancer of the upper aerodigestive tract: A case-control in Uruguay, *Oral Oncol* **36**(1): 47–53 (2000).
23. Giovannucci, E., Tomatoes, tomato-based products, lycopene, and cancer: Review of the epidemiologic literature, *J Natl Cancer Inst* **91**(4): 317 (1999).
24. El-Rouby, D.H., Histological and immunohistochemical evaluation of the chemopreventive role of lycopene in tongue carcinogenesis induced by 4-nitroquinoline-1-oxide, *Arch Oral Biol* **56**(7): 664–671 (2011).
25. Livny, O., I. Kaplan, R. Reifen, S. Polak-Charcon, Z. Madar, and B. Schwartz, Oral cancer cells differ from normal oral epithelial cells in tissue like organization and in response to lycopene treatment: An organotypic cell culture study, *Nutr Cancer* **47**(2): 195–209 (2003).
26. Heberand, D. and Q.Y. Lu, Overview of mechanisms of action of lycopene, *Exp Biol Med (Maywood)* **227**(10): 920–923 (2002).
27. Wright, A.J.A., D.A. Hughes, A.L. Bailey, and S. Southon, Beta-carotene and lycopene, but not lutein, supplementation changes the plasma fatty acid profile of healthy male non-smokers, *J Lab Clin Med* **134**(6): 592–598 (1999).
28. Fuhrman, B., A. Elis, and M. Aviram, Hypocholesterolemic effect of lycopene and β-carotene is related to suppression of cholesterol synthesis and augmentation

of LDL receptor activity in macrophages, *Biochem Biophys Res Commun* **233**(3): 658–662 (1997).
29. Heber, D. and V. Go, Gene-nutrient interaction and the xenobiotic hypothesis of cancer, *Nutritional Oncology*: 613–618 (1999).
30. Heber, D., Colorful cancer prevention: α-carotene, lycopene, and lung cancer, *Am J Clin Nutr* **72**(4): 901–902 (2000).
31. Seeram, N.P., L.S. Adams, S.M. Henning, Y. Niu, Y. Zhang, M.G. Nair, and D. Heber, *In vitro* antiproliferative, apoptotic and antioxidant activities of punicalagin, ellagic acid and a total pomegranate tannin extract are enhanced in combination with other polyphenols as found in pomegranate juice, *J Nutr Biochem* **16**(6): 360–367 (2005).
32. Baligaand, M.S. and J.J. Dsouza, Amla (*Emblica officinalis Gaertn*), a wonder berry in the treatment and prevention of cancer, *Eur J Cancer Prev* **20**(3): 225–239 (2011).
33. Narayananand, B.A. and G.G. Re, IGF-II down regulation associated cell cycle arrest in colon cancer cells exposed to phenolic antioxidant ellagic acid, *Anticancer Res* **21**(1A): 359–364 (2001).
34. Weissand, J.F. and M.R. Landauer, Protection against ionizing radiation by antioxidant nutrients and phytochemicals, *Toxicology* **189**(1–2): 1–20 (2003).
35. Hosseinimehr, S.J., Trends in the development of radioprotective agents, *Drug Discov Today* **12**(19–20): 794–805 (2007).
36. Jagetia, G., M. Baliga, K. Malagi, and M. Sethukumar Kamath, The evaluation of the radioprotective effect of Triphala (an ayurvedic rejuvenating drug) in the mice exposed to γ-radiation, *Phytomed* **9**(2): 99–108 (2002).
37. Kaur, S., H. Michael, S. Arora, P.L. Härkönen, and S. Kumar, The *in vitro* cytotoxic and apoptotic activity of triphala — An Indian herbal drug, *J Ethnopharmacol* **97**(1): 15–20 (2005).
38. Garodia, P., H. Ichikawa, N. Malani, G. Sethi, and B.B. Aggarwal, From ancient medicine to modern medicine: Ayurvedic concepts of health and their role in inflammation and cancer, *J Soc Integr Oncol* **5**(1): 25–37 (2007).
39. Aggarwal, B.B., H. Ichikawa, P. Garodia, P. Weerasinghe, G. Sethi, I.D. Bhatt, M.K. Pandey, S. Shishodia, and M.G. Nair, From traditional Ayurvedic medicine to modern medicine: Identification of therapeutic targets for suppression of inflammation and cancer, *Expert Opin Ther Targets* **10**(1): 87–118 (2006).
40. Khan, K., Roles of Emblica officinalis in medicine — A review, *Bot Res Int* **2**(4): 218–228 (2009).
41. Zhang, L.Z., W.H. Zhao, Y.J. Guo, G.Z. Tu, S. Lin, and L. Xin, Studies on chemical constituents in fruits of Tibetan medicine *Phyllanthus emblica*, *Zhongguo Zhong Yao Za Zhi* **28**(10): 940 (2003).

42. Habib-ur-Rehman, K.A. Yasin, M.A. Choudhary, N. Khaliq, Atta-ur-Rahman, M.I. Choudhary, and S. Malik, Studies on the chemical constituents of *Phyllanthus emblica, Nat Prod Res* **21**(9): 775–781 (2007).
43. Mirunaliniand, S. and M. Krishnaveni, Therapeutic potential of Phyllanthus emblica (amla): The Ayurvedic wonder, *J Basic Clin Physiol Pharmacol* **21**(1): 93–105 (2010).
44. Kawase, M., N. Motohashi, K. Satoh, H. Sakagami, H. Nakashima, S. Tani, Y. Shirataki, T. Kurihara, G. Spengler, K. Wolfard, and J. Molnár, Biological activity of persimmon (*Diospyros kaki*) peel extracts, *Phytother Res* **17**(5): 495–500 (2003).
45. Lee, Y.A., E.J. Cho, and T. Yokozawa, Protective effect of persimmon (Diospyros kaki) peel proanthocyanidin against oxidative damage under H_2O_2-induced cellular senescence, *Biol Pharm Bull* **31**(6): 1265–1269 (2008).
46. Simon, J.J., Phytochemicals and cancer, *J Chiropr Med* **1**(3): 91–96 (2002).
47. Nomura, A.M., R.G. Ziegler, G.N. Stemmermann, P.H. Chyou, and N.E. Craft, Serum micronutrients and upper aerodigestive tract cancer, *Cancer Epidemiol Biomarkers Prev* **6**(6): 407–412 (1997).
48. Galeone, C., C. Pelucchi, F. Levi, E. Negri, S. Franceschi, R. Talamini, A. Giacosa, and C. La Vecchia, Onion and garlic use and human cancer, *Am J Clin Nutr* **84**(5): 1027–1032 (2006).
49. Fleischauerand, A.T. and L. Arab, Garlic and cancer: A critical review of the epidemiologic literature, *J Nutr* **131**(3s): 1032S–1040S (2001).
50. Kimand, J.Y. and O. Kwon, Garlic intake and cancer risk: An analysis using the Food and Drug Administration's evidence-based review system for the scientific evaluation of health claims, *Am J Clin Nutr* **89**(1): 257–264 (2009).
51. Zheng, W., W.J. Blot, X.O. Shu, Y.T. Gao, B.T. Ji, R.G. Ziegler, and J.F. Fraumeni Jr., Diet and other risk factors for laryngeal cancer in Shanghai, China, *Am J Epidemiol* **136**(2): 178–191 (1992).
52. Zheng, W., W.J. Blot, X.O. Shu, E.L. Diamond, Y.T. Gao, B.T. Ji, and J.F. Fraumeni Jr., A population-based case-control study of cancers of the nasal cavity and paranasal sinuses in Shanghai, *Int J Cancer* **52**(4): 557–561 (1992).
53. Hu, J., O. Nyren, A. Wolk, R. Bergstrom, J. Yuen, H.O. Adami, L. Guo, H. Li, G. Huang, X. Xu, *et al.* Risk factors for oesophageal cancer in northeast China, *Int J Cancer* **57**(1): 38–46 (1994).
54. Gerhauser, C., Cancer chemoprevention and nutriepigenetics: State of the art and future challenges, *Top Curr Chem* **329**: 73–132 (2013).
55. Asgarpanahand, J. and B. Ghanizadeh, Pharmacologic and medicinal properties of *Allium hirtifolium Boiss, Afr J Pharm Pharacol* **6**(25): 1809–1814 (2012).

56. Hark, L., K. Ashton, and D. Deen, *The Nurse Practitioner's Guide to Nutrition, Wiley-Blackwell* (2012).
57. Le Bonand, A.M. and M.H. Siess, Organosulfur compounds from *Allium* and the chemoprevention of cancer, *Drug Metab Drug Interact* **17**(1–4): 51–80 (2011).
58. Yang, K., H. Tang, and Q. Su, Apoptosis of nasopharyngeal carcinoma cells line CNE1 induced by diallyl disulfide, *J Nanhua Univ (Medical Edition)* **3**: 306–309 (2008).
59. Fleischauer, A.T., C. Poole, and L. Arab, Garlic consumption and cancer prevention: Meta-analyses of colorectal and stomach cancers, *Am J Clin Nutr* **72**(4): 1047–1052 (2000).
60. ElAttar, T.M. and A.S. Virji, Modulating effect of resveratrol and quercetin on oral cancer cell growth and proliferation, *Anticancer Drugs* **10**(2): 187–193 (1999).
61. Chow, S.E., J.S. Wang, S.F. Chuang, Y.L. Chang, W.K. Chu, W.S. Chen, and Y.W. Chen, Resveratrol-induced p53-independent apoptosis of human nasopharyngeal carcinoma cells is correlated with the downregulation of ΔNp63, *Cancer Gene Ther* **17**(12): 872–882 (2010).
62. Huang, T.T., H.C. Lin, C.C. Chen, C.C. Lu, C.F. Wei, T.S. Wu, F.G. Liu, and H.C. Lai, Resveratrol induces apoptosis of human nasopharyngeal carcinoma cells via activation of multiple apoptotic pathways, *J Cell Physiol* **226**(3): 720–728 (2011).
63. Zhang, Q., X. Tang, Q.Y. Lu, Z.F. Zhang, J. Brown, and A.D. Le, Resveratrol inhibits hypoxia-induced accumulation of hypoxia-inducible factor-1alpha and VEGF expression in human tongue squamous cell carcinoma and hepatoma cells, *Mol Cancer Ther* **4**(10): 1465–1474 (2005).
64. Berta, G.N., P. Salamone, A.E. Sprio, F. Di Scipio, L.M. Marinos, S. Sapino, M.E. Carlotti, R. Cavalli, and F. Di Carlo, Chemoprevention of 7,12-dimethylbenz[a]-anthracene (DMBA)-induced oral carcinogenesis in hamster cheek pouch by topical application of resveratrol complexed with 2-hydroxypropyl-beta-cyclodextrin, *Oral Oncol* **46**(1): 42–48 (2010).
65. Zhang, M., X. Zhou, and K. Zhou, Resveratrol inhibits human nasopharyngeal carcinomaell growth via blocking pAkt/p70S6K signaling pathways, *Int J Mol Med* **31**(3): 621–627 (2013).
66. Hu, F.W., L.L. Tsai, C.H. Yu, P.N. Chen, M.Y. Chou, and C.C. Yu, Impairment of tumor-initiating stem-like property and reversal of epithelial–mesenchymal transdifferentiation in head and neck cancer by resveratrol treatment, *Mol Nutr Food Res* **56**(8): 1247–1258 (2012).

67. Lee, T.K., R.T. Poon, J.Y. Wo, S. Ma, X.Y. Guan, J.N. Myers, P. Altevogt, and A.P. Yuen, Lupeol suppresses cisplatin-induced nuclear factor-kappaB activation in head and neck squamous cell carcinoma and inhibits local invasion and nodal metastasis in an orthotopic nude mouse model, *Cancer Res* **67**: 8800–8809 (2007).
68. Shrotriya, S., G. Deep, M. Gu, M. Kaur, A.K. Jain, S. Inturi, R. Agarwal, and C. Agarwal, Generation of reactive oxygen species by grape seed extract causes irreparable DNA damage leading to G2/M arrest and apoptosis selectively in head and neck squamous cell carcinoma cells, *Carcinogenesis* **33**: 848–858 (2012).
69. Carteaand, M.E. and P. Velasco, Glucosinolates in Brassica foods: Bioavailability in food and significance for human health, *Phytochem Rev* **7**: 213–229 (2008).
70. Hayes, J.D., M.O. Kelleher, and I.M. Eggleston, The cancer chemopreventive actions of phytochemicals derived from glucosinolates, *Eur J Nutr* **47**(2): 73–88 (2008).
71. Rask, L., E. Andreasson, B. Ekbom, S. Eriksson, B. Pontoppidan, and J. Meijer, Myrosinase: Gene family evolution and herbivore defense in Brassicaceae, *Plant Mol Biol* **42**(1): 93–113 (2000).
72. Xu, Y., J. Zhang, and W.G. Dong, Indole-3-carbinol (I3C)-induced apoptosis in nasopharyngeal cancer cells through Fas/FasL and MAPK pathway, *Med Oncol* **28**(4): 1343–1348 (2011).
73. Zhu, W., W. Li, G. Yang, Q. Zhang, M. Li, and X. Yang, Indole-3-carbinol inhibits nasopharyngeal carcinoma, *Int J Toxicol* **29**(2): 185–192 (2010).
74. Takada, Y., M. Andreeff, and B.B. Aggarwal, Indole-3-carbinol suppresses NF-κB and IκBα kinase activation, causing inhibition of expression of NF-κB-regulated antiapoptotic and metastatic gene products and enhancement of apoptosis in myeloid and leukemia cells, *Blood* **106**(2): 641–649 (2005).
75. Huang, M.T., Y.R. Lou, J.G. Xie, W. Ma, Y.P. Lu, P. Yen, B.T. Zhu, H. Newmark, and C.T. Ho, Effect of dietary curcumin and dibenzoylmethane on formation of 7,12-dimethylbenz[a]anthracene-induced mammary tumors and lymphomas/leukemias in Sencar mice, *Carcinogenesis* **19**(9): 1697–1700 (1998).
76. Shen, G., T.O. Khor, R. Hu, S. Yu, S. Nair, C.T. Ho, B.S. Reddy, M.T. Huang, H.L. Newmark, and A.N.T. Kong, Chemoprevention of familial adenomatous polyposis by natural dietary compounds sulforaphane and dibenzoylmethane alone and in combination in ApcMin/+ mouse, *Cancer Res* **67**(20): 9937–9944 (2007).
77. Singh, S.V., S.K. Srivastava, S. Choi, K.L. Lew, J. Antosiewicz, D. Xiao, Y. Zeng, S.C. Watkins, C.S. Johnson, and D.L. Trump, Sulforaphane-induced cell death

in human prostate cancer cells is initiated by reactive oxygen species, *J Biol Chem* **280**(20): 19911–19924 (2005).
78. Fimognariand, C. and P. Hrelia, Sulforaphane as a promising molecule for fighting cancer, *Mut Res* **635**(2-3): 90 (2007).
79. Zhang, Y. and L. Tang, Discovery and development of sulforaphane as a cancer chemopreventive phytochemical, *Acta Pharmacol Sin* **28**(9): 1343–1354 (2007).
80. Yao, H., H. Wang, Z. Zhang, B.H. Jiang, J. Luo, and X. Shi, Sulforaphane inhibited expression of hypoxia-inducible factor-1α in human tongue squamous cancer cells and prostate cancer cells, *Int J Cancer* **123**(6): 1255–1261 (2008).
81. Kingsley, K., K. Truong, E. Low, C.K. Hill, S.B. Chokshi, D. Phipps, M.A. West, M.A. Keiserman, and C.J. Bergman, Soy protein extract (SPE) exhibits differential *in vitro* cell proliferation effects in oral cancer and normal cell lines, *J Diet Suppl* **8**(2): 169–188 (2011).
82. Alhasan, S.A., J.F. Ensley, and F.H. Sarkar, Genistein induced molecular changes in a squamous cell carcinoma of the head and neck cell line, *Int J Oncol* **16**(2): 333–338 (2000).
83. Russo, P., A. Del Bufalo, and A. Cesario, Flavonoids acting on DNA topoisomerases: Recent advances and future perspectives in cancer therapy, *Curr Med Chem* **19**(31): 5287–5293 (2012).
84. Liu, Y., J. Dai, C. Xu, Y. Lu, Y. Fan, X. Zhang, C. Zhang, and Y. Chen, Greater intake of fruit and vegetables is associated with lower risk of nasopharyngeal carcinoma in Chinese adults: A case-control study, *CCC* **23**(4): 589–599 (2012).

7

Anticancer Activities of Fruits and Vegetables Against Liver and Pancreatic Cancers

Farid A. Badria, Diaaeldin M. Elimam and Ahmed S. Ibrahim*

INTRODUCTION

Hepatocellular carcinoma (HCC) and pancreatic carcinoma (PC) are two of the most common cancers in the world. It has been reported that the annual mortality rates from liver and pancreatic malignancies are 700,000 and 266,000, respectively.[1] It has been shown that the typical treatment options for these cancers have limited efficacy and marked patient-to-patient variation in therapeutic outcomes. In most cases, surgical resection and organ transplantation remain the only curative treatment options and they can be very expensive and invasive procedures. Therefore, natural components in edible fruits and vegetables can provide a safe, effective, and economic therapeutic option that is of prime importance.

Extensive research over the past decade has been dominated by multiple synthetic chemotherapeutic drugs that are non-invasive but display low selectivity and hence deadly adverse effects. Moreover, given the variable success of these drugs, a targeted drug development strategy would be selective,

*Corresponding author: Farid A. Badria, Ph.D., Professor, Pharmacognosy Department, Mansoura University, Mansoura 35516, Egypt. Tel: (+20) 122-354-2193, Fax: (+20) 50-236-3641, Email: faridbadria@gmail.com.

less toxic, and more fruitful for rational and successful transition of preclinical discoveries to the clinical realm. These therapies can be discovered by unraveling the etiology of these malignancies which is multi-factorial. Various factors are known to be involved in their progression, including genetic instability, gene expression abnormality, aberrant growth factors and signal transduction, production of inflammatory cytokines, and oxidative stress. Since all of these appear simultaneously either in HCC or PC, therapeutic strategies should be integrated appropriately.

The use of natural products as an alternative to conventional therapy in healing and treatment of various diseases has been on the rise in the last few decades. Fruits and vegetables are the only foods which collectively have been consistently associated with risk reduction in several kinds of cancer including liver and pancreatic malignancies.[2–4] The protective effects of high fruit and vegetable consumption are attributed to their active micronutrients (e.g., vitamins and minerals) and non-nutritive components that are known as phytochemicals. These natural components exhibit wide therapeutic index, act on mechanistically biological pathways, and target events that occur in hepatic or pancreatic malignant cells exclusively, thus they will not be as harmful to normal cells, representing a revolution in cancer therapy. However, the exact mechanism that explains their protective role in fighting these malignancies is still controversial and complex and thus has to be dissected out. In this chapter, the reader will get a clear roadmap of what has been accomplished so far in the field. This necessarily entails a description of how hepatic and pancreatic cancer cells work at the cellular as well as at organism levels, target-oriented strategies in HCC and PC therapy, and how natural compounds in fruits and vegetables fit into this mechanism-based approach with the aim of increasing their value in cancer treatment beyond what has previously been demonstrated.

CELLULAR SIGNALING PATHWAYS INVOLVED IN CARCINOGENESIS

In healthy liver or pancreatic tissues, the cells stay where they are, adhering to each other in structures that characterize the tissue and assist in its function. In addition, cells are programmed to commit suicide peacefully when cellular machinery is damaged beyond repair, or when they are old or no longer needed. This death is called programmed cell death or apoptosis.

Within this community, cells are differentiated, each performing a special function necessary for the survival of the entire community of cells. In order to perform their unique functions effectively, cells must react to situations in their surrounding environment as well as communicate with each other. Communication takes place either indirectly, via exchange of messenger compounds such as hormones and growth factors, or directly, via cell-to-cell contact. With the help of proper communication, appropriate cells proliferate when new cells are needed, and when enough new cells have been produced, cell division stops.[5] However, some types of internal or even external stress causes a change in the genetic code of the cell, initiating the precancerous state. HCC or PC, like any other cancer, develops when there is a mutation to the cellular machinery that causes the cell to replicate at a higher rate and/or results in the cell avoiding apoptosis. This original cancer cell divides to generate a population of cancer cells. As they divide, they accumulate malignant characteristics, such as the tendency to invade and metastasize. Furthermore, they acquire other characteristics to assure survival, such as the capacity to evade the immune system, and to induce the growth of new blood vessels through the process called angiogenesis. From the above scenario, the seven clusters of procancer events classified by Boik can be applied here for either HCC or PC; these include the following[6]:

(1) Induction of genetic instability;
(2) Abnormal expression of genes;
(3) Abnormal signal transduction;
(4) Abnormal cell-to-cell communication;
(5) Induction of angiogenesis;
(6) Invasion and metastasis; and
(7) Immune evasion.

Induction of Genetic Instability

The majority of HCCs emerge in the background of a chronic liver disease caused by viral infection, alcohol intake, or exposure to chemical carcinogens such as aflatoxin B1 (AFB1).[7] Likewise, the consistent risk factor for PC is the chronic pancreatitis induced by alcohol abuse, cigarette smoking, or other diseases such as obesity and diabetes.[8] All these underlying pathogenic stimuli initiate a state of oxidative stress and free radical overproductions that subsequently induces a spectrum of genetic and epigenetic alterations in several cancer-related genes. These genes are basically grouped into two general categories: tumor suppressor genes (growth inhibitory) and proto-oncogenes (growth promoting). Like other solid tumors, it has been widely accepted that hepatic and pancreatic carcinogenesis are multi-step processes requiring the accumulation of genetic alterations which involve activation of proto-oncogenes and inactivation of tumor suppressor genes, leading to the uncontrolled proliferation of progeny cells. However, the incidence of genetic alterations is relatively rare and is limited to a subset of few cancer-specific genes, while epigenetic changes that involve aberrant methylation of genes occur far more frequently. Various lines of evidence have shown that the most commonly mutated genes in the majority of HCCs and PCs regardless of the etiologies are tumor suppressor genes (TSGs), *TP53* and *p16*; oncogenes, *c-MYC*, *cyclin D1*, and *K-ras* (the most common genetic abnormality in pancreatic cancer); and other cancer-associated genes, such as *CTNNB*1, a gene encoding adherens junctions necessary for the creation and maintenance of epithelial cell layers.[9,10]

The term epigenetic refers to all stable changes of phenotypic traits that are not coded in the DNA sequence itself, including DNA methylation, histone modification, and microRNA. Unlike classical mutations, these epigenetic changes are reversible. DNA methylation by DNA methyltransferase (DNMT) is a major epigenetic mechanism characterized primarily by the attachment of a methyl (CH_3) group to the cytosine base at CpG sites, usually enriched in the promoters of genes and therefore silenced. This is particularly true of some TSGs. Methylation of certain TSGs, such as the *SOCS-1*, *GADD45b*, *STAT1*, *APC*, and *TP53* genes, has reportedly been observed in HCC as well as in PC. On the contrary, global hypomethylation of DNA leads to alterations in the expression of proto-oncogenes that facilitate chromosomal instability and ultimately contributes to carcinogenesis.[11] Taken together, such widespread genomic alterations cause disruption of normal cellular signaling and finally lead to the acquisition of a malignant phenotype seen in HCC or PC. However, the origin of these genomic or epigenomic alterations remains a critical missing link. If such a link is established, clinical interventions with agents that target these early features would provide long-term protection against these cancers.

Recently, oxidative stress and generation of free radical have been recognized as potential culprit mechanisms contributing to the above-mentioned gene mutations.[12] This input has originated partly in studies showing that chromosomal abnormalities could be induced in cultured pancreatic ductal epithelium from normal organ donors by chronic exposure to dilute hydrogen peroxide.[13] These initial observations have been supported by studies demonstrating AB1, the most commonly occurring and potent of the aflatoxins, is associated with a specific AGG to AGT transversion mutation at codon 249 of the *p53* gene in human HCC through reactive oxygen species (ROS).[14] This concept was further reinforced by additional genetically studies that tracked genetic mutations through the human equivalent of about 5,000 years showing oxidative DNA damage is a primary cause of the process of mutation.[15] The primary finding of that study is that a predominant number of genetic mutations are linked to guanine, one of the four basic nucleotides known to be particularly sensitive to oxidative damage.[15] Following this further, it has been reported that epigenetic silencing of TSGs was mediated by ROS that stimulate DNA methyltransferase upregulation with increased expression and activity, and this silencing was reversed by treatment with antioxidants.[16] All of this seemingly overwhelming evidence has sculpted the concept of oxidative stress as underlying cause of genetic mutations associated with either HCC or PC development. Thus, clinical interventions with agents that target these early features of oxidative stress would provide long-term preventive benefits from genetic alterations responsible for HCC or PS occurrence.

The body maintains a variety of antioxidants as a multilevel defense against ROS and free-radical damage. These include the enzymes, such as superoxide dismutase, catalase, and glutathione peroxidase, and antioxidants synthesized in the body, such as glutathione. In human tissues of liver and pancreas, DNA damages occur frequently by cellular processes generating ROS and, typically, cells work to repair the vast majority of these damages by cellular antioxidant enzymes. However, because of the continual bombardment of DNA by free radicals, the body must replenish antioxidant supply through the diet containing antioxidants such as flavonoids, vitamins C and E, and beta-carotene. As such, several epidemiological studies support a protective role for dietary antioxidants by reporting that populations who consume inadequate amounts of fresh fruits and vegetables are at a higher risk for developing liver and pancreatic carcinoma.[3,4]

Fruit and vegetable components that mitigate HCC and PC genetic and epigenetic mutations

There are two ways for natural components in fruits and vegetables to reduce HCC/PC genetic mutations: directly by acting as ROS scavengers and indirectly by targeting the epigenetic modifiers. Only a few studies have so far investigated the direct causal relationship between dietary antioxidant and HCC or PC genetic mutations. Among these studies was one that demonstrated the suppression of β-catenin mutation in rat HCCs by auraptene (AUR), an antioxidant agent isolated from citrus fruit.[17] The paucity of data in this field due to most of antioxidant researches rely on end points of survival times and anticarcinogenic activity and do not look for preventive measures. Additionally, the incidence of HCC or PC genetic alterations is relatively rare when compared to epigenetic changes. Moreover, classical mutations and epigenetic changes are closely linked suggesting that by reducing abnormal methylation, mutations may also be reduced. Therefore, a more recent indirect approach involves targeting the epigenetic modifiers, DNA methyltransferase, has been proposed.

Recently, natural compounds, such as epigallocatechin gallate (EGCG, in green tea and pomegranates), have been shown to alter epigenetic mechanisms, in a way beyond their antioxidant properties.[17] EGCG induces apoptosis in human HCC HepG2 cells via upregulating miR-16 while inhibiting invasion of AsPC-1 human pancreatic adenocarcinoma cells through the modulation of histone deacetylase activity.[18,19]

Abnormal Expression of Genes

HCC or PC development and progression are caused by altered expression of thousands of cancer-related genes including genes involved in cell cycle regulation and apoptosis. The expression of these genes is controlled by several transcription factors whose abnormal activity and quantity in cancer cells. These abnormalities favor the production of proteins that allow cancer cells to proliferate, invade, and metastasize, as well as avoid apoptosis.[6] Therefore, HCC or PC can be inhibited by normalizing the activity and quantity of those transcription factors that control the expression of these genes. Although many transcription factors have been described as regulators of cancer-related gene expression, the most attention has focused on three that play a crucial role in HCC and PC genesis: the p53 protein, NF-κB (nuclear factor-kappa B), and AP-1 (activator protein-1).

p53 acts predominantly as a transcription factor, regulating the expression of more than 100 target genes initiating apoptosis, cell cycle arrest, DNA repair, cellular senescence, as well as differentiation. Deregulation of all these processes contributes to neoplastic transformation in p53-deficient hepatocytes or pancreatic cells.[20] Numerous approaches are being taken to reconstitute the expression of p53 in tumors and to use the function of the p53 pathway as an indicator of prognosis and response to therapy. The ability of p53 to induce cell cycle arrest depends on three critical target genes: p21, 14-3-3 sigma, and GADD45 (growth arrest and DNA damage-inducible protein 45). Moreover, p53 targets genes involved in the execution of apoptosis that can be divided in two classes. The first class is the components of extrinsic cell death signaling pathway triggered by death receptors (DRs), members of the tumor necrosis factor (TNF) receptor (R) superfamily, after receptor–ligand interaction. The TNF-R family members CD95/Fas/Apo-1, DR4, and DR5 (also known as TRAIL-R1 and R2) were all reported to be transcriptionally induced by p53.[21]

The second class of p53 target genes relevant to apoptosis induction under extreme stress and severe DNA damage, is the central components of the cell-intrinsic mitochondria-mediated cell death pathway. The intrinsic apoptotic pathway dominated by the Bcl-2 family proteins. The Bcl-2 family proteins are composed of three classes: antiapoptotic proteins Bcl-2 and Bcl-x_L, pro-apoptotic proteins Bax, Bak, and Bcl-x_L, and pro-apoptotic "BH3-only" proteins Bid (BH3-interacting death agonist), Bad, Noxa, and Puma. In the regulation of the intrinsic pathway, pro-apoptotic gene products such as Bax, Bid, Puma, and Noxa, localize to the mitochondria promoting the loss of mitochondrial membrane potential and the release of cytochrome c, resulting in the formation of the apoptosome complex with Apaf-1 and caspase 9.[22]

The p53 protein contains 10 different cysteine residues, and although disulfide bonds do not actually form between these cysteine residues, a similar type of bond does form, based on the insertion of zinc atoms between the sulfur atoms. These bonds, which help to maintain the active three-dimensional structure of the protein, are redox-sensitive and are altered by oxidants.[6] Indeed, Sun and Oberley have shown that free radicals reacted with cysteine and changed the structure of the p53 protein, making it inactive.[23] Moreover, Mdm2 has been identified as an important negative regulator of the p53 tumor suppressor. It functions both as an E3 ubiquitin ligase that recognizes the N-terminal trans-activation domain of the p53 and as an inhibitor of p53 transcriptional activation. It has been shown that some cases of HCC or PC show no p53 mutations, but have an overexpressed *MDM2* gene.[24] Consequently, it is believed that blocking the interaction of p53 with MDM2 is a potential effective strategy for of HCC or PC treatment.

Like the p53 protein, the NF-κB and AP-1 protein, which are redox-sensitive transcription factors, bind to several genes and are thus multi-functional. Constitutively activated NF-κB transcription factor has been associated with several aspects of HCC and PC tumorigenesis, including promoting cancer cell proliferation, preventing apoptosis, and increasing a tumor's angiogenic and metastatic potential. NF-κB controls cell proliferation by stimulating the transcription of genes that encode G1 cyclins.[25] This factor also activates the transcription of several genes that are known to block the induction of apoptosis including cellular inhibitors of apoptosis (cIAPs), caspase-8/FADD, and members of the Bcl2 family (such as Bcl-x_L).[26] Another important component of tumor growth is angiogenesis, a process that requires both migratory and invasive capabilities of vascular epithelial cells. Recently, NF-κB activation was found to stimulate angiogenesis, possibly by inducing expression of IL-8 and vascular endothelial growth factor (VEGF). In addition, NF-κB sites in pancreatic adenocarcinoma and HCC were identified in the promoters of genes that encode several matrix metalloproteinases (MMPs), proteolytic enzymes that promote tumor invasion of surrounding tissue.[27,28]

Activation of NF-κB is mediated through the production of ROS which is known to be increased in HCC milieu. NF-κB exists in the cytosol as a preformed trimeric complex, p50/p65 associated with an inhibitory protein known as IκB. Oxidants trigger a change in the cell that results in phosphorylation of the IκB subunit. After IκB is phosphorylated, a process of the proteolytic digestion of this subunit is activated. When the inhibitor subunit is dislodged from the p60/p65 heterodimer, the activator NF-κB can migrate to the nucleus and bind to DNA, thereby initiating transcription.[29]

Likewise, AP-1 is a transcription factor regulates the expression of several genes involved in human tumorigenesis in response to a variety of stimuli, including ROS. It composed of fos and jun proteins that in turn control a number of cellular processes including differentiation, proliferation, and apoptosis in PC and HCC.[30,31]

Collectively, HCCs and/or PCs gain a survival advantage by producing non-functional p53 proteins and by producing excessive amounts of NF-κB and AP-1.

Fruits and vegetable components that normalize abnormal gene expression in HCC and PC

There are two different situations to be considered when we discuss about the effects of fruit and vegetable components on the *p53* gene: when it is not mutated and when it is. Both situations can occur within the same tumor. In HCCs or PCs with normal *p53* genes, natural compounds can stimulate the expression of that gene, leading to apoptosis. This has been reported for melatonin, which is commonly found in fruits and vegetables including tomatoes, grape skins, tart cherries, and walnuts.[6,32]

In addition, natural compounds may also be useful in assuring that the p53 protein, once produced, is functional. Although there are few studies on this possibility, it is reasonable to expect that p53 functionality could be increased by using compounds that target MDM2, a well-characterized regulatory protein for the p53 (e.g., ginsenosides).[6,33]

On the other hand, natural compounds that inhibit NF-κB and AP-1 activity can be grouped into two groups: those act through antioxidant means and those act through non-antioxidant ones. Antioxidants as inhibitors of NF-κB and AP-1 in treating HCC or PC have been reported *in vitro* by a number of different natural components found in fruits and vegetables: EGCG, resveratrol, vitamin A.[34–36] The primary means by which non-antioxidant compounds inhibit NF-κB and AP-1 activity is by inhibiting the NF-κB upstream signaling pathway involving Ras and mitogen-activated protein kinases (MAPKs).[37]

Abnormal Signal Transduction

Current evidence indicates that during hepatocarcinogenesis, two main pathogenic mechanisms prevail: (1) cirrhosis associated with hepatic regeneration after tissue damage caused by hepatitis infection, and (2) mutations occurring in single or multiple oncogenes or TSGs. Both mechanisms have been linked with alterations in several important cellular signaling pathways caused by overexpression and/or dysregulation of growth factors, their receptors, or mutations in downstream signaling proteins that ultimately lead to modulation of transcription factor activities involved in cell proliferation and/or apoptosis (e.g., NF-κB).[38] A selection of the relevant signaling pathways altered in HCC and PC is briefly discussed here. These include the epidermal growth factor (EGF), insulin-like growth factor (IGF), hepatocyte growth factor/c-MET, RAS/RAF/MEK/ERK, phosphatidylinositol-3 kinase (PI3K)/Akt/mammalian target of rapamycin (mTOR), and WNT/β-catenin pathways.[38]

EGF signaling is one of the most thoroughly evaluated signaling cascades in human HCC as well as in PC.[39,40] EGF was ranked among the top upregulated genes used to identify HCC patients at high risk of developing a recurrence (*de novo* HCC) after surgical resection.[40]

Another pathway involved in proliferation control that is found abnormally activated in HCC and PC is the IGF system. The biological actions of the axis comprise a complex network of molecules whose main components are two high-affinity mitogenic ligands: IGF1 and IGF2. The type 1 IGF receptor (IGF1R) has tyrosine kinase activity, the type 2 IGF receptor (IGF2R) is involved in the internalization and degradation of IGF2, and at least six high-affinity IGF binding proteins (IGFBPs), which modulate the amount and bioactivity of locally available IGFs. Despite its role in normal physiology, the IGF axis is involved in the pathogenesis of several human malignancies, including those of the pancreas and liver.[41,42] In HCC, the most frequently described aberrant feature concerning this pathway is overexpression of IGF2 and aberrant activation of IGF1R in early stage HCC.[43,44]

Unlike the EGF and IGF signaling pathways, the interplay of HGF and its receptor, the MET tyrosine kinase, induces disruption of intercellular links and allows hepatocyte and pancreatic epithelium to migrate from their primary location to adjacent surroundings.[45,46] In HCC, several investigators had identified overexpression of MET (20–48%) when compared to surrounding non-tumoral tissue. The HGF/MET system is involved in reactivation of the invasive program during tumor progression and metastasis. Moreover, there is compelling evidence of anti-neoplasic activity (i.e., decreased proliferation, migration, and invasion) following MET downregulation in experimental models of HCC.[45]

The cellular receptors for aforementioned growth factors are protein tyrosine kinases (PTKs). Receptor PTKs consist of an extracellular receptor domain, a transmembrane domain, and an intracellular tyrosine kinase domain. Upon EGFR, IGFR, or MET activation, extracellular signals can be transduced through either the Akt or MAPK signaling pathways. Molecules belonging to both signaling cascades (e.g., Akt or KRAS) have been identified as *bona fide* oncogenes in human HCC and PC.[47] The RAS cascade transduces extracellular signals initiated by growth factor receptor activation that in turn activate RAF, MEK, ERK, and NF-κB, and result in proliferative and anti-apoptotic signals. However, Akt has been described as a predictor of tumor recurrence after surgical resection in a large cohort of Japanese HCC patients,[48] suggesting a possible implication in the invasive phenotype. mTOR complex 1 (MTORC1) is one of the most important molecules downstream Akt that plays a pivotal role in human HCC.[49] The anti-neoplasic properties of mTOR inhibitors (e.g., rapamycin and its analogs) in experimental models of HCC establish the proof-of-principle to conduct clinical trials evaluating mTOR inhibitors in human HCC.

Lastly, Wnt/β-catenin is a developmental pathway that is commonly known for its fundamental role in embryogenesis, which aids the cell in differentiation, proliferation, and apoptosis. However, the aberrant activation of this pathway is a major event in human HCC and PC that accelerates cell proliferation and promotes tumor formation. In the absence of Wnt signaling, cytoplasmic β-catenin complexes with the tumor suppressors: adenomatosis polyposis coli (APC) and Axin1, as well as the glycogen synthase kinase-3β (GSK-3β). In this complex, GSK-3β phosphorylates β-catenin, targeting it for ubiquitination and subsequent degradation. In the event that Wnt signaling receptors are engaged, conformational changes in the Axin complex cause the release of β-catenin, which then localizes to the nucleus and activates the transcription of *Myc*, *cyclin D1*, and *COX-2* amongst others several genes related to cell differentiation and proliferation.[50,51]

Fruits and vegetable components that normalize abnormal signal transduction in HCC and PC

The specific HCC and PC aberrancies in signaling pathways that are targeted by dietary fruits and vegetable components can be conceptualized as membrane-bound receptor kinases (HGF/c-Met, human EFGR, and IGFR pathways), and intracellular signaling kinases (RAS-MAPK, PI3k/Akt/mTOR, and Wnt/β-catenin pathways). These pathways are of interest from a therapeutic perspective as targeting them may help to reverse, delay, or prevent tumorigenesis. A number of natural compounds have been reported to normalize abnormal signal transduction *in vitro*, and some of these inhibit it in animals, the prospects of doing so in humans look hopeful.

Natural compounds that inhibit the over-activity receptor tyrosine kinases seen in HCC or PC include EGCG,[52] luteolin,[53] and genistein.[54] The movement of a signal from receptor tyrosine kinases toward the nucleus relies on several proteins (including RAS proteins and MAPK enzymes). Therefore, HCC or PC genesis can be inhibited by a signal transduction interference-based approach using natural compounds for this purpose. Given the way RAS proteins work, there are two conceivable ways their activity can be inhibited. The first is to inhibit the downstream signaling (MAPKs) that occurs after RAS activation, or to reduce production of the lipid tail necessary for the protein to function.[6] Quercetin has been reported to modulate MAPK pathways to induce cell death in human HCC cells.[55] Moreover, the EGCG inhibition of pancreatic cancer orthotopic tumor growth, angiogenesis, and metastasis was associated with inhibition of ERK pathway, a MAPK.[56] However, geraniol, an acyclic dietary monoterpene, was shown to inhibit the growth of HepG2 human HCC cells by decreasing 3-hydroxymethylglutaryl coenzyme A (HMG-CoA) reductase, the major rate-limiting enzyme in RAS lipid tail production.[57]

The other two possible pathways involved in passing a signal from outside the cell toward the nucleus are Akt and β-catenin, which are pivotal in promoting HCC or PC growth and survival. In HCC and PC, both quercetin and EGCG, respectively, mitigated survival and angiogenesis through inhibition of PI3K/Akt pathway.[58]

Abnormal Cell-to-Cell Communication

Efficient cell-to-cell communications are essential to coordinate the activity of the myriad of cells making up the liver and pancreas. At the same time, they are crucial to healthy cell turnover, which prevents aggressive cancer cells from taking over. These cell-to-cell communications are facilitated through the action of gap junction channels through which cells exchange ions and small molecules. Gap junctions are collections of transmembrane channels that communicate directly between contacting cells, and are regulated by E-cadherin, a calcium-dependent intercellular adhesion molecule. Each gap junction unit is composed of a hexamer of structural protein subunits called connexins. The major gap junction protein in human livers and pancreas is connexin 32 (Cx32).[59,60]

Additionally, a frequent characteristic of HCC and PC is the reduced or the absent expression of E-cadherin.[61,62] In parallel with E-cadherin lack of function, detachment from the basal lamina is often observed as a prerequisite to cell invasion. A major E-cadherin-binding protein, β-catenin, plays a critical role in Wnt signaling and in tumorigenesis. E-cadherin-binding sequesters β-catenin to the cell membrane, where β-catenin signaling is inhibited. Decreased E-cadherin expression in liver and tumor is associated with the cytoplasmic/nuclear redistribution of β-catenin, with decreased cell adhesion, increased cell growth and motility, and with poor prognosis.[63,64] All these findings support the notion that cell-to-cell communications are impaired in human HCC or PC.

Fruit and vegetable components that restore normal cell-to-cell communications in HCC and PC

Despite the complexities in cell-to-cell communications, many natural compounds help to restore normal communication in more than one way.

Improved activity of E-cadherin as well as improved gap junction communication are the most prominent effects of natural compounds in inhibiting HCC. Retinoic acid (RA) is a natural derivative of vitamin A that regulates important biological processes including cell proliferation and differentiation. *In vitro* studies have shown that RA is effective in inhibiting growth of HCC cells through inhibiting ERK and β-catenin signaling pathways together with increasing E-cadherin and Cx32 expression.[65] Similarly, EGCG inhibits invasion of AsPC-1 human pancreatic adenocarcinoma cells by increasing E-cadherin expression.[19]

Induction of Angiogenesis

Angiogenesis plays an important role in HCC and PC biology. Because tumor masses rapidly outgrow their available blood supply, their local environment becomes hypoxic and low in necessary nutrients. Thus, to survive, tumors must stimulate the formation of new blood vessels, angiogenesis, to supply the tumor with oxygen and nutrients and provides access to the circulation for metastasizing cells. As such, antiangiogenic therapies may severely limit tumor growth and metastasis. While HCC is a highly vascularized tumor, PC is not a grossly vascular tumor. However, angiogenesis in HCC, PC, and other solid tumors is based on the same fundamental principles of activation, proliferation, and migration of resting endothelial cells (ECs) in adjacent blood vessels.[66–68] The angiogenic cascade consists of genetic changes and local hypoxia in tumors leading to the release of angiogenic factors from cancerous cells, binding of angiogenic factors to receptors on ECs leading to their activation, loosening of interendothelial cell contacts, and degradation of the basement membrane by proteases secreted from activated ECs. The degradation of basement membrane allows the bud to grow as well as EC migration and proliferation. Adhesion molecules and integrins then help to pull the sprouting blood vessels forward and join their ends to form a new capillary vessel that finally organized into a network of blood vessels.[69]

However, blood vessels formed during HCC angiogenesis are incompletely covered by pericytes and often leaky due to the lack of a complete basement membrane around them. In addition, this new blood vessel formation is frequently inadequate to support the entire tumor, and regions of necrosis are frequently observed within solid tumors. As a consequence, despite the presence of the new blood vessels, many regions within a tumor remain hypoxic. Hypoxia in the center of growing tumors leads to intracellular stabilization of hypoxia-inducible factor (HIF)-1α, the key transcription factor in hypoxic tissues that induces the expression of several hypoxia response genes, such as VEGF. This process triggers the angiogenic switch characterized by high expression of endogenous proangiogenic factors and low expression of antiangiogenic factors in tumor cells, simultaneously. Angiogenic factors include VEGF; eicosanoids such as PGE2 that derive from omega-6 fatty acids; tumor necrosis factor (TNF); fibrin; basic fibroblast growth factor (bFGF); and histamine.[68,69]

The two signaling pathways, VEGF/KDR and angiopoietin/Tie2, were clarified to be activated in HCC tissues. VEGF is 50,000 times more active than histamine in enhancing vascular permeability. Increased vascular permeability is a very important requirement for angiogenesis and in fact may be its rate-limiting step.[6] Furthermore, VEGF, one of the strongest stimulatory angiogenic factors that is more expressed in endothelial cells within the tumor than in the non-tumoral hepatic parenchyma. The increased VEGF levels could be at least in part due to increased secretion of inflammatory mediators via the COX pathway in tumor tissues. Overexpression of COX-2 in neoplastic cells and tumor neovasculature has been described in HCC.[70] COX-2 catalyzes the conversion of arachidonic acid into prostaglandins and thromboxanes that promote cell survival as well as the release of angiogenic factors including NO and VEGF. The effects of VEGF are mediated mainly through two cell surface receptor tyrosine kinases: Flt-1 (or VEGFR-1) and KDR/Flk-1 (or VEGFR-2). In normal hepatic parenchyma, Flt-1 is expressed on endothelial cells within portal tracts and on macrophages while KDR/Flk-1 is expressed on sinusoidal endothelial cells. Both receptors, but especially KDR/Flk-1, are expressed on endothelial cells of HCC vessels.[68,71]

Besides VEGF, angiopoietins 1 and 2, which belong to the numerous factors involved in the angiogenic switch, have been specifically implicated in HCC. Angiopoietins 1 and 2 bind to the same tyrosine kinase receptor Tie2 on endothelial cells. Angiopoietin 1 stabilizes vessels by promoting the recruitment of pericytes and smooth muscle cells, whereas angiopoietin 2, which is a competitive antagonist of angiopoietin 1, reduces vascular stability at sites of remodeling. The expression of angiopoietin 2 is increased in HCC, particularly with high vascularity.[72]

While PC is not grossly vascular, it exhibits foci of micro-angiogenesis that overexpress the pro-angiogenic factor, VEGF together with VEGFR-2. This is evidence by the observation that high VEGFR-2 levels are associated with a worse prognosis in this disease.[73] Therefore, mechanisms that target VEGF and the various pathways that enhance the angiogenic process in PC may ultimately be of great therapeutic benefit in patients with unresectable disease as well as following surgery to prevent disease recurrence.

Furthermore, tumor expansion and building of private tumor vessels require the breakdown of the surrounding basal membrane and extracellular matrix (ECM). The loosening of this matrix requires the intervention of multiple enzymes like urokinase, tissue plaminogen activator (tPA), and MMPs. This loosening uncovers angiogenic factors embedded in the matrix. MMP-9 is considered to be a major component in the angiogenic switch by liberating matrix-sequestered VEGF.[74]

All these specific characteristics of tumor vessel have an impact on diagnostic and therapeutic strategies in tumors. For example, leakiness of tumor vessels leads to increased interstitial fluid pressure which compromises the delivery of drugs into tumor tissue or the diffusion of contrast agents for imaging.

Fruit and vegetable components that attenuate HCC and PC angiogenesis

Specific molecular and cellular targets have been identified for fruit and vegetable components in the context of tumor angiogenesis. These include angiogenic growth factor production and receptor activation. Kim *et al.*[75] showed that apigenin can decrease the releasing amounts of VEGF and MMP-8, which are closely relevant to angiogenic activity in HCC (HUH-7) cells. EGCG and other green tea derivatives have also been demonstrated to have antiangiogenic properties against both HCC as well as PC lines.[56,76] Zhang *et al.*[76] demonstrated that green tea extract and EGCG significantly inhibited HIF-1α and VEGF expression at both mRNA and protein levels. The mechanisms of green tea extract and EGCG inhibition of hypoxia-induced HIF-1α protein accumulation involve the blocking of both PI3K/Akt and

ERK1/2 signaling pathways and the enhancing of HIF-1α protein degradation through the proteasome system.[76]

Invasion and Metastasis

Invasion, the spread of cancer cells into adjacent tissues, along with metastasis, the spread of cells to distant sites, are two of the distinguishing traits of malignancy, representing potential obstacles in cancer therapy. They are interrelated processes in which cancer cells must invade the connective tissue surrounding blood vessels (the basement membrane) for metastasis to be successful.[6] These two processes remain a major cause of poor prognosis and death in cancer patients. Cell migration, cell adhesion, and proteolytic degradation of tissue barriers such as the ECM and basement membrane are the hallmarks of invasion and metastasis. The microenvironment of HCC or PC is composed of hepatic or pancreatic stellate cells, fibroblasts, invading inflammatory/immune cells (including regulatory and cytotoxic T cells and tumor-associated macrophages), endothelial cells (ECs), pericytes adjacent to the ECs, and extensive ECM components.[77,78] These components of the microenvironment interact with one another and with tumor cells directly or indirectly in order to acquire an abnormal phenotype that arises subsequently to genetic and epigenetic deregulation.

During the early stage of carcinogenesis, HCC or PC is predominantly well differentiated, and they proliferate slowly. However, HCC or PC becomes progressively dedifferentiated with tumor enlargement, and most advanced cases have high proliferation activity. During this stage, the tumors progress to give rise to intra-tissue metastasis as well as extra-tissue metastasis in which some hepatocytes or pancreatic cells undergo a fundamental change in morphology, adopting a mesenchymal architecture in a process called epithelial–mesenchymal transition (EMT), which is concomitant with the acquisition of a motile phenotype.[79,80] EMT is a key event in the tumor invasion process, whereby epithelial cell layers lose cell–cell contacts through upregulating N-cadherin and downregulation of E-cadherin, then undergo a dramatic remodeling of the cytoskeleton. Various factors in HCC or PC microenvironment are known to induce EMT including, inflammatory cytokines, HGF, HIF, and increased ROS in mitochondria induced by hypoxia. Due to the normal absence of membrane barriers to physically separate hepatocytes from the hepatic sinusoids permits easy entry of motile neoplastic hepatocytes into the vascular system by transmigration through ECM as a single cell. Hepatocyte migration is largely driven by F-actin restructuring in Rho/ROCK signaling-dependent manner. With F-actin constant state of flux, new monomers being added at the barbed or plus end and depolymerization at the pointed or minus end, allowing hepatocytes or pancreatic cells to migrate directionally.[81,82] Metastatic cells travel through the blood and lymphatic circulation systems then adhere to the wall of a blood vessel at the metastatic sites via intercellular adhesion molecule (ICAM; chiefly ICAM-1). Fibrin, a product of thrombin's enzymatic activity, helps tumor cells to aggregate with each other while migrating in the blood, thereby forming a larger clump that easily lodge in a capillary bed. Moreover, the excessive fibrin production surrounding tumor cells enhances their stickiness and facilitates their arrest at metastatic sites.[6] The arrested cells exit the blood vessel and, by invading through the basement membrane, penetrate, and re-express E-cadherin and other epithelial markers having a crucial role in epithelial cell–cell adhesion via a process that is referred to as mesenchymal-to-epithelial transition (MET), then attach to the target tissue's basal matrix. This allows the cancer cell to pull itself forward into the tissue. The attachment is mediated by cell-surface receptors known as integrins, which bind to components of the ECM. Integrins are crucial for cell invasion and migration, not only for physically tethering cells to the matrix, but also for sending and receiving molecular signals that regulate these processes.[83] Recently, the focal adhesion kinase (FAK) has been established as a key component of the signal transduction pathways triggered by integrins. FAK had been reported to be overexpressed in HCC and PC, and the expression of FAK in invasive or metastatic cells is significantly higher than that in non-invasive or non-metastatic cells.[84,85] Therefore, FAK seems to be an important pharmacologic target site.

HCC or PC invasion and metastasis also involve ECM-degrading proteinase activity to allow cell migration. The strength and structure of the ECM is provided by collagen fibers linked together by glycosaminoglycan (GAG) chains. To break free of the ECM, tumor cells produce enzymes that degrade these ECM components. These enzymes include glycosidases such as heparanase, which break apart GAG chains, and proteases such as MMPs, which break apart protein structures. Among MMPs, the type IV collagenases, such as MMP-2 and MMP-9, have been most strongly linked to HCC and pancreatic tumor-cell invasion.[86] One of the prime components of the intracellular signaling pathways responsible for MMP-2 and MMP-9 induction is transcription factor NF-κB. Apart from MMPs, cysteine proteases and serine proteases such as urokinase-type plasminogen activator (uPA) have also been involved in the invasion and metastasis of cancer cells by initiating pericellular proteolysis of the ECM and inducing cell migration.[87,88]

Fruits and vegetable components that minimizes HCC and PC invasion and metastasis

A wide variety of nutraceuticals derived from fruits and vegetables had been shown to inhibit HCC or PC spread by targeting one or more steps in the invasion or metastasis processes.

Butein, a polyphenolic compound obtained from cashews, was recently shown to inhibit migration and invasion of SK-HEP-1 human HCC cells, through the reversal of EMT.[89] The human HCC cell line SK-HEP-1 is invasive and expresses the gelatinase activity required for migration and invasion. Likewise, luteolin, isolated from olive fruit and leaves, inhibited HCC invasion via interfering with the HGF-mediated EMT in MAPK/ERKs and PI3K/Akt dependent pathways.[53]

S-allylcysteine (SAC), a water-soluble organosulfur compounds derived from *Allium* vegetables, restored the expression of E-cadherin in metastatic HCC cell line, MHCC97L cells, suggesting its anti-metastatic effect on HCC.[90] Similarly, EGCG inhibited EMT in PC by upregulating the expression of E-cadherin and inhibiting the expression of N-cadherin.[56] Berberine has been reported to suppress HCC tumor migration and invasion by impeding Rho/ROCK-dependent F-actin polymerization.[81] The recent study has identified EGCG, the major polyphenolic compound in green tea, as a potent inhibitor of the thrombin/proteinase-activated receptor (PAR1/PAR4) invasive signaling axis in HCC cells as a previously unrecognized mode of action for EGCG in cancer cells.[91] The other way to slow HCC or PC spread is to strengthen connective tissue by inhibiting

ECM degradation so that the ability of cancer cells to invade neighboring tissue is reduced. A number of natural compounds present in fruits and vegetables typically used to hinder cancer cells invasion to connective tissue by inhibiting the enzymes secreted from cancer cells to dissolve the extracellular matrix of connective tissue which normally blocks their migration. Caffeic acid, an active component of the propolis obtained from honeybee hives present in a variety of fruits, vegetables, and seasonings, predominantly in the form of ester conjugates, exerts anti-HCC metastatic potential through inhibition of MMP-2 and MMP-9 expression, possibly by targeting NF-κB.[92] At the same target, catechin gallate, a phenolic compound obtained from the red pine, inhibited the invasion and migration of SK-HEP-1 human HCC cells, which strongly correlated with reduced expression of MMP-2 and MMP-9.[93] Similarly, both vanillin, obtained from the cured pods (fruits) of the vanilla plant *Vanilla planifolia* (family: Orchidaceae), and emodin-containing vegetable powder (rhubarb, senna), have been shown as potent anti-invasive agents that suppress the MMP-9 enzymatic activity via NF-κB signaling pathway in HCC and PC, respectively.[94,95] Moreover, resveratrol exerts anti-invasive activity against HCC cells through downregulation of MMP-2, MMP-9, and upregulation of tissue inhibitor of metalloproteinases (TIMP-1 and TIMP-2).[96] MMP/TIMP imbalances in favor of MMPs were found to correlate with capsule invasion, metastatic dissemination, and poor outcome in HCC. Both [6]-shogaol and [6]-gingerol, two active compounds in ginger (*Zingiber officinale*), possess anti-invasive activity against highly metastatic HCC (Hep3B) cells via downregulation of (MMPs) as well as (uPA).[97]

Immune Evasion

Immune evasion is now recognized as a key feature in HCC and PC progression. Numerous mechanisms of tumor immune evasion have been described and they have collectively been linked to dysfunction of the host's immune system as well as to tumor-related factors. Dysfunction of the host's immune has been attributed to the existence of regulatory T cells (Tregs) that suppress immune responses, and to the systemic defects of dendritic cells derived from tumor patients, while tumor-related mechanisms have been attributed to the secretion of immunosuppressive mediators such as PGE2, transforming growth factor-beta (TGF-β), and

IL-10, and the resistance to apoptosis. Immunosuppressive cytokines inhibit effector T cell responses and promote the production of Tregs.

It was recently shown that the increased prevalence of Tregs has been induced in pancreatic adenocarcinoma *in vivo* and is dependent on TGF-β secretion by the tumor cells.[98] Moreover, tumor cells can convert immature dendritic cells into TGF-β-secreting cells, inducing Treg proliferation.[99] These findings support the concept that the tumor induces an increase of Tregs via TGF-β secretion, which results in an inhibition of the immune response against the tumor. Moreover, pancreatic tumor cells have adopted inhibitory mechanisms, the TGF-β2 and TGF-β type I receptor/ALK5-dependent auto-induction of forkhead transcription factor (Foxp3), which enables the tumor cells *in vitro* to suppress effector T cells via direct inhibition of their proliferation rather than indirectly through Treg.[100]

In HCC, tumor immune evasion has been associated with IL-10-mediated suppression of circulating dendritic cell subsets in HCC patients.[101] In addition, HCC immune evasion has been associated with acquiring apoptosis resistance either by downregulation of pro-apoptotic molecules or by decrease the expression of the death receptor, CD95.[102,103]

Fruit and vegetable components that target HCC and PC immune evasion

Vegetable sugars obtained from Radix Glycyrrhizae polysaccharide has been shown to downregulate the population of Treg cells and decrease lymph node Foxp3 and IL-10 mRNA expression in H22 hepatocarcinoma bearing mice. In addition, GP treatment decreased IL-10 and TGF-β levels in serum of H22 tumor-bearing mice.[104] Moreover, protein-bound polysaccharide (PSK) from pumpkin fruits suppressed the metastasis of line-10 hepatocarcinoma in the lung by activating the neutrophils.[105] In another study, in which intraperitoneal resveratrol significantly reduced the growth of implanted HCC, it was found to have enhanced host's immune response by promoting the cytotoxicity of peritoneal macrophages against HCC cells.[106]

Additionally, pancreatic cancer gemcitabine (GEM) chemoresistance has been demonstrated to be associated with enhanced NF-κB activation and anti-apoptotic protein synthesis. Treatment with omega-3-containing fruits such as kiwifruit is specifically associated with inhibition of proliferation in these pancreatic cell lines irrespective of varied chemoresistance resistance.[107]

CONCLUSION

In hepatic and pancreatic carcinogenesis, multiple signaling transduction pathways important for cell proliferation and differentiations are deregulated. Advancement in molecular biology has increased our understanding of these anomalies and identified a large number of molecular targets, against which a large number of anticancer agents had been evaluated. Despite advancement in anticancer therapeutics, treatment options remain limited and prognosis poor for patients with these malignancies. As such, the molecularly targeted agents held significant promise in liver or pancreas cancers for many reasons, including the better-tolerated toxicity profiles and they target known molecular aberrancies. Ideally, any potential agent should have minimal side effects, be nontoxic to non-malignant cells, acceptable to patients, inexpensive, and sufficiently bioavailable. During the past decade, nutraceuticals have drawn considerable attention because they are efficient, safe, economic, and readily available, and have multi-targeted potential. Cohort studies from Taiwan and Japan observed a significant inverse association between vegetable and fruits consumption and risk of HCC.[3] Based on available evidence, the World Cancer Research Fund (WCRF) concluded that there was limited suggestive evidence for the protective effect of fruit against liver cancer and limited non-conclusive evidence for vegetables.[108] Similarly, many case control studies have suggested that higher consumption of fruit and vegetables is associated with a lower risk of pancreatic cancer, whereas cohort studies do not support such an association.[109] Reasons for these discrepancies are likely multi-factorial, including the wrong target, problems in delivery, the existence of resistance or redundant molecular pathways, and failure to identify the susceptible molecular phenotype. Moreover, many of these cellular pathways overlap, showing a high degree of redundancy within the system. Therefore, targeting a single molecule might ultimately have little or no effect, resulting in the need for either combination therapy or multi-targeted therapy.[87] In this review, we have focused primarily on the classes of targets and corresponding active components present in fruits and vegetables that may have potential impact on the life of hepatic or pancreatic cancer patients in the near future (Table 7.1). As this review has shown, the future of nutraceuticals as a cancer-fighting weapon seems promising as proposed in Fig. 7.1.

Table 7.1: Molecular targets of fruit and vegetable components in HCC/PC prevention.

No	Major active constituents	Fruit/vegetable	Proposed mechanism(s)	Cancer type(s)
1	Allicin	*Allium sativum* (Garlic)	(2)	HCC/PC
2	Allyl isothiocyanate	Mustard, horseradish	(6)	HCC
3	Apigenin	Parsley and celery	(5)	HCC
4	Auraptene (AUR)	Citrus fruits	(1)	HCC
5	Berberine	Berberis (e.g., Oregon grape, barberry, and tree turmeric), *Hydrastis canadensis* (Amur cork tree), and *Tinospora cordifolia*	(6)	HCC
6	Butein	Found in *Toxicodendron vernicifluum* (or formerly *Rhus verniciflua*)	(6)	HCC
7	Caffeic acid	Abundant in all plants (key intermediate in the biosynthesis)	(5), (6)	HCC
8	Catechin gallate	Green tea, buckwheat, and in grape	(6)	HCC
9	Epigallocatechin gallate (EGCG)	Green tea and *Punica pomegranata* (pomegranate)	(1)–(6)	HCC/PC
10	Evodiamine	Fruits of Wuzhuyu	(2)	HCC
11	Genistein	Lupin, fava beans, soybeans, kudzu, and psoralea	(3), (5)–(7)	HCC
12	Geraniol	Rose oil, palmarosa oil, and citronella oil	(3)	HCC
13	[6]-gingerol	*Zingiber officinale* (fresh ginger)	(5), (6)	HCC
14	Ginsenosides	Ginseng species	(2)	HCC/PC

(*Continued*)

Table 7.1: (*Continued*)

No	Major active constituents	Fruit/vegetable	Proposed mechanism(s)	Cancer type(s)
15	Luteolin	Celery, green pepper, thyme, chamomile, carrots, olive oil, peppermint, rosemary, navel oranges, and oregano	(3), (6)	HCC
16	Lycopene	Tomatoes, red carrots, red bell peppers, watermelons, and papayas	(6)	HCC
17	Melatonin	Tomatoes, banana, grape skins, tart cherries, and walnuts	(2)	HCC/PC
18	Omega-3 fatty acids	Kiwi fruit, fish oils, algal oil, squid oil, and plant oils such as echium oil and flaxseed oil	(7)	HCC/PC
19	Phytoalexin	Grape skin and leaf	(3)	HCC
20	PSK(krestin) (*polysaccharide*-Kureha)	Mushroom trametes versicolor, pumpkin fruits	(7)	HCC/PC
21	Quercetin	Black and green tea, onion, red grapes, citrus fruit, tomato, broccoli and other leafy green vegetables	(2), (3), (5)	HCC/PC
22	RA Carotenoids (converted to Vit. A)	Many dark-green or dark-yellow plants (including the famous carrot)	(2), (4)	HCC/PC
23	Resveratrol	Red grapes	(2), (3), (5)–(7)	HCC/PC
24	S-allylcysteine (SAC)	*Allium sativum* (garlic)	(6)	HCC
25	[6]-shogaol	*Zingiber officinale* (ginger)	(6)	HCC
26	Vanillin	Pods of *Vanilla planifola*, a vining orchid native to Mexico	(6)	HCC

Notes: (1) Induction of genetic instability; (2) Abnormal expression of genes; (3) Abnormal signal transduction; (4) Abnormal cell-to-cell communication; (5) Induction of angiogenesis; (6) Invasion and metastasis; and (7) Immune evasion.

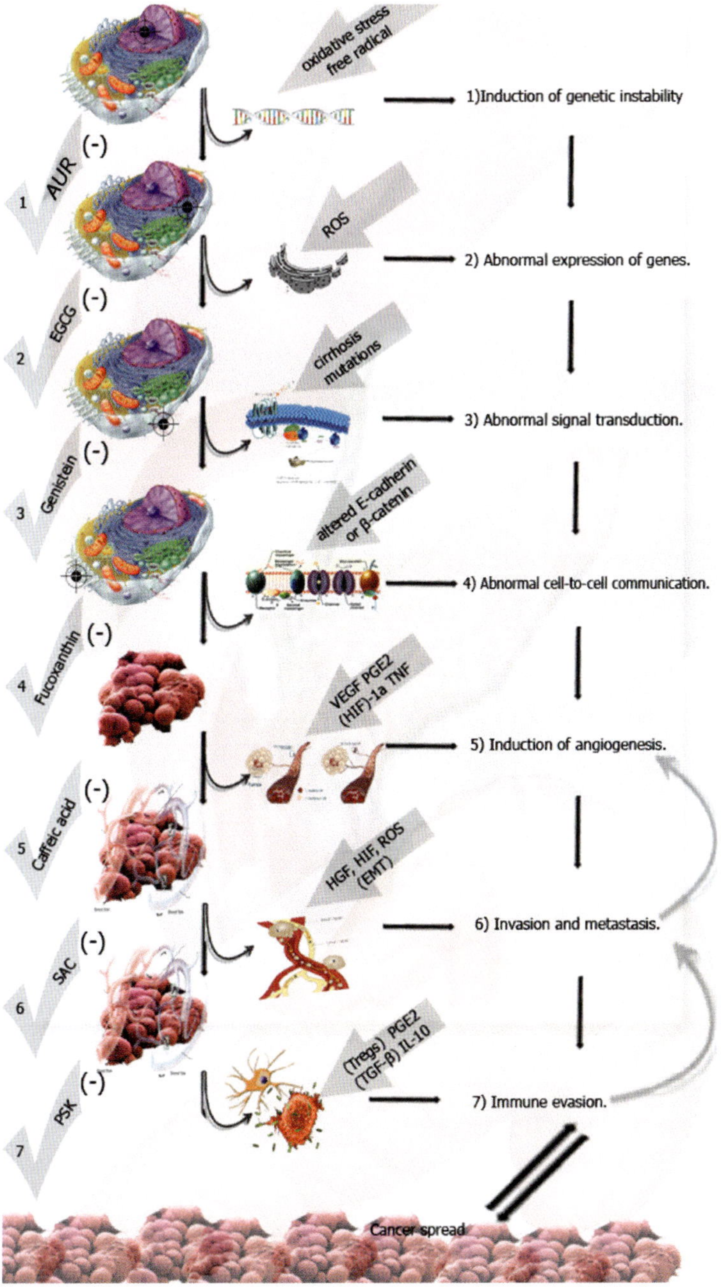

Figure 7.1: Seven clusters of procancer events occuring in hepatocellular carcinoma (HCC) or pancreatic carcinoma (PC) and proposed anticancer mechanisms of fruits and vegetables.

Some nutraceuticals have already progressed from the bench to the bedside either alone or in combination with existing therapy. Problems regarding validation of biomarkers, agent delivery, side effects, and patient selection are barriers that need to be overcome to determine the likely effectiveness of such agents in clinical practice.

ACKNOWLEDGMENTS

We apologize to authors whose works are not cited here due to space limitations. This work was financially supported by the PI of the liver research lab, Prof. Farid A. Badria, Faculty of Pharmacy, Mansoura University, Mansoura 35166, Egypt.

REFERENCES

1. Jemal, A., F. Bray, M.M. Center, J. Ferlay, E. Ward, and D. Forman, Global cancer statistics, *CA Cancer J Clin* **61**(2): 69–90 (2011).
2. Vainio, H. and E. Weiderpass, Fruit and vegetables in cancer prevention, *Nutr Cancer* **54**(1): 111–142 (2006).
3. Kurahashi, N., M. Inoue, M. Iwasaki, Y. Tanaka, M. Mizokami, and S. Tsugane, Vegetable, fruit and antioxidant nutrient consumption and subsequent risk of hepatocellular carcinoma: A prospective cohort study in Japan, *Br J Cancer* **100**(1): 181–184 (2009).
4. Chan, J.M., F. Wang, and E.A. Holly, Vegetable and fruit intake and pancreatic cancer in a population-based case-control study in the San Francisco bay area, *Cancer Epidemiol Biomarkers Prev* **14**(9): 2093–2097 (2005).
5. Guthrie, M., When a cell goes bad — how cancer starts, www.cancure.org/Cancer_cells.html.
6. Boik, J., *Natural Compound in Cancer Therapy*, Princeton: MN, Oregon Medical Press, 2001.
7. Forner, A., J.M. Llovet, and J. Bruix, Hepatocellular carcinoma, *Lancet* **379**(9822): 1245–1255 (2012).
8. Whitcomb, D.C., Inflammation and Cancer V. Chronic pancreatitis and pancreatic cancer, *Am J Physiol Gastrointest Liver Physiol* **287**(2): G315–G319 (2004).
9. Teufel, A., F. Staib, S. Kanzler, A. Weinmann, H. Schulze-Bergkamen, and P.R. Galle, Genetics of hepatocellular carcinoma, *World J Gastroenterol* **13**(16): 2271–2282 (2007).

10. Greer, J.B., D.C. Whitcomb, and R.E. Brand, Genetic predisposition to pancreatic cancer: A brief review, *Am J Gastroenterol* **102**(11): 2564–2569 (2007).
11. Kuroki, T., Y. Tajima, and T. Kanematsu, Role of hypermethylation on carcinogenesis in the pancreas, *Surg Today* **34**(12): 981–986 (2004).
12. Georgakilas, A.G., Oxidative stress, DNA damage and repair in carcinogenesis: Have we established a connection?, *Cancer Lett* **327**(1–2): 3–4 (2012).
13. Moskovitz, A.H., N.J. Linford, T.A. Brentnall, M.P. Bronner, B.E. Storer, J.D. Potter, R.H. Bell Jr, and P.S. Rabinovitch, Chromosomal instability in pancreatic ductal cells from patients with chronic pancreatitis and pancreatic adenocarcinoma, *Genes Chromosomes Cancer* **37**(2): 201–206 (2003).
14. Wild, C.P. and R. Montesano, A model of interaction: Aflatoxins and hepatitis viruses in liver cancer aetiology and prevention, *Cancer Lett* **286**(1): 22–28 (2009).
15. Denver, D.R., P.C. Dolan, L.J. Wilhelm, W. Sung, J.I. Lucas-Lledo, D.K. Howe, S.C. Lewis, K. Okamoto, W.K. Thomas, M. Lynch, and C.F. Baer, A genome-wide view of *Caenorhabditis elegans* base-substitution mutation processes, *Proc Natl Acad Sci USA* **106**(38): 16310–16314 (2009).
16. Lim, S.O., J.M. Gu, M.S. Kim, H.S. Kim, Y.N. Park, C.K. Park, J.W. Cho, Y.M. Park, and G. Jung, Epigenetic changes induced by reactive oxygen species in hepatocellular carcinoma: Methylation of the E-cadherin promoter, *Gastroenterology* **135**(6): 2128–2140 (2008).
17. Hara, A., K. Sakata, Y. Yamada, T. Kuno, N. Kitaori, T. Oyama, Y. Hirose, A. Murakami, T. Tanaka, and H. Mori, Suppression of beta-catenin mutation by dietary exposure of auraptene, a citrus antioxidant, in N,N-diethylnitrosamine-induced hepatocellular carcinomas in rats, *Oncol Rep* **14**(2): 345–351 (2005).
18. Tsang, W.P. and T.T. Kwok, Epigallocatechin gallate up-regulation of miR-16 and induction of apoptosis in human cancer cells, *J Nutr Biochem* **21**(2): 140–146 (2010).
19. Kim, S.O. and M.R. Kim, (−)-Epigallocatechin 3-gallate inhibits invasion by inducing the expression of Raf kinase inhibitor protein in AsPC1 human pancreatic adenocarcinoma cells through the modulation of histone deacetylase activity, *Int J Oncol* **42**(1): 349–358 (2013).
20. Bellamy, C.O., A.R. Clarke, A.H. Wyllie, and D.J. Harrison, p53 deficiency in liver reduces local control of survival and proliferation, but does not affect apoptosis after DNA damage, *FASEB J* **11**(7): 591–599 (1997).
21. Michalak, E., A. Villunger, M. Erlacher, and A. Strasser, Death squads enlisted by the tumour suppressor p53, *Biochem Biophys Res Commun* **331**(3): 786–798 (2005).

22. Jendrossek, V., The intrinsic apoptosis pathways as a target in anticancer therapy, *Curr Pharm Biotechnol* **13**(8): 1426–1438 (2012).
23. Sun, Y. and L.W. Oberley, Redox regulation of transcriptional activators, *Free Radic Biol Med* **21**(3): 335–348 (1996).
24. Qiu, S.J., S.L. Ye, Z.Q. Wu, Z.Y. Tang, and Y.K. Liu, The expression of the *mdm2* gene may be related to the aberration of the *p53* gene in human hepatocellular carcinoma, *J Cancer Res Clin Oncol* **124**(5): 253–258 (1998).
25. Cao, Y., G. Bonizzi, T.N. Seagroves, F.R. Greten, R. Johnson, E.V. Schmidt, and M. Karin, IKKalpha provides an essential link between RANK signaling and cyclin D1 expression during mammary gland development, *Cell* **107**(6): 763–775 (2001).
26. Karin, M. and A. Lin, NF-kappaB at the crossroads of life and death, *Nat Immunol* **3**(3): 221–227 (2002).
27. Karin, M., Y. Cao, F.R. Greten, and Z.W. Li, NF-κB in cancer: From innocent bystander to major culprit, *Nat Rev Cancer* **2**(4): 301–310 (2002).
28. Huang, S., J.B. Robinson, A. Deguzman, C.D. Bucana, and I.J. Fidler, Blockade of nuclear factor-kappaB signaling inhibits angiogenesis and tumorigenicity of human ovarian cancer cells by suppressing expression of vascular endothelial growth factor and interleukin 8, *Cancer Res* **60**(19): 5334–5339 (2000).
29. Gloire, G., S. Legrand-Poels, and J. Piette, NF-kappaB activation by reactive oxygen species: Fifteen years later, *Biochem Pharmacol* **72**(11): 1493–1505 (2006).
30. Shin, S., T. Asano, Y. Yao, R. Zhang, F.X. Claret, M. Korc, K. Sabapathy, D.G. Menter, J.L. Abbruzzese, and S.A. Reddy, Activator protein-1 has an essential role in pancreatic cancer cells and is regulated by a novel Akt-mediated mechanism, *Mol Cancer Res* **7**(5): 745–754 (2009).
31. Guo, L.L., S. Xiao, and Y. Guo, Activation of transcription factors NF-kappaB and AP-1 and their relations with apoptosis associated-proteins in hepatocellular carcinoma, *World J Gastroenterol* **11**(25): 3860–3865 (2005).
32. Martin-Renedo, J., J.L. Mauriz, F. Jorquera, O. Ruiz-Andres, P. Gonzalez, and J. Gonzalez-Gallego, Melatonin induces cell cycle arrest and apoptosis in hepatocarcinoma HepG2 cell line, *J Pineal Res* **45**(4): 532–540 (2008).
33. Wang, W., E.R. Rayburn, Y. Zhao, H. Wang, and R. Zhang, Novel ginsenosides 25-OH-PPD and 25-OCH3-PPD as experimental therapy for pancreatic cancer: Anticancer activity and mechanisms of action, *Cancer Lett* **278**(2): 241–248 (2009).
34. Nishikawa, T., T. Nakajima, M. Moriguchi, M. Jo, S. Sekoguchi, M. Ishii, H. Takashima, T. Katagishi, H. Kimura, M. Minami, Y. Itoh, K. Kagawa, and T. Okanoue, A green tea polyphenol, epigalocatechin-3-gallate, induces apoptosis

of human hepatocellular carcinoma, possibly through inhibition of Bcl-2 family proteins, *J Hepatol* **44**(6): 1074–1082 (2006).
35. Yu, H.B., H.F. Zhang, X. Zhang, D.Y. Li, H.Z. Xue, C.E. Pan, and S.H. Zhao, Resveratrol inhibits VEGF expression of human hepatocellular carcinoma cells through a NF-kappa B-mediated mechanism, *Hepatogastroenterology* **57**(102–103): 1241–1246 (2010).
36. Yan, T.D., H. Wu, H.P. Zhang, N. Lu, P. Ye, F.H. Yu, H. Zhou, W.G. Li, X. Cao, Y.Y. Lin, J.Y. He, W.W. Gao, Y. Zhao, L. Xie, J.B. Chen, X.K. Zhang, and J.Z. Zeng, Oncogenic potential of retinoic acid receptor-gamma in hepatocellular carcinoma, *Cancer Res* **70**(6): 2285–2295 (2010).
37. Wang, W., J.L. Abbruzzese, D.B. Evans, L. Larry, K.R. Cleary, and P.J. Chiao, The nuclear factor-kappa B RelA transcription factor is constitutively activated in human pancreatic adenocarcinoma cells, *Clin Cancer Res* **5**(1): 119–127 (1999).
38. Whittaker, S., R. Marais, and A.X. Zhu, The role of signaling pathways in the development and treatment of hepatocellular carcinoma, *Oncogene* **29**(36): 4989–5005 (2010).
39. Hoshida, Y., A. Villanueva, M. Kobayashi, J. Peix, D.Y. Chiang, A. Camargo, S. Gupta, J. Moore, M.J. Wrobel, J. Lerner, M. Reich, J.A. Chan, J.N. Glickman, K. Ikeda, M. Hashimoto, G. Watanabe, M.G. Daidone, S. Roayaie, M. Schwartz, S. Thung, H.B. Salvesen, S. Gabriel, V. Mazzaferro, J. Bruix, S.L. Friedman, H. Kumada, J.M. Llovet, and T.R. Golub, Gene expression in fixed tissues and outcome in hepatocellular carcinoma, *N Engl J Med* **359**(19): 1995–2004 (2008).
40. Papageorgio, C. and M.C. Perry, Epidermal growth factor receptor-targeted therapy for pancreatic cancer, *Cancer Invest* **25**(7): 647–657 (2007).
41. Sachdev, D. and D. Yee, Disrupting insulin-like growth factor signaling as a potential cancer therapy, *Mol Cancer Ther* **6**(1): 1–12 (2007).
42. Tomizawa, M., F. Shinozaki, T. Sugiyama, S. Yamamoto, M. Sueishi, and T. Yoshida, Insulin-like growth factor-I receptor in proliferation and motility of pancreatic cancer, *World J Gastroenterol* **16**(15): 1854–1858 (2010).
43. Breuhahn, K., T. Longerich, and P. Schirmacher, Dysregulation of growth factor signaling in human hepatocellular carcinoma, *Oncogene* **25**(27): 3787–3800 (2006).
44. Tovar, V., C. Alsinet, A. Villanueva, Y. Hoshida, D.Y. Chiang, M. Sole, S. Thung, S. Moyano, S. Toffanin, B. Minguez, L. Cabellos, J. Peix, M. Schwartz, V. Mazzaferro, J. Bruix, and J.M. Llovet, IGF activation in a molecular subclass of hepatocellular carcinoma and pre-clinical efficacy of IGF-1R blockage, *J Hepatol* **52**(4): 550–559 (2010).

45. Takayama, H., W.J. LaRochelle, R. Sharp, T. Otsuka, P. Kriebel, M. Anver, S.A. Aaronson, and G. Merlino, Diverse tumorigenesis associated with aberrant development in mice overexpressing hepatocyte growth factor/scatter factor, *Proc Natl Acad Sci USA* **94**(2): 701–706 (1997).
46. Zender, L., A. Villanueva, V. Tovar, D. Sia, D.Y. Chiang, and J.M. Llovet, Cancer gene discovery in hepatocellular carcinoma, *J Hepatol* **52**(6): 921–929 (2010).
47. Furukawa, T., W.P. Duguid, M. Kobari, S. Matsuno, and M.S. Tsao, Hepatocyte growth factor and Met receptor expression in human pancreatic carcinogenesis, *Am J Pathol* **147**(4): 889–895 (1995).
48. Nakanishi, K., M. Sakamoto, S. Yamasaki, S. Todo, and S. Hirohashi, Akt phosphorylation is a risk factor for early disease recurrence and poor prognosis in hepatocellular carcinoma, *Cancer* **103**(2): 307–312 (2005).
49. Villanueva, A., D.Y. Chiang, P. Newell, J. Peix, S. Thung, C. Alsinet, V. Tovar, S. Roayaie, B. Minguez, M. Sole, C. Battiston, S. Van Laarhoven, M.I. Fiel, A. Di Feo, Y. Hoshida, S. Yea, S. Toffanin, A. Ramos, J.A. Martignetti, V. Mazzaferro, J. Bruix, S. Waxman, M. Schwartz, M. Meyerson, S.L. Friedman, and J.M. Llovet, Pivotal role of mTOR signaling in hepatocellular carcinoma, *Gastroenterology* **135**(6): 1972–1983 (2008).
50. Clevers, H., Wnt/beta-catenin signaling in development and disease, *Cell* **127**:469–480, 2006.
51. Kumar, M., X. Zhao, and X.W. Wang, Molecular carcinogenesis of hepatocellular carcinoma and intrahepatic cholangiocarcinoma: One step closer to personalized medicine?, *Cell Biosci* **1**(1): 5 (2011).
52. Shimizu, M., Y. Shirakami, H. Sakai, H. Tatebe, T. Nakagawa, Y. Hara, I.B. Weinstein, and H. Moriwaki, EGCG inhibits activation of the insulin-like growth factor (IGF)/IGF-1 receptor axis in human hepatocellular carcinoma cells, *Cancer Lett* **262**(1): 10–18 (2008).
53. Lee, W.J., L.F. Wu, W.K. Chen, C.J. Wang, and T.H. Tseng, Inhibitory effect of luteolin on hepatocyte growth factor/scatter factor-induced HepG2 cell invasion involving both MAPK/ERKs and PI3K-Akt pathways, *Chem Biol Interact* **160**(2): 123–133 (2006).
54. Wu, B.W., Y. Wu, J.L. Wang, J.S. Lin, S.Y. Yuan, A. Li, and W.R. Cui, Study on the mechanism of epidermal growth factor-induced proliferation of hepatoma cells, *World J Gastroenterol* **9**(2): 271–275 (2003).
55. Granado-Serrano, A.B., M.A. Martin, L. Bravo, L. Goya, and S. Ramos, Quercetin modulates NF-kappa B and AP-1/JNK pathways to induce cell death in human hepatoma cells, *Nutr Cancer* **62**(3): 390–401 (2010).

56. Shankar, S., L. Marsh, and R.K. Srivastava, EGCG inhibits growth of human pancreatic tumors orthotopically implanted in Balb C nude mice through modulation of FKHRL1/FOXO3a and neuropilin, *Mol Cell Biochem* **372**(1–2): 83–94 (2013).
57. Polo, M.P. and M.G. de Bravo, Effect of geraniol on fatty-acid and mevalonate metabolism in the human hepatoma cell line Hep G2, *Biochem Cell Biol* **84**(1): 102–111 (2006).
58. Granado-Serrano, A.B., M.A. Martin, L. Bravo, L. Goya, and S. Ramos, Quercetin induces apoptosis via caspase activation, regulation of Bcl-2, and inhibition of PI-3-kinase/Akt and ERK pathways in a human hepatoma cell line (HepG2), *J Nutr* **136**(11): 2715–2721 (2006).
59. Nicholson, B., R. Dermietzel, D. Teplow, O. Traub, K. Willecke, and J.P. Revel, Two homologous protein components of hepatic gap junctions, *Nature* **329**(6141): 732–734 (1987).
60. Meda, P., M.S. Pepper, O. Traub, K. Willecke, D. Gros, E. Beyer, B. Nicholson, D. Paul, and L. Orci, Differential expression of gap junction connexins in endocrine and exocrine glands, *Endocrinology* **133**(5): 2371–2378 (1993).
61. Wei, Y., J.T. Van Nhieu, S. Prigent, P. Srivatanakul, P. Tiollais, and M.A. Buendia, Altered expression of E-cadherin in hepatocellular carcinoma: Correlations with genetic alterations, beta-catenin expression, and clinical features, *Hepatology* **36**(3): 692–701 (2002).
62. Winter, J.M., A.H. Ting, F. Vilardell, E. Gallmeier, S.B. Baylin, R.H. Hruban, S.E. Kern, and C.A. Iacobuzio-Donahue, Absence of E-cadherin expression distinguishes noncohesive from cohesive pancreatic cancer, *Clin Cancer Res* **14**(2): 412–418 (2008).
63. Liu, J., Z. Lian, S. Han, M.M. Waye, H. Wang, M.C. Wu, K. Wu, J. Ding, P. Arbuthnot, M. Kew, D. Fan, and M.A. Feitelson, Downregulation of E-cadherin by hepatitis B virus X antigen in hepatocellullar carcinoma, *Oncogene* **25**(7): 1008–1017 (2006).
64. Prange, W., K. Breuhahn, F. Fischer, C. Zilkens, T. Pietsch, K. Petmecky, R. Eilers, H.P. Dienes, and P. Schirmacher, Beta-catenin accumulation in the progression of human hepatocarcinogenesis correlates with loss of E-cadherin and accumulation of p53, but not with expression of conventional WNT-1 target genes, *J Pathol* **201**(2): 250–259 (2003).
65. Ionta, M., M.C. Rosa, R.B. Almeida, V.M. Freitas, P. Rezende-Teixeira, and G.M. Machado-Santelli, Retinoic acid and cAMP inhibit rat hepatocellular carcinoma cell proliferation and enhance cell differentiation, *Braz J Med Biol Res* **45**(8): 721–729 (2012).

66. Semela, D. and J.F. Dufour, Angiogenesis and hepatocellular carcinoma, *J Hepatol* **41**(5): 864–880 (2004).
67. Itakura, J., T. Ishiwata, H. Friess, H. Fujii, Y. Matsumoto, M.W. Buchler, and M. Korc, Enhanced expression of vascular endothelial growth factor in human pancreatic cancer correlates with local disease progression, *Clin Cancer Res* **3**(8): 1309–1316 (1997).
68. Coultas, L., K. Chawengsaksophak. and J. Rossant, Endothelial cells and VEGF in vascular development, *Nature* **438**(7070): 937–945 (2005).
69. Bae, S.H., E.S. Jung, Y.M. Park, B.S. Kim, B.K. Kim, D.G. Kim, and W.S. Ryu, Expression of cyclooxygenase-2 (COX-2) in hepatocellular carcinoma and growth inhibition of hepatoma cell lines by a COX-2 inhibitor, NS-398, *Clin Cancer Res* **7**(5): 1410–1418 (2001).
70. Semela, D. and J.F. Dufour, Angiogenesis and hepatocellular carcinoma, *J Hepatol* **41**(5): 864–880 (2004).
71. Yamaguchi, R., H. Yano, Y. Nakashima, S. Ogasawara, K. Higaki, J. Akiba, D.J. Hicklin, and M. Kojiro, Expression and localization of vascular endothelial growth factor receptors in human hepatocellular carcinoma and non-HCC tissues, *Oncol Rep* **7**(4): 725–729 (2000).
72. Torimura, T., T. Ueno, M. Kin, R. Harada, E. Taniguchi, T. Nakamura, R. Sakata, O. Hashimoto, M. Sakamoto, R. Kumashiro, M. Sata, O. Nakashima, H. Yano, and M. Kojiro, Overexpression of angiopoietin-1 and angiopoietin-2 in hepatocellular carcinoma, *J Hepatol* **40**(5): 799–807 (2004).
73. Buchler, P., H.A. Reber, M.W. Buchler, H. Friess, and O.J. Hines, VEGF-RII influences the prognosis of pancreatic cancer, *Ann Surg* **236**(6): 738–749 (2002).
74. Egeblad, M. and Z. Werb, New functions for the matrix metalloproteinases in cancer progression, *Nat Rev Cancer* **2**(3): 161–174 (2002).
75. Kim, B.R., Y.K. Jeon, and M.J. Nam, A mechanism of apigenin-induced apoptosis is potentially related to anti-angiogenesis and anti-migration in human hepatocellular carcinoma cells, *Food Chem Toxicol* **49**(7): 1626–1632 (2011).
76. Zhang, Q., X. Tang, Q. Lu, Z. Zhang, J. Rao, and A.D. Le, Green tea extract and (−)-epigallocatechin-3-gallate inhibit hypoxia- and serum-induced HIF-1alpha protein accumulation and VEGF expression in human cervical carcinoma and hepatoma cells, *Mol Cancer Ther* **5**(5): 1227–1238 (2006).
77. Yang, J.D., I. Nakamura, and L.R. Roberts, The tumor microenvironment in hepatocellular carcinoma: Current status and therapeutic targets, *Semin Cancer Biol* **21**(1): 35–43 (2011).

78. Kleeff, J., P. Beckhove, I. Esposito, S. Herzig, P.E. Huber, J.M. Lohr, and H. Friess, Pancreatic cancer microenvironment, *Int J Cancer* **121**(4): 699–705 (2007).
79. Jou, J. and A.M. Diehl, Epithelial-mesenchymal transitions and hepatocarcinogenesis, *J Clin Invest* **120**(4): 1031–1034 (2010).
80. Nakajima, S., R. Doi, E. Toyoda, S. Tsuji, M. Wada, M. Koizumi, S.S. Tulachan, D. Ito, K. Kami, T. Mori, Y. Kawaguchi, K. Fujimoto, R. Hosotani, and M. Imamura, N-cadherin expression and epithelial-mesenchymal transition in pancreatic carcinoma, *Clin Cancer Res* **10**(12 Pt. 1): 4125–4133 (2004).
81. Wang, N., Y. Feng, E.P. Lau, C. Tsang, Y. Ching, K. Man, Y. Tong, T. Nagamatsu, W. Su, and S. Tsao, F-actin reorganization and inactivation of rho signaling pathway involved in the inhibitory effect of Coptidis Rhizoma on hepatoma cell migration, *Integr Cancer Ther* **9**(4): 354–364 (2010).
82. Zhang, K., D. Chen, X. Jiao, S. Zhang, X. Liu, J. Cao, L. Wu, and D. Wang, Slug enhances invasion ability of pancreatic cancer cells through upregulation of matrix metalloproteinase-9 and actin cytoskeleton remodeling, *Lab Invest* **91**(3): 426–438 (2011).
83. Hood, J.D. and D.A. Cheresh, Role of integrins in cell invasion and migration, *Nat Rev Cancer,* **2**(2): 91–100 (2002).
84. Cai, L., J. Han, X. Zhuo, Y. Xiong, J. Dong, and X. Li, Overexpression and significance of focal adhesion kinase in hepatocellular carcinoma and its relationship with HBV infection, *Med Oncol* **26**(4): 409–414 (2009).
85. Ucar, D.A., L.H. Dang, and S.N. Hochwald, Focal adhesion kinase signaling and function in pancreatic cancer, *Front Biosci (Elite Ed)* **3**: 750–756 (2011).
86. Maatta, M., Y. Soini, A. Liakka, and H. Autio-Harmainen, Differential expression of matrix metalloproteinase (MMP)-2, MMP-9, and membrane type 1-MMP in hepatocellular and pancreatic adenocarcinoma: implications for tumor progression and clinical prognosis, *Clin Cancer Res* **6**(7): 2726–2734 (2000).
87. Gupta, S.C., J.H. Kim, S. Prasad, and B.B. Aggarwal, Regulation of survival, proliferation, invasion, angiogenesis, and metastasis of tumor cells through modulation of inflammatory pathways by nutraceuticals, *Cancer Metastasis Rev* **29**(3): 405–434 (2010).
88. Zheng, Q., Z.Y. Tang, Q. Xue, D.R. Shi, H.Y. Song, and H.B. Tang, Invasion and metastasis of hepatocellular carcinoma in relation to urokinase-type plasminogen activator, its receptor and inhibitor, *J Cancer Res Clin Oncol* **126**: 641–646 (2000).
89. Ma, C.Y., W.T. Ji, F.S. Chueh, J.S. Yang, P.Y. Chen, C.C. Yu, and J.G. Chung, Butein inhibits the migration and invasion of SK-HEP-1 human hepatocarcinoma

cells through suppressing the ERK, JNK, p38, and uPA signaling multiple pathways, *J Agric Food Chem* **59**(16): 9032–9038 (2011).

90. Ng, K.T., D.Y. Guo, Q. Cheng, W. Geng, C.C. Ling, C.X. Li, X.B. Liu, Y.Y. Ma, C.M. Lo, R.T. Poon, S.T. Fan, and K. Man, A garlic derivative, S-allylcysteine (SAC), suppresses proliferation and metastasis of hepatocellular carcinoma, *PLoS One* **7**(2): e31655 (2012).
91. Kaufmann, R., P. Henklein, and U. Settmacher, Green tea polyphenol epigallocatechin-3-gallate inhibits thrombin-induced hepatocellular carcinoma cell invasion and p42/p44-MAPKinase activation, *Oncol Rep* **21**(5): 1261–1267 (2009).
92. Lee, K.W., N.J. Kang, J.H. Kim, K.M. Lee, D.E. Lee, H.J. Hur, and H.J. Lee, Caffeic acid phenethyl ester inhibits invasion and expression of matrix metalloproteinase in SK-Hep1 human hepatocellular carcinoma cells by targeting nuclear factor kappa B, *Genes Nutr* **2**(4): 319–322 (2008).
93. Lee, S.J., K.W. Lee, H.J. Hur, J.Y. Chun, S.Y. Kim, and H.J. Lee, Phenolic phytochemicals derived from red pine (*Pinus densiflora*) inhibit the invasion and migration of SK-Hep-1 human hepatocellular carcinoma cells, *Ann NY Acad Sci* **1095**: 536–544 (2007).
94. Liang, J.A., S.L. Wu, H.Y. Lo, C.Y. Hsiang, and T.Y. Ho, Vanillin inhibits matrix metalloproteinase-9 expression through down-regulation of nuclear factor-kappaB signaling pathway in human hepatocellular carcinoma cells, *Mol Pharmacol* **75**(1): 151–157 (2009).
95. Liu, A., L. Sha, Y. Shen, L. Huang, X. Tang, and S. Lin, Experimental study on anti-metastasis effect of emodin on human pancreatic cancer, *Zhongguo Zhong Yao Za Zhi* **36**(22): 3167–3171 (2011).
96. Weng, C.J., C.F. Wu, H.W. Huang, C.H. Wu, C.T. Ho, and G.C. Yen, Evaluation of anti-invasion effect of resveratrol and related methoxy analogues on human hepatocarcinoma cells, *J Agric Food Chem* **58**(5): 2886–2894 (2010).
97. Weng, C.J., C.F. Wu, H.W. Huang, C.T. Ho, and G.C. Yen, Anti-invasion effects of 6-shogaol and 6-gingerol, two active components in ginger, on human hepatocarcinoma cells, *Mol Nutr Food Res* **54**(11): 1618–1627 (2010).
98. Liyanage, U.K., P.S. Goedegebuure, T.T. Moore, C.T. Viehl, T.A. Moo-Young, J.W. Larson, D.M. Frey, J.P. Ehlers, T.J. Eberlein, and D.C. Linehan, Increased prevalence of regulatory T cells (Treg) is induced by pancreas adenocarcinoma, *J Immunother* **29**(4): 416–424 (2006).
99. Ghiringhelli, F., P.E. Puig, S. Roux, A. Parcellier, E. Schmitt, E. Solary, G. Kroemer, F. Martin, B. Chauffert, and L. Zitvogel, Tumor cells convert immature myeloid

dendritic cells into TGF-beta-secreting cells inducing CD4+CD25+ regulatory T cell proliferation, *J Exp Med* **202**(7): 919–929 (2005).

100. Hinz, S., L. Pagerols-Raluy, H.H. Oberg, O. Ammerpohl, S. Grussel, B. Sipos, R. Grutzmann, C. Pilarsky, H. Ungefroren, H.D. Saeger, G. Kloppel, D. Kabelitz, and H. Kalthoff, Foxp3 expression in pancreatic carcinoma cells as a novel mechanism of immune evasion in cancer, *Cancer Res* **67**(17): 8344–8350 (2007).
101. Geng, L., J. Deng, G. Jiang, P. Song, Z. Wang, Z. Jiang, M. Zhang, and S. Zheng, B7-H1 up-regulated expression in human hepatocellular carcinoma tissue: Correlation with tumor interleukin-10 levels, *Hepatogastroenterology* **58**(107–108): 960–964 (2011).
102. Lee, S.H., M.S. Shin, H.S. Lee, J.H. Bae, H.K. Lee, H.S. Kim, S.Y. Kim, J.J. Jang, M. Joo, Y.K. Kang, W.S. Park, J.Y. Park, R.R. Oh, S.Y. Han, J.H. Lee, S.H. Kim, J.Y. Lee, and N.J. Yoo, Expression of Fas and Fas-related molecules in human hepatocellular carcinoma, *Hum Pathol* **32**(3): 250–256 (2001).
103. Liu, Z., M. Cheng and M. Cao, Potential targets for molecular imaging of apoptosis resistance in hepatocellular carcinoma, *Biomed Imaging Interv J* **7**(1): e5 (2011).
104. He, X., X. Li, B. Liu, L. Xu, H. Zhao, and A. Lu, Down-regulation of Treg cells and up-regulation of TH1/TH2 cytokine ratio were induced by polysaccharide from Radix Glycyrrhizae in H22 hepatocarcinoma bearing mice, *Molecules* **16**(10): 8343–8352 (2011).
105. Ishihara, Y., T. Fujii, H. Iijima, K. Saito, and K. Matsunaga, The role of neutrophils as cytotoxic cells in lung metastasis: Suppression of tumor cell metastasis by a biological response modifier (PSK), *In Vivo* **12**(2): 175–182 (1998).
106. Liu, H.S., C.E. Pan, W. Yang, and X.M. Liu, Antitumor and immunomodulatory activity of resveratrol on experimentally implanted tumor of H22 in Balb/c mice, *World J Gastroenterol* **9**(7): 1474–1476 (2003).
107. Hering, J., S. Garrean, T.R. Dekoj, A. Razzak, A. Saied, J. Trevino, T.A. Babcock, and N.J. Espat, Inhibition of proliferation by omega-3 fatty acids in chemoresistant pancreatic cancer cells, *Ann Surg Oncol* **14**(12): 3620–3628 (2007).
108. Wiseman, M., The second World Cancer Research Fund/American Institute for Cancer Research expert report. Food, nutrition, physical activity, and the prevention of cancer: A global perspective, *Proc Nutr Soc* **67**(3): 253–256 (2008).
109. Vrieling, A., B.A. Verhage, F.J. van Duijnhoven, M. Jenab, K. Overvad, A. Tjonneland, A. Olsen, F. Clavel-Chapelon, M.C. Boutron-Ruault, R. Kaaks,

S. Rohrmann, H. Boeing, U. Nothlings, A. Trichopoulou, T. John, Z. Dimosthenes, D. Palli, S. Sieri, A. Mattiello, R. Tumino, P. Vineis, C.H. van Gils, P.H. Peeters, D. Engeset, E. Lund, L. Rodriguez Suarez, P. Jakszyn, N. Larranaga, M.J. Sanchez, M.D. Chirlaque, E. Ardanaz, J. Manjer, B. Lindkvist, G. Hallmans, W. Ye, S. Bingham, K.T. Khaw, A. Roddam, T. Key, P. Boffetta, E.J. Duell, D.S. Michaud, E. Riboli, and H.B. Bueno-de-Mesquita, Fruit and vegetable consumption and pancreatic cancer risk in the European Prospective Investigation into Cancer and Nutrition, *Int J Cancer* **124**(8): 1926–1934 (2009).

8

Cancer Preventive and Therapeutic Properties of Fruits and Vegetables Against Lung Cancer

*Kunnathur Murugesan Sakthivel, Javadi Monisha, Ajaikumar B. Kunnumakkara and Chandrasekharan Guruvayoorappan**

INTRODUCTION

Lung cancer is the most common cancer worldwide, killing approximately 1.38 million people globally every year. It has also been estimated that approximately 1.61 million people around the world are diagnosed with lung cancer annually.[1] As per the current histological lung cancer classification proposed by the World Health Organization (WHO) in 1981, lung cancers can be divided into two broad groups: small cell lung cancer (SCLC), accounting for 20–25% of bronchogenic carcinomas, and non-small cell lung cancer (NSCLC), accounting for almost all of the remaining cases. SCLC is a highly aggressive form of lung cancer and almost always occurs in smokers than in non-smokers. It is rapidly growing, and roughly 60% of patients have widespread metastatic disease at the time of diagnosis. NSCLC is the most common type of lung cancer, and further divided histologically into three main subtypes: adenocarcinoma,

*Corresponding author: Chandrasekharan Guruvayoorappan, Ph.D., Assistant Professor, Department of Biotechnology, Karunya University, Karunya Nagar, Coimbatore-641114, Tamil Nadu, India. Tel: (+91) 98-9433-7418, Email: gurukarunya@gmail.com.

squamous cell lung carcinoma, and large cell lung carcinoma. Approximately one-fourth of all lung cancers show no symptoms of the disease and are detected incidentally with chest imaging. Symptoms and signs can result from local tumor progression (cause severe cough and sometimes dyspnea), regional spread (cause pleuritic chest pain or dyspnea), or distant metastases which is eventually cause symptoms that vary by location include the lungs, liver, brain, and adrenal glands. Paraneoplastic syndromes and constitutional symptoms may occur at any stage of the disease. Although symptoms are not specific to different types of lung cancer, certain complications may be more likely with different types.[2] The clinical behavior of NSCLC is highly variable and depends on histologic type. It has been estimated that 40% of lung cancer patients show metastatsis outside of the chest at the time of diagnosis.

THERAPEUTIC APPROACHES IN LUNG CANCER

Therapeutic approaches in lung cancer, such as chemotherapy, radiotherapy, and surgery have been widely used. The current National Comprehensive Cancer Network (NCCN) guidelines recommend several options for first- and second-line therapies for treating NSCLC based on a better understanding of the molecular origins and evolution of the disease.[3] The survival of patients with relapsed/progressive NSCLC remains poor. Currently for treatment of SCLC, cisplatin, etoposide, and celecoxib are generally recommended agents, whereas anthracycline, doxorubicin, epirubicin, topotecan, irinotecan, paclitaxel, and gemcitabine are applied either alone or in combination with others. Erlotinib and gefitinib, which target EGFR (epidermal growth factors and their receptor), cisplatin, and carboplatin are often used for cancer therapy in patients with advanced/metastatic NSCLC in combination with other anticancer agents such as gemcitabine, paclitaxel, docetaxel, etoposide, or vinorelbine.[4,5]

Several epidemiological studies have identified numerous factors associated with the risk of lung cancer. Quite a number of important risk factors for lung cancer are known, including cigarette smoke (the most well-established risk factor), exposure to second-hand cigarette smoke, radon gas, asbestos, and other chemicals and particles such as arsenic, beryllium, cadmium, vinyl chloride, nickel, chromates, etc.[6] Remarkably, lung cancer in non-smokers has been described in detail, and the frequency has been increasing in the past five years in certain geographical regions than in others (Asia > North America > Europe). A 'never smoker' is commonly defined as an individual who has smoked less than 100 cigarettes over his or her lifetime. An estimated 10–25% of lung cancers worldwide occur in "never smokers," more frequently in women possibly due to exposure to environmental tobacco smoke and also exposure to workplace environmental carcinogens. In 2010, Clement-Duchene *et al.*[7] found that 63% of lung cancers in a French cohort of 67 never smoking lung cancer patients were due to environmental tobacco smoke and occupational exposure to carcinogens. Of these, 78.6% of women were exposed to environmental tobacco smoke versus 21.4% of men. Within recent years, several advanced technologies have been developed to diagnose the lung cancer even in the preneoplastic stage. Currently, we have tools for early diagnose of lung cancer like low-dose helical CT, it is easy to diagnose small cell lung cancers and fluorescence bronchoscopy in high-risk populations (i.e., heavy smokers) is able to diagnose preneoplastic bronchial lesions. These advanced diagnostic technologies combined with the developments of more specific targeted therapeutic agents, which can block different steps of biological pathways for lung carcinogenesis, will give rise to new optimism for the novel approaches of chemoprevention in lung cancer.

ROLE OF FRUITS AND VEGETABLES IN THE PREVENTION OF LUNG CANCER

The role for plant foods in the maintenance of health has been known for several thousand years. Consumption of fruits and vegetables is important for human health because these foods are the primary sources of many essential nutrients and contain phytochemicals that may lower risk of chronic disease include cancer. Fruits and vegetables can provide the bulk of the pharmacopoeia. In 1991, Steinmetz and Potter[8] summarized the available (largely case control) data on cancer, vegetables, and fruit, concluding that the evidence was consistent with higher consumption being associated with a lower risk of many cancers. The 1997 World Cancer Research Fund (WCRF) report, reviewed the available literature to the end of 1996, concluded that vegetables and fruits were probably or convincingly associated with a lower risk of cancers of mouth, oesophagus, lung, stomach, colorectum (vegetables only), larynx, pancreas, breast, and bladder. Controversially, for lung cancer, some of cohort studies suggest, if any association, a lower risk for women but not men; by far the largest study (n = 500,000) shows a reduced risk associated with fruit consumption, but not vegetables. Block *et al.*[9] reviewed about 200 studies of the consumption of fruits and vegetables and the incidence of cancer. One hundred and twenty-eight of 156 studies show statistically significant protective effect of fruits and vegetables and different cancers. For most cancers, people in the lower quartile (one-fourth of the population) who consumed the least amount of fruits and vegetables had about twofold increase in the risk of cancer compared to those in the upper quartile who ate the most fruits and vegetables. Even in lung cancer, after accounting for smoking, increased fruits and vegetables consumption shows a reduced risk for this disease (20–33%).

The association between diet and lung cancer has been extensively reconnoitered in epidemiological studies and there is much information to support an association between the fruits and vegetables consumption and reduced risk of lung cancer. Plenteous effort has been expended to identify the specific components of the fruits and vegetables that may be responsible for lowering lung cancer risk. From the early 1980s, in the United States and other countries, several government agencies have promoted programs on cancer prevention, and dietary guidelines have been established in order to reduce the risk of cancer. So far, several molecules were studied as potential "chemoprotective agents" and more than 50 bioactive compounds are being tested in clinical trials. Considerably, in many studies, attention has been given to β-carotene, lutein, lycopene, and other micronutrients such as selenium, isothiocyanates, vitamin E (α-tocopherol), allyl sulfur compounds (onions and garlic), and green tea polyphenols because of its potent antioxidant properties. Reports focused on cooking practices has shown increased risk of lung cancer has been noted as a significance of regular intake of heterocyclic amines, which are produced when meats are cooked at high temperatures. Recent epidemiological studies on diet and lung cancer support the hypothesis that regular intake of dietary products can modulate the risk of lung cancer.

In traditional medicine, several fruits and vegetables have been used frequently to treat lung-related disorders with folk remedies and medicines (including lung cancer). It is important to understand their unique mechanisms of action for the development of therapeutically useful agents for treating cancer. Analysis of the molecular mechanisms whereby fruits and vegetables exert anticancer activity has resulted in the development of many targeted therapeutic drugs for cancer treatment. Molecular methodologies provide a viewing platform for early diagnosis and screening of high-risk individuals, determination of prognosis, and identification of innovative treatments. Although the precise mechanism of action remains unknown, several evidences are emerging, indicating modulatory effects on apoptosis, cell proliferation, immune responses, antioxidative processes, xenobiotic metabolism, and COX-2 expression.[10] The angiogenesis- and metastasis-related factors such as VEGF and MMPs, along with cell proliferation- and survival-related factors such as Akt, NF-κB, Ras, MAPKs, and EGFR, are importantly considered as target molecules for lung cancer therapy.[11]

Although it is hard to identify with assurance, cancer preventive compounds in fruits and vegetables, experimental data, and human observational studies showing the protective effects of major nutritional antioxidants prompted five large intervention trials to be initiated in the 1990s to determine the potential of specific antioxidant supplements in reducing cancer risk. A study in China, the United States, and Finland tested the protective effects of various combined micronutrients (vitamin E, vitamin A, and β-carotene) in various combinations on reducing lung cancer risk in smokers and non-smokers.[12] Table 8.1 shows a list of lung cancer preventive compounds present in fruits and vegetables and their mechanisms of action.

COMPOUNDS PRESENT IN FRUITS AND VEGETABLES THAT PREVENT LUNG CANCER

Carotenoids

Carotenoids are lipophilic compounds with polyisoprenoid structures, a family of pigmented compounds (yellow-orange-red pigments) found in all higher plants and microorganisms, but not in animals. Animals cannot synthesize carotenoids, so their presence is due to dietary intake. Fruits and vegetables constitute the major sources of carotenoids in human diet.

Table 8.1: Phytochemicals isolated from fruits and vegetables for lung cancer chemoprevention and their mechanisms of action.

No	Phytochemicals	Sources	Mechanism of action
1	EGCG (catechins)	Grapes	• Cell cycle arrest • Induce apoptosis • Reduces cell adhesion and migration • Inhibition of cell invasion, metastasis, and angiogenesis
2	Quercetin	Apples, grapes, lemons, tomatoes, and onions	• Antioxidant activity • Cell cycle arrest • Induces apoptosis and necrosis • Inhibits cell migration and invasion • Inhibits angiogenesis • Induces cell differentiation • Anti-inflammatory activity
3	Kaempferol	Broccoli and man-goes	• Cell cycle arrest • Induces apoptosis • Antioxidant activity • Inhibits angiogenesis • Inhibits cell migration
4	Isorhamnetin	Apples and pear fruit	• Induces apoptosis • Induces necrosis • Inhibitor of angiogenesis
5	Silibinin	*Silybum marianum* fruits	• Cell cycle arrest • Induces apoptosis • Induces cell differentiation • Reduces invasion • Inhibitor of angiogenesis
6	Baicalein	*Oroxylum indicum* fruits	• Cell cycle arrest • Induces apoptosis • Suppresses cell adhesion and migration
7	Lycopene and vitamin C	Tomatoes, cabbage, and cauliflowers	• Strong antioxidants • Inhibit lymphocytes — DNA oxidative damage

(*Continued*)

Table 8.1: (*Continued*)

No	Phytochemicals	Sources	Mechanism of action
8	β-elemene	Ginger	• Triggers apoptosis in NSCLC cells through a mitochondrial release of the cytochrome c-mediated apoptotic pathway
9	Fisetin (3,7,3,4-tetrahydroxyflavone)	Strawberries, apples, grapes, onions, and cucumbers	• Inhibits cell proliferation • Free radical scavenging activity • Strong antioxidant activity
10	Geraniin	Emblica fruit (*Phyllanthus emblica*)	• Immunomodulatory and antioxidant activities
11	Magniferin	Mangoes	• Inhibits cell proliferation • Antioxidant property
12	Resveratrol	Grapes	• Inhibition of STAT-3 and NF-κB-dependent transcription, and suppression of Bcl-x_L expression
13	Pyrogallol	*Embilica officinalis*	• Induce apoptosis
14	Sulforaphane	Broccoli	• Cell cycle arrest • Apoptosis induction

Carotenoids are thought to be responsible for the beneficial properties of fruits and vegetables in preventing human diseases including cancer and other chronic diseases. More than 600 carotenoids have so far been identified in nature. However, only about 40 are present in a typical human diet. The major carotenoids in the fruits and vegetables are represented by β-carotene (carrots, spinach, cantaloupe, green broccoli, tomato), α-carotene (carrots), lycopene (tomato, watermelon guava, grape fruit, papaya, and apricot), lutein (papaya), and cryptoxanthin (spinach, green broccoli, and green peas). β-carotene has been the most studied carotenoid with respect to disease prevention particularly cancer. Many preclinical studies showed that these carotenoids inhibits lung cancer cell proliferation, survival, invasion, and metastasis of different lung cancer cells and carcinogen-induced lung tumorigenesis by modulating the expression of different proteins that are involved in different signaling pathways in lung cancer.[13–16] In addition, based on epidemiological studies, a positive link is suggested between higher dietary intake and tissue concentrations of carotenoids and lower risk lung cancer. Evidence from observational epidemiologic studies demonstrates inverse association between the incidence of lung cancer and a high consumption of fruits and vegetables (which are rich in carotenoids). Männistö *et al.* showed that intake of dietary carotenoids such as α-carotene, lutein/zeaxanthin, lycopene, and β-cryptoxanthin was inversely associated with lung cancer risk in humans.[17] In addition, the Japan Collaborative Cohort (JACC) study showed that higher serum levels of carotenoids such as α- and β-carotenes play a role in preventing death from lung cancer among the Japanese.[18] Therefore, it can be concluded that there is an inverse relation between dietary consumption of carotenoids and lung cancer risk.

Flavonoids

Flavonoids are another example of chemopreventive compounds presenting a double-edged characteristic. The intake of these phenolic compounds that are widely present in fruits as well as vegetables, have been reported to be associated with many beneficial properties, such as antioxidant, antiviral, anti-inflammatory, hepatoprotective active, prevention of cardiovascular diseases, and antitumoral activities. Hence, flavonoids are frequently ingested in relatively large amounts as dietary factors for health maintenance. In the last decade, studies have attempted to understand the molecular mechanism involved in flavonoids action. Studies showed that quercetin inhibits the growth in different human lung cancer cells such as A549, H1299, and H460 lung carcinoma cells[19,20] by downregulating the COX-2, iNOS, survivin, P450, NF-κB, and MEK–ERK pathways, inducing the expression of death receptor 5 (DR5), p53, glutathione S-transferase (GSTM1, GSTM2, GSTT2, and GSTP1), etc.[21–23] Studies showed that quercetin prevented benzo[a]pyrene-induced DNA damages, pulmonary precancerous pathologic lesions,[24] and N-nitrosodiethylamine-induced lung tumorigenesis by decreasing lipid peroxidation and increasing GSH levels.[25] Other flavonoids which show anticancer activities against lung cancer are kaempferol and fisetin. The kaempferol compound induces apoptosis in lung cancer cells by inhibiting the MEK–ERK pathway[26] and inducing antioxidant enzymes.[27] Fisetin is known to inhibit benzo(a)pyrene-induced lung carcinogenesis in mice by the induction of antioxidant enzymes.[28]

However, not all flavonoids and their actions are necessarily beneficial. The dual role of this substance by producing either toxic or beneficial effects seems to depend on doses and/or the experimental cell type. According to the FDA (Food and Drug administration), nearly 30 flavonoid trials are in course and have advanced up to Phases II and III with tests performed in volunteers. The majority of flavonoids clinical trials are still under test in Phase I or II. For instance, EGCG, quercetin, kaempferol, isorhamnetin, silibinin, and baicalein were the main flavonoid targets for trials in distinct phases for lung cancer.[29]

Vitamins

Vitamin A

Due to their ability to regulate cell proliferation and diffrentiation, the derivatives of vitamin A or retinoids have been regarded as a potentially useful class of agents from the very beginning of chemoprevention research. Many studies showed that vitamin A and retinoids inhibit lung cancer cell proliferation, tumor growth, invasion, and metastasis in animals, and enhances the immune system in lung cancer patients. In 1985, Palgi *et al.*[30] critically reviewed 16 studies (eight dietary studies and eight serum studies) which showed a relationship between lung cancer and vitamin A intake. Three dietary studies showed a negative association between vitamin A intake and lung cancer risk, and the reduction in risk was found to be greatest in persons in the higher socio-economic strata. These studies show that consumption of carrots and milk (daily) lowers lung cancer risk (three studies); high intake of dietary vitamin A inhibited the development of squamous and small cell carcinoma of the lung in smokers (four studies); and lower levels of serum vitamin A was associated with lung cancer patients than in controls. In 2011, Fritz *et al.* reviewed and analyzed 248 studies from six electronic data bases (Pubmed, EMBASE, CINAHL, AltHealthWatch, the Cochrane Library, and the National Library of Science and Technology) about the beneficial effect of vitamin A and retinoid derivatives in lung cancer risk, and they showed that synthetic rexinoid bexarotene significantly increased survival of lung cancer patients.[31] Therefore, it is clear that the intake of vitamin A has some beneficial effect in the prevention and treatment of lung cancer.

Vitamin C

Vitamin C (ascorbic acid) is a water-soluble antioxidant that is an essential nutrient for humans. All fruits and vegetables contain vitamin C, with high concentrations found in citrus fruits, cruciferous vegetables, and dark leafy greens. The dietary reference intake (DRI) estimated that the average requirements of vitamin C for women and men are 60 and 75 mg/day, respectively. A number studies have shown that vitamin C inhibits proliferation of lung cancer cells, and demonstrates synergism with tea polyphenols by modulating different signaling pathways.[32–35] Studies have also shown that combination of ascorbic acid and α-tocopherol prevented smoke-induced lung squamous metaplasia in ferrets,[36] and a combination of vitamin C and vitamin K3 inhibited tumor growth and metastasis of Lewis lung carcinoma xenograft in mice.[37] In the 1970s, Linus Pauling promoted the use of vitamin C to prevent the common cold, and later for the treatment of cancer including lung cancer. His results remain controversial, but popular interest in vitamin C remains high. Bandara *et al.*,[38] in the state of New York, found that there is a direct relationship between vitamin C uptake and lung cancer for men. Recently, Iowa Women's Health Study (34,708 postmenopausal women; aged 55–69; 16-years follow-up) reported that supplementation of vitamin C reduced the lung cancer risk in women.[39] Overall, it can be concluded that vitamin C reduces the risk for lung cancer.

Vitamin E (α-tocopherol)

Vitamin E (tocopherols and tocotrienols) present in green leafy vegetables and fruits is an antioxidant fat-soluble vitamin that plays an important role in protecting the cell membrane from oxidation. In the clinical investigations of vitamin E, α-tocopherol is used most often because of its high biological activity. There is much information available about the lung cancer chemopreventive properties of vitamin E. It has been shown that vitamin E inhibits cell proliferation and survival and induces apoptosis in different lung cancer cells in laboratory experimental conditions; it also inhibits lung cancer cells-induced tumors in animals and enhances the apoptotic activity of paclitaxel and parthenolide in lung cancer cells.[40–43] As aforementioned, this compound in combination with ascorbic acid also inhibits smoke-induced lung squamous metaplasia in ferrets.[36] Studies suggested that this compound inhibits generation of free radicals and reduces the expression of COX-2 and inflammatory genes that play an important role in lung tumorigenesis. In addition to preclinical studies, clinical studies also proved the effect of vitamin E intake on reduced lung cancer risk. In 2010, Ju *et al.* reviewed four case-control studies and three cohort studies involving the role of vitamin E in reduced lung cancer risk. Out of the four case-control studies, three studies showed lower serum concentrations of α-tocopherol in lung cancer patients compared to controls. Of the three cohort studies, two studies showed a significant inverse association between vitamin E and risk of lung cancer in current smokers, which demonstrated the protective effects of vitamin E supplementation against insult from cigarette smoking.[44] Recent studies showed that tocotrienols — the natural analogs of vitamin E — inhibits cell growth, migration, and invasion, and induces apoptosis in NSCLC cells by suppressing activation of NF-κB, Notch-1, Hes-1, and Bcl-2, and increasing cleaved caspase-3 and PARP expressions.[43,45] Although certain populations may benefit from taking vitamin E for lung cancer prevention, further research is needed to identify exactly what patient populations will benefit from vitamin E supplementation and the optimal dose that will be beneficial.

Selenium

Selenium is a trace element found in selenoenzymes, including glutathione peroxidase (GPx), an antioxidant enzyme for detoxification of hydrogen peroxide, and thioredoxin reductase (TrxR), an enzyme involved in the reduction of protein disulfides. The trace element selenium that resembles sulfur in its various forms was first associated with cancer protection in the late 1960s. Several years later, epidemiological evidence also pointed to preventive capacities of selenium. Preclinical studies using cell culture indicated that selenium can decrease cell proliferation, migration, promote cell cycle arrest, and induce apoptosis in cancer cells.[46] Pretreatment of this compound inhibits formaldehyde-induced genotoxicity in A549 cell lines.[47] In animals, it has been shown that dietary selenium inhibits pulmonary cell proliferation[48] and cigarette smoke-induced lung tumorigenesis.[49] It has also been shown that different selenium-containing compounds also possess anticancer properties against lung cancer. For example, methylseleninic acid inhibits spontaneous metastasis of Lewis lung carcinoma in mice;[50] selenium-containing analogs of suberoylanilide hydroxamic acid (SAHA) induce cytotoxicity in lung cancer cells;[51] and ethaselen (a selenium-containing thioredoxin reductase inhibitor) sensitizes non-small cell lung cancer to radiotherapy.[52] A randomized controlled trial to prevent skin cancer in 1,312 patients suggested that supplementation with selenium (l-selenomethionine) was associated with a reduction in the risk of developing lung and prostate cancer. Recent studies have shown that a low selenium level is increase the risk for lung and laryngeal cancers[53] and plasma levels of selenium is reduced in NSCLC patients undergoing radiotherapy.[54] These studies suggest that selenium supplementation reduces the risk for lung cancer.

Alkaloids

The first isolations of alkaloids in the nineteenth century followed the reintroduction into medicine of a number of alkaloid-containing drugs to treat various types of cancers. Alkaloids are a group of naturally occurring compounds containing nitrogen in a heterocyclic ring present in wide group of fruits and vegetables. β-carbolines are biologically active alkaloids that occur in naturally occurring fruits such as bananas, pineapples, oranges, grapes, kiwis, and vegetables such as tomatoes. β-carboline derivatives, namely, harmine, kauluamine, and cantin-6-one alkaloids showed significant cytotoxic activity *in vitro* against the NSCLC PA-801 cell line.[55] Glycoalkaloid-rich green tomato (*Solanum lycopersicum*) extracts have shown inhibition of human lung adenocarcinoma A549 cells. α-chaconine isolated from *Solanum tuberosum* Linn, is a glycoalkaloid present in potato sprouts. Scientific reports demonstrated its anticarcinogenic properties. α-chaconine inhibited lung metastasis in human lung adenocarcinoma A549 cells by downregulating the expression of matrix metalloproteinase-2

(MMP-2) and MMP-9 activities and by suppression of phosphoinositide-3-kinase (PI3K)/Akt/NF-κB signaling pathway. Similarly, α-tomatine, a glycoalkaloid from *Lycopersicon esculentum* (green tomato) has shown anti-metastatic effect in NCI-H460 human NSCLC cells. Based on the above information, the use of alkaloids as anti-lung cancer agents is very promising, but more research and clinical trials are necessary before final recommendations on specific alkaloids can be made.[56–58]

Folic Acid

Folic acid is a water-soluble vitamin B present naturally in fruits (papaya and bananas) and vegetables (rich in broccoli, lettuce, cantaloupe, and cabbage). A meta-analysis on eight cohort studies found no significant association between dietary folate and total folate intake and lung cancer risk. However, a subsequent study suggests that there may be a link between increased folate intake and an increase in lung cancer. The New York State Cohort study has reported that folic acid has a protective effect in lung cancer risk in men, but not in women, particularly squamous cell carcinomas.[59] It has also been shown that folate intake protects against lung cancer in smokers.[60] Overall, people who have a healthy folic acid intake generally have a lower risk of developing lung cancer.

Phytoestrogens

Phytoestrogens are non-steroidal compounds which bind with estrogen receptors. Most phytoestrogens exist in the diet as inactive compounds and after consumption it undergo enzymatic conversion in the gastrointestinal tract, resulting in the formation of compounds with a steroidal structure similar to that of estrogens. Phytoestrogens are subdivided into three main classes: isoflavones, lignans, and cumestrans. The isoflavones and the lignans are the two main groups of hormone-like diphenolic dietary phytoestrogens. Isoflavones are the most common form, and most extensively investigated phytoestrogen. The two major forms of isoflavones, genistein and daidzein, are formed from the precursors genistin and daidzin and are found in a variety of sources including soy products, soybeans, chickpeas, and red clover. Lignans are derived from carrots, spinach, broccoli, and other vegetables. The lignan metabolites, enterolactone and enterodiol, are formed from the precursors matairesinol and secoisolariciresinol. Coumesterol is the predominant estrogenic phytoestrogen in the cumestran group and is mainly found in beans, peas, clover, spinach, and sprouts.

A fourth group of plant-derived steroidal compounds that is believed to have estrogenic properties are the phytosterols, which are derived from the intestinal absorption of vegetable oils, margarines, and certain fruits and vegetables. Although structurally similar to cholesterol, phytosterols (which include β-sitosterol, campesterol, and stigmasterol) could affect levels of endogenous hormones through alterations in bile acid metabolism and estrogen reabsorption or by acting as substrates for synthesis of steroid hormones.[61] Many studies showed the potential of these phytoestrogens in preventing lung cancer. For example, phytoestrogens like genistein and barbigerone inhibit lung cancer cell proliferation, survival, invasion, and metastasis in different experimental conditions.[62–65] In addition, many studies showed the potential of phytoestrogens in preventing lung cancer in humans. Matthew *et al.*[66] showed in a case study, reductions in risk of lung cancer tended to increase with each increasing quartile of phytoestrogen intake. In addition, the Shanghai Women's Health Study suggests that there is a reduced risk of lung cancer with increased consumption of soy food mainly in non-smoking women. This study analyzed the protective effect of soy food against lung cancer in 71,550 women recruited into this study from 1997–2000. The identified 370 incident lung cancer cases in a mean follow-up period of 9.1 years. After adjustment for potential confounders, soy food intake was inversely associated with subsequent risk of lung cancer predominately among women with later age of menopause and with aggressive lung cancer.[67] The studies conducted in Japanese women also show that there is a reduced risk of getting lung cancer with high plasma concentrations of genestein.[68] In addition, the Japan Public Health Center-based Prospective Study shows that there is an inverse relation between isoflavone uptake and risk for lung cancer.[69]

These data provide further support for the limited but growing epidemiologic evidence that estrogens and phytoestrogens are associated with a decrease in risk of lung cancer, especially in never and current smokers. However, confirmation of these findings is still required in large-scale hypothesis driven prospective studies.

Isothiocyanates

Isothiocyanates are natural compounds found in edible cruciferous vegetables such as broccoli, watercress, Brussels sprouts, cabbage, Japanese radish, and cauliflower. They have been shown to play a significant role in cancer chemopreventive activity of these vegetables. Some of the isothiocyanates extracted from these cruciferous vegetables include phenethyl isothiocyanate (PEITC), benzyl isothiocyanate (BITC), and sulforaphane (SFN). Recently Wu *et al.*[70] demonstrated that BITC and PEITC inhibited highly metastatic L9981 NSCLC proliferation, migration, and invasion by modulating/inhibiting the metastasis-related genes involved in Akt/NFκB pathway. Similarly, another report showed the chemopreventive role of sulforaphane by upholding the GSH redox cycle in pre-and post-initiation phases of benzo[a]pyrene-induced lung carcinogenesis.[71] The proposed mechanism of isothiocyanates in cancer chemoprevention are the inhibition of Phase I enzymes of the cytochrome P450 family involved in the activation of carcinogen and/or induction of phase II detoxifying enzymes, such as glutathione S-transferases, quinone reductase, and UDP-glucuronosyltransferases. Recent studies have shown that isothiocyanates inhibit the growth of several types of cultured human cancer cells, induce cancer cell apoptosis and cell cycle arrest, regulate the activation of transcription factors STAT3, NF-κB, and Nrf2, inhibit MAPK and PKC activities, and downregulate estrogen receptors.[71]

Nevertheless, understanding the precise mechanism of these compounds may provide important information for their possible application in the prevention and therapy of cancer. Currently, many studies are being conducted to evaluate the effects of isothiocyanates in human subjects; this could potentially facilitate clinical development of isothiocyanates for lung cancer prevention and therapy.[71]

PREVENTION RATIONALE: MECHANISMS OF ACTION

Based on preclinical and clinical studies, several mechanisms have been proposed by which fruits and vegetables and their protective nutrients act in the prevention of lung cancer (Fig. 8.1). The possible mechanisms for

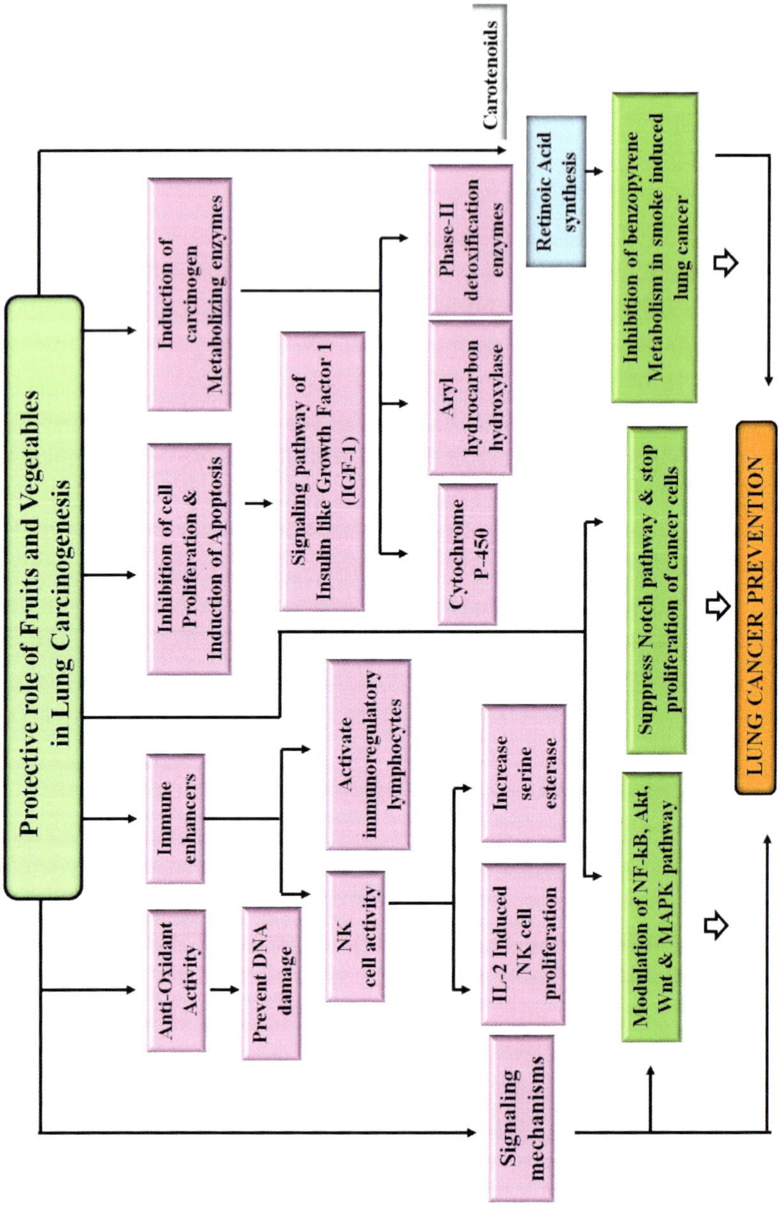

Figure 8.1: Proposed mechanisms of action of fruits and vegetables and their components in the prevention of lung cancer.

this beneficial property of fruits and vegetables and their nutrients on lung carcinogenesis are outlined here: (1) antioxidant properties; (2) immune system modulation; (3) induction of carcinogen-metabolizing enzymes; (4) inhibition of cell proliferation; (5) induction of apoptosis; (6) suppression of insulin-like growth factor 1 (IGF-1) — stimulated cell proliferation by inducing insulin-like growth factor-binding protein (IGFBP); (7) carotenoids, precursors of retinoic acid (RA), inhibit benzopyrene metabolism; and (8) interaction with signaling pathways associated with lung carcinogenesis.

Antioxidant Property

The major risk factor for lung cancer is cigarette smoking, which is the most common among other carcinogens. The major constituents of cigarette smoke include free radicals and reactive oxygen species, polycyclic aromatic hydrocarbons like benzo[a]pyrene, and nitrosamines such as 4-(methylnitrosamino)-1-(3-pyridyl)-1-butanone (NNK).[72] DNA damage caused by the reactive oxygen species has a major role in the development of carcinogenesis. To circumvent this condition, potent antioxidants like carotenoids abundant in fruits and vegetables can provide protective role. An *in vivo* study on lycopenes present in tomato demonstrated decreased damage to DNA, low-density lipoprotein oxidation, and lipid peroxidation.[73] Subsequent *in vitro* studies showed the relation between β-carotene, α-tocopherol, and ascorbic acid that resulted in the protection from oxidative damage. Combination of these antioxidants may play a role in the complex signaling interaction for prevention of DNA damage.

Immune System Modulation

Carotenoids, mainly β-carotene, supplementation has proven to enhance the natural killer (NK) cell activity as depletion of NK cell activity has been suggested to play a partial role in the increased incidence of cancer with growing age. A possible mechanism proposed is that after 72 h of β-carotene administration, there was a significant increase in the peripheral blood mononuclear cells (PBMCs) expressing the IL-2 receptor. IL-2, a growth factor, then binds to this receptor, resulting in upregulation of

NK cell proliferation. Another possible mechanism involves the carotenoid-induced upregulation of NK cell proteins involved in target cell lysis, such as perforin and granzymes (serine esterases).[74] In addition to the increased production of NK cells, there has been marked increase in immunomodulatory effects. Similarly, Bendich *et al.* reported that animals fed carotenoids had increased mitogenesis of T and B lymphocytes.[75]

Induction of Carcinogen-Metabolizing Enzymes

Several microsomal enzymes have shown to efficiently metabolize and detoxify carcinogens leading to lung cancer. Cytochrome P450 and aryl hydrocarbon hydroxylase (AHH) are involved in the metabolism and detoxification of benzo[a]pyrene and other polycyclic aromatic hydrocarbons found in cigarette smoke. Dietary components such as β-carotene found in fruits and vegetables have been proven to increase the activity of the carcinogen-metabolizing enzymes mainly in humans.

Another proposed model for the detoxification of the carcinogens is Phase II detoxification. Enzymes such as NAD(P)H, quinine oxidoreductase (NQO1), and γ-glutamylcysteine synthetase (GCS) detoxify many harmful substances by converting them to hydrophilic metabolites. Induction of the Phase II detoxification systems are mediated through *cis*-regulatory DNA sequences which are known as antioxidant-responsive elements. Transcription factors such as nuclear factor E2-related factor 2 (Nrf2) and active antioxidant responsive element (ARE) play a key role in induction of antioxidant and detoxifying genes.[76]

Inhibition of Cell Differentiation and Promotion of Apoptosis

Cell proliferation and differentiation are controlled by mitogens called the insulin-like growth factors (IGFs). IGF binding protein (IGFBP-3) regulates cell proliferation by shunning IGF-1 from its receptor, thereby inhibiting mitogenic activity. Lower levels of IGF-1 and IGFBP-3 have been implicated in the pathogenesis of lung cancer.[77] Studies conducted on animal models demonstrated that the administration of lycopene supplements was associated with an increase in plasma levels of IGFBP-3, which in turn decreased the proliferating cell nuclear antigen (PCNA) and phosphorylation of BAD.[78] Another study showed that the combination of β-carotene, α-tocopherol, and ascorbic acid plays an important role in apoptosis by regulating Bax levels during lung carcinogenesis.[79]

Interaction with Signaling Pathways

Six decades ago, studies pointed out the potential of flavonoids in cancer therapy. In last 10 years, several groups have shown that the biological effect of flavonoids is linked to their ability to modulate signaling pathways. For instance, flavonoids like EGCG, kaempferol, and quercetin can modulate different components of the NF-κB pathway, thereby inhibiting the translocation of this factor to the nucleus and activating target genes. This pathway plays important roles in the control of cell growth and apoptosis. The other two pathways targeted by flavonoids like kaempferol, quercetin, and isorhamnetin are the Akt and MAPK pathways, which are critical in mammalian cell survival signaling, and they have been shown to be activated in various cancers including lung cancer.

Another important signaling pathway involved in lung cancer is the Notch pathway, which is abnormally activated and leads to increased proliferation of cancers cells. Quercetin can decrease levels of the Notch 2 protein, hence leading to a reduction in proliferation rate of cancer cells. The Wnt pathway is key to many cellular processes; it controls embryonic axis formation, cell fate, proliferation, migration, tissue architecture, and organogenesis during development and play homeostatic roles in adult life. Ectopic expression of Wnt5a enhances motility of malignant cells and tumor invasion in lung cancer. In this regard, small molecules synthesized or from natural origins, like flavonoids, have been identified as potential modulators of the Wnt/β-catenin signaling pathway.[80]

Many studies have reported the effect of quercetin which controls the Wnt pathway directly by affecting components of the pathway in several types of cells. In 2005, Park and co-workers showed that quercetin interferes with the binding of Tcf complexes to DNA in colon cancer cells.[81] Consistently, another report showed that quercetin inhibits the expression of cyclin D1 and survivin as well as the Wnt/β-catenin signaling pathway. Currently, quercetin has been considered a Wnt pathway inhibitor, being used in similar studies as a negative control for modulation of this pathway.[82] From these findings, the molecular mechanism of fruits and vegetables and interaction of their active components with various signaling pathways are emphasized. Nevertheless, more research is still needed in this area to highlight their potential as therapeutic agents in fighting and preventing lung cancer.

EPIDEMIOLOGICAL STUDIES

Quite a number of epidemiological studies have reported the prevention of lung cancer by fruits and vegetables; however, in this chapter, we have highlighted only few studies which will be of considerable importance to assess the incidence and occurrence of lung cancer in the near future.

The strongest risk factor for lung cancer is attributed to cigarette smoking. However, the percentage of non-smokers affected with lung cancer is comparable to smokers, indicating the impact of environmental, genetic, and other miscellaneous factors in the development of lung cancer. Patients who never had a history of smoking and are not smoking were categorized as non-smokers and the rest as smokers. Evidences clearly indicate gender disparity among the people affected with lung cancer.[83] The histology of lung cancer differs in different parts of the world. In India, the most common histology is adenocarcinoma and squamous cell carcinoma rather than small and large cell carcinoma. However, the occurrence of large cell carcinoma and small cell carcinoma in India is comparatively lower than that in developed countries.[84]

Globally, from 1998–2002, the most predominant type of histology found among males is the squamous cell carcinoma, which accounted for 39.6% in the United Kingdom, 45.7% in Korea, and 40.8% in France. Among females, adenocarcinoma accounted for 44.3% of the population in France, 58.7% in Korea, and 23.5% in the United Kingdom. Twelve studies, including eight prospective cohort studies and four case control studies, conducted in several countries including the United States, Finland, the Netherlands, Spain, and Greece reported the association between intake of fruits and vegetables rich in flavonoids and lung cancer incidence. None of the flavonoid (flavonols, flavones, and catechins) studies considered lung cancer mortality.[85] Most of the studies reported a significantly lower risk of lung cancer with a high intake of flavonoids, whereas one study reported a significantly increased risk of lung cancer.[86] Therefore, more well-designed cohort and case-control studies are essential to strengthen the evidence on effects of long-term exposure to physiological doses of dietary flavonoids present in fruits and vegetables. A total of 16 cohort studies reported an association between dietary intake of carotenoids and lung cancer. Ten studies were conducted in the United States, four in Europe, and one each in Canada and Singapore. Eight studies included only men, three included only women, and five included both men and women. The protective role that carotenoids may play against lung cancer was studied by systematically evaluating a large, diverse body of epidemiologic evidences.[87] There was an overall statistically significant inverse association with lung cancer. Although β-carotene has been shown to be beneficial in preclinical and epidemiological studies, controversial results from large clinical trials have been disappointing.

Overall, epidemiological studies, *in vitro* tissue culture studies, animal studies, and now several human intervention studies are demonstrating that increased intake of β-carotene will result in preventing or reducing the risk of several cancers. The mechanism of action of β-carotene suggests that in *in vivo* conditions, this compound acts as a potent antioxidant and protect cells against oxidative damage and thereby prevent or reduce the risk of lung cancer. Further studies are needed to obtain more concrete proof and to gain better understanding of the mechanisms involved. Updated information from the European Prospective Investigation into Cancer and Nutrition (EPIC) on fruits and vegetables intake and lung cancer risk strengthened the scientific evidence on the role of fruit and vegetable consumption in primary lung cancer prevention. In the whole study population, fruit consumption was significantly inversely associated with lung cancer risk, while no association was found for vegetable consumption. In current smokers, however, lung cancer risk significantly decreased with higher vegetable consumption. Cancer incidence decreased with higher consumption of apples and pears (entire cohort) as well as root vegetables (smokers). In addition to an overall inverse association with fruit consumption, the results of this study add evidence for a significant inverse association of vegetable consumption and lung cancer incidence in smokers.[88]

CONCLUSION

The general nutritional principles indicate that the healthy diets should include at least moderate amounts of fruit and vegetables, sufficient to prevent deficiencies of any nutrients, especially micronutrients such as vitamin C, folic acid, and selenium, which are mostly supplied by fruits and vegetables. It is well known that a number of substances in fruits and vegetables may contribute to the reduction of lung cancer risk. Lung cancer risk was modestly lower with a higher consumption of both fruits and vegetables, particularly with a diet rich in carotenoids-, flavonoids-, vitamins-, folic acid-, phytoestrogens-, and isothiocyanates-based products. Moreover, as suggested by many cohort and case-control studies, the reduction in lung cancer risk with the intake of fruits and vegetables was observed to be greater in women than in men worldwide. This may be due to several risk factors including smoking and consumption of alcohol by men, which will increase lung cancer incidence and correspondingly, there is another statement that the consumption of fruits reduces lung cancer risk more than if vegetables were consumed. Thus it is essential in conducting a large international cohort study that takes advantage of the complexities of these difficulties mentioned above and to characterize the strength of the association of fruits and vegetables with lung cancer. Even though there are some limitations and concerns regarding case control studies to associate the effect of fruits and vegetables consumption on lung cancer, the overall data obtained so far highlight and add some weight to the hypothesis that a daily intake of fruits and vegetables is associated with a reduced risk of cancer mortality, specifically cancers of the lung.

REFERENCES

1. "Lung Carcinoma: Tumors of the Lungs: Merck Manual Professional." *pulmonary_disorders/tumors_of_the_lungs /lung_carcinoma.* N.p., n.d. Web. 4 Sept. 2013.
2. Stoppler, M.C., Lung cancer, causes, types, and treatment, retrieved from Medicine Net Inc., 2009. [Online] URL http://www.medicinenet.com/lung cancer (2009).
3. Bonomi, P.D., Implications of key trials in advanced non-small cell lung cancer, *Cancer* **116**(5): 1155–1164 (2010).
4. NCCN Clinical Practice Guidelines in Oncology (NCCN Guidelines). Non-small cell lung cancer, National Comprehensive Cancer, Network 2012.2 (2012).

5. Langer, C.J., T. Mok, and P.E. Postmus, Targeted agents in the third-/fourth-line treatment of patients with advanced (stage III/IV) non-small cell lung cancer (NSCLC), *Cancer Treat Rev* **39**(3): 252–260 (2012).
6. Heintz, N.H., Y.M. Janssen-Heininger, and B.T. Mossman, Asbestos, lung cancers, and mesotheliomas: From molecular approaches to targeting tumor survival pathways, *Am J Respir Cell Mol Biol* **42**(2): 133–139 (2010).
7. Clément-Duchêne, C., J.M. Vignaud, A. Stoufflet, O. Bertrand, A. Gislard, L. Thiberville, G. Grosdidier, Y. Martinet, J. Benichou, P. Hainaut, and C. Paris, Characteristics of never smoker lung cancer including environmental and occupational risk factors, *Lung Cancer* **67**(2): 144–150 (2010).
8. Steinmetz, K.A. and J.D. Porter, Vegetables, fruits and cancer, I. Epidemiology, *Cancer Cont* **2**(5): 325–327 (1991).
9. Block, G., B. Patterson, and A. Subar, Fruit, vegetables, and cancer prevention: A review of the epidemiological evidence, *Nutr Cancer* **18**(1): 1–29 (1992).
10. Palozza, P., S. Serena, F. Di Nicuolo, and G. Calviello, Modulation of apoptotic signaling by carotenoids in cancer cells, *Arch Biochem Biophys* **430**(1): 104–109 (2004).
11. Jeong, S.J., W. Koh, B. Kim, and Sung-Hoon Kim, Are there new therapeutic options for treating lung cancer based on herbal medicines and their metabolites? *J Ethnopharmacol* **138**(3): 652–661 (2011).
12. Greenwald, P., C.K. Clifford, and J. Milner, A diet and cancer prevention, *Eur J of Cancer* **37**(8): 948–965 (2001).
13. Hecht, S.S., P.M. Kenney, M. Wang, N. Trushin, S. Agarwal, A.V. Rao, and P. Upadhyaya, Evaluation of butylated hydroxyanisole, myo-inositol, curcumin, esculetin, resveratrol and lycopene as inhibitors of benzo[a]pyrene plus 4-(methylnitrosamino)-1-(3-pyridyl)-1-butanone-induced lung tumorigenesis in A/J mice, *Cancer Lett* **137**(2): 123–130 (1999).
14. Liu, C., F. Lian, D.E. Smith, R.M. Russell, and X.D. Wang, Lycopene supplementation inhibits lung squamous metaplasia and induces apoptosis via up-regulating insulin-like growth factor-binding protein 3 in cigarette smoke-exposed ferrets, *Cancer Res* **63**(12): 3138–3144 (2003).
15. Liu, C., R.T. Bronson, R.M. Russell, and X.D. Wang, β-cryptoxanthin supplementation prevents cigarette smoke-induced lung inflammation, oxidative damage, and squamous metaplasia in ferrets, *Cancer Prev Res (Phila)* **4**(8): 1255–1266 (2011).
16. Iskandar, A.R., C. Liu, D.E. Smith, K.Q. Hu, S.W. Choi, L.M. Ausman, and X.D. Wang, β-cryptoxanthin restores nicotine-reduced lung SIRT1 to normal levels and inhibits nicotine-promoted lung tumorigenesis and emphysema in A/J mice, *Cancer Prev Res (Phila)* **6**(4): 309–320 (2013).

17. Männistö, S., S.A. Smith-Warner, D. Spiegelman, D. Albanes, K. Anderson, P.A. van den Brandt, J.R. Cerhan, G. Colditz, D. Feskanich, J.L. Freudenheim, E. Giovannucci, R.A. Goldbohm, S. Graham, A.B. Miller, T.E. Rohan, J. Virtamo, W.C. Willett, and D.J. Hunter, Dietary carotenoids and risk of lung cancer in a pooled analysis of seven cohort studies, *Cancer Epidemiol Biomarkers Prev* **13**(1): 40–48 (2004).
18. Ito, Y., K. Wakai, K. Suzuki, A. Tamakoshi, N. Seki, M. Ando, Y. Nishino, T. Kondo, Y. Watanabe, K. Ozasa, and Y. Ohno, JACC Study Group, Serum carotenoids and mortality from lung cancer: A case-control study nested in the Japan Collaborative Cohort (JACC) study, *Cancer Sci* **94**(1): 57–63 (2003).
19. Kuo, P.C., H.F. Liu, and J.I. Chao, Survivin and p53 modulate quercetin-induced cell growth inhibition and apoptosis in human lung carcinoma cells, *J Biol Chem* **279**(53): 55875–55885 (2004).
20. Youn, H., J.C. Jeong, Y.S. Jeong, E.J. Kim, and S.J. Um, Quercetin potentiates apoptosis by inhibiting nuclear factor-kappaB signaling in H460 lung cancer cells, *Biol Pharm Bull* **36**(6): 944–951 (2013).
21. Banerjee, T., A. Van der Vliet, and V.A. Ziboh, Downregulation of COX-2 and iNOS by amentoflavone and quercetin in A549 human lung adenocarcinoma cell line, *Prostaglandins Leukot Essent Fatty Acids* **66**(5–6): 485–492 (2002).
22. Nguyen, T.T., E. Tran, T.H. Nguyen, P.T. Do, T.H. Huynh, and H. Huynh, The role of activated MEK–ERK pathway in quercetin-induced growth inhibition and apoptosis in A549 lung cancer cells, *Carcinogenesis* **25**(5): 647–659 (2004).
23. Lam, T.K., M. Rotunno, J.H. Lubin, S. Wacholder, D. Consonni, A.C. Pesatori, P.A. Bertazzi, S.J. Chanock, L. Burdette, A.M. Goldstein, M.A. Tucker, N.E. Caporaso, A.F. Subar, and M.T. Landi, Dietary quercetin, quercetin–gene interaction, metabolic gene expression in lung tissue and lung cancer risk, *Carcinogenesis* **31**(4): 634–642 (2010).
24. Jin, N.Z., Y.P. Zhu, J.W. Zhou, L. Mao, R.C. Zhao, T.H. Fang, and X.R. Wang, Preventive effects of quercetin against benzo[a]pyrene-induced DNA damages and pulmonary precancerous pathologic changes in mice, *Basic Clin Pharmacol Toxicol* **98**(6): 593–598 (2006).
25. Khanduja, K.L., R.K. Gandhi, V. Pathania, and N. Syal, Prevention of N-nitrosodiethylamine-induced lung tumorigenesis by ellagic acid and quercetin in mice, *Food Chem Toxicol* **37**(4): 313–318 (1999).
26. Nguyen, T.T., E. Tran, C.K. Ong, S.K. Lee, P.T. Do, T.T. Huynh, T.H. Nguyen, J.J. Lee, Y. Tan, C.S. Ong, and H. Huynh, Kaempferol-induced growth inhibition and apoptosis in A549 lung cancer cells is mediated by activation of MEK–MAPK, *J Cell Physiol* **197**(1): 110–121 (2003).

27. Leung, H.W., C.J. Lin, M.J. Hour, W.H. Yang, M.Y. Wang, and H.Z. Lee, Kaempferol induces apoptosis in human lung non-small carcinoma cells accompanied by an induction of antioxidant enzymes, *Food Chem Toxicol* **45**(10): 2005–2013 (2007).
28. Ravichandran, N., G. Suresh, B. Ramesh, and G.V. Siva, Fisetin, a novel flavonol attenuates benzo(a)pyrene-induced lung carcinogenesis in Swiss albino mice, *Food Chem Toxicol* **49**(5): 1141–1147 (2011).
29. Tang, N.P., B. Zhou, B. Wang, R.B. Yu, and J. Ma, Flavonoids intake and risk of lung cancer: A meta-analysis, *Jpn J Clin Oncol* **39**(6): 352–359 (2009).
30. Palgi, A., Vitamin A and lung cancer: A perspective, *Nutr Cancer* **6**(2): 105–120 (1985).
31. Fritz, H., D. Kennedy, D. Fergusson, R. Fernandes, S. Doucette, K. Cooley, A. Seely, S. Sagar, R. Wong, and D. Seely, Vitamin A and retinoid derivatives for lung cancer: A systematic review and meta analysis, *PLoS One* **6**(6): e21107 (2011).
32. Li, W., J.X. Wu, and Y.Y. Tu, Synergistic effects of tea polyphenols and ascorbic acid on human lung adenocarcinoma SPC-A-1 cells, *J Zhejiang Univ Sci B* **11**(6): 458–464 (2010).
33. Dey, N., D.J. Chattopadhyay, and I.B. Chatterjee, Molecular mechanisms of cigarette smoke-induced proliferation of lung cells and prevention by vitamin C, *J Oncol* **2011**: 561862 (2011).
34. Vuyyuri, S.B., J. Rinkinen, E. Worden, H. Shim, S. Lee, and K.R. Davis, Ascorbic acid and a cytostatic inhibitor of glycolysis synergistically induce apoptosis in non-small cell lung cancer cells, *PLoS One* **8**(6): e67081 (2013).
35. Gao, Y., W. Li, L. Jia, B. Li, Y.C. Chen, and Y. Tu, Enhancement of (−)-epigallocatechin-3-gallate and theaflavin-3-3′-digallate induced apoptosis by ascorbic acid in human lung adenocarcinoma SPC-A-1 cells and esophageal carcinoma Eca-109 cells via MAPK pathways, *Biochem Biophys Res Commun* **438**(2): 370–374 (2013).
36. Kim, Y., N. Chongviriyaphan, C. Liu, R.M. Russell, and X.D. Wang, Combined α-tocopherol and ascorbic acid protects against smoke-induced lung squamous metaplasia in ferrets, *Lung Cancer* **75**(1): 15–23 (2012).
37. Chen, M.F., C.M. Yang, C.M. Su, J.W. Liao, and M.L. Hu, Inhibitory effect of vitamin C in combination with vitamin K3 on tumor growth and metastasis of Lewis lung carcinoma xenografted in C57BL/6 mice, *Nutr Cancer* **63**(7): 1036–1043 (2011).
38. Bandera, E.V., J.L. Freudenheim, J.R. Marshall, M. Zielezny, R.L. Priore, J. Brasure, M. Baptiste, and S. Graham, Diet and alcohol consumption and

lung cancer risk in the New York State Cohort (United States), *Cancer Causes Control* **8**(6): 828–840 (1997).

39. Lee, D.H., and D.R. Jacobs Jr., Interaction among heme iron, zinc, and supplemental vitamin C intake on the risk of lung cancer: Iowa Women's Health Study, *Nutr Cancer* **52**(2): 130–137 (2005).
40. Lambert, J.D., G. Lu, M.J. Lee, J. Hu, J. Ju, and C.S. Yang, Inhibition of lung cancer growth in mice by dietary mixed tocopherols, *Mol Nutr Food Res* **53**(8): 1030–1035 (2009).
41. Li, G.X., M.J. Lee, A.B. Liu, Z. Yang, Y. Lin, W.J. Shih, and C.S. Yang, δ-tocopherol is more active than α- or γ-tocopherol in inhibiting lung tumorigenesis *in vivo*, *Cancer Prev Res (Phila)* **4**(3): 404–413 (2011).
42. Gill, K.K., A. Kaddoumi, and S. Nazzal, Mixed micelles of PEG(2000)-DSPE and vitamin-E TPGS for concurrent delivery of paclitaxel and parthenolide: Enhanced chemosenstization and antitumor efficacy against non-small cell lung cancer (NSCLC) cell lines, *Eur J Pharm Sci* **46**(1–2): 64–71 (2012).
43. Zarogoulidis, P., A. Cheva, K. Zarampouka, H. Huang, C. Li, Y. Huang, N. Katsikogiannis, and K. Zarogoulidis, Tocopherols and tocotrienols as anticancer treatment for lung cancer: Future nutrition, *J Thorac Dis* **5**(3): 349–352 (2013).
44. Ju, J., S.C. Picinich, Z. Yang, Y. Zhao, N. Suh, A.N. Kong, and C.S. Yang, Cancer-preventive activities of tocopherols and tocotrienols, *Carcinogenesis* **31**(4): 533–542 (2010).
45. Ji, X., Z. Wang, F.H. Sarkar, and S.V. Gupta, Delta-tocotrienol augments cisplatin-induced suppression of non-small cell lung cancer cells via inhibition of the Notch-1 pathway, *Anticancer Res* **32**(7): 2647–2655 (2012).
46. Song, H., J. Kim, H.K. Lee, H.J. Park, J. Nam, G.B. Park, Y.S. Kim, D. Cho, and D.Y. Hur, Selenium inhibits migration of murine melanoma cells via down-modulation of IL-18 expression, *Int Immunopharmacol* **11**(12): 2208–2213 (2011).
47. Shi, Y.Q., X. Chen, J. Dai, Z.F. Jiang, N. Li, B.Y. Zhang, and Z.B. Zhang, Selenium pretreatment attenuates formaldehyde-induced genotoxicity in A549 cell lines, *Toxicol Ind Health* [Epub ahead of print] (2012).
48. Li, J., J.C. Tharappel, S.G. Han, A.H. Cantor, E.Y. Lee, C.G. Gairola, and H.P. Glauert, Effect of dietary selenium and cigarette smoke on pulmonary cell proliferation in mice, *Toxicol Sci* **111**(2): 247–253 (2009).
49. Glauert, H.P., J.B. Martin, J. Li, J.C. Tharappel, S.G. Han, H.D. Gillespie, A.H. Cantor, E.Y. Lee, and C. Gary Gairola, Dietary selenium fails to influence

cigarette smoke-induced lung tumorigenesis in A/J mice, *Cancer Lett* **334**(1): 127–132 (2013).

50. Yan, L. and L.C. DeMars, Dietary supplementation with methylseleninic acid, but not selenomethionine, reduces spontaneous metastasis of Lewis lung carcinoma in mice, *Int J Cancer* **31**(6): 1260–1266(2012).
51. Karelia, N., D. Desai, J.A. Hengst, S. Amin, S.V. Rudrabhatla, and J. Yun, Selenium-containing analogs of SAHA induce cytotoxicity in lung cancer cells, *Bioorg Med Chem Lett* **20**(22): 6816–6819 (2010).
52. Wang, L., J.N. Fu, J.Y. Wang, C.J. Jin, X.Y. Ren, Q. Tan, J. Li, H.W. Yin, K. Xiong, T.Y. Wang, X.M. Liu, and H.H. Zeng, Selenium-containing thioredoxin reductase inhibitor ethaselen sensitizes non-small cell lung cancer to radiotherapy, *Anticancer Drugs* **22**(8): 732–740 (2011).
53. Jaworska, K., S. Gupta, K. Durda, M. Muszyńska, G. Sukiennicki, E. Jaworowska, T. Grodzki, M. Sulikowski, P. Woloszczyk, J. Wójcik, J. Lubiński, C. Cybulski, T. Dębniak, M. Lener, A.W. Morawski, K. Krzystolik, S.A. Narod, P. Sun, J. Lubiński, and A. Jakubowska, A low selenium level is associated with lung and laryngeal cancers, *PLoS One* **8**(3): e59051 (2013).
54. Zeng, Y.C., M. Xue, F. Chi, Z.G. Xu, G.L. Fan, Y.C. Fan, M.H. Zheng, W.Z. Zhong, S.L. Wang, Z.Y. Zhang, X.D. Chen, L.N. Wu, X.Y. Jin, W. Chen, Q. Li, X.Y. Zhang, Y.P. Xiao, R. Wu, and Q.Y. Guo, Serum levels of selenium in patients with brain metastases from non-small cell lung cancer before and after radiotherapy, *Cancer Radiother* **16**(3): 179–182 (2012).
55. Cao, R., W. Pens, Z. Wang, and A. Xu, Beta-Carboline Alkaloids: Biochemical and pharmacological functions, *Curr Med Chem* **14**(4): 479–500 (2007).
56. Choi, S.H., S.H. Lee, H.J. Kim, I.S. Lee, N. Kozukue, C.E. Levin, and M. Friedman, Changes in free amino acid, phenolic, chlorophyll, carotenoid, and glycoalkaloid contents in tomatoes during 11 stages of growth and inhibition of cervical and lung human cancer cells by green tomato extracts, *J Agricult Food Chem* **58**(13): 7547–7556 (2010).
57. Shih, Y.W., P.S. Chen, C.H. Wu, Y.F. Jeng, and C.J. Wang, α-chaconine-reduced metastasis involves a PI3K/Akt signaling pathway with downregulation of NF-κB in human lung adenocarcinoma A549 cells, *J Agricult Food Chem* **55**(26): 11035–11043 (2007).
58. Shieh, J.M., T.H. Cheng, M.D. Shi, P.F. Wu, Y. Chen, S.C. Ko, and Y.W. Shih, α-tomatine suppresses invasion and migration of human non-small cell lung cancer NCI-H460 cells through inactivating FAK/PI3K/Akt signaling pathway and reducing binding activity of NF-κB, *Cell Biochem Biophys* **60**(3): 297–310 (2011).

59. Ebbing, M., K.H. Bønaa, O. Nygård, E. Arnesen, P.M. Ueland, J.E. Nordrehaug, K. Rasmussen, I. Njølstad, H. Refsum, D.W. Nilsen, A. Tverdal, K. Meyer, and S.E. Vollset, Cancer incidence and mortality after treatment with folic acid and vitamin B12, *J Am Med Assoc* **302**(19): 2119–2216 (2009).
60. Voorrips, L.E., R.A. Goldbohm, H.A. Brants, G.A. van Poppel, F. Sturmans, R.J. Hermus, and P.A. van den Brandt, A prospective cohort study on antioxidant and folate intake and male lung cancer risk, *Cancer Epidemiol Biomarkers Prev* **9**(4): 357–365 (2000).
61. Gallo, D., G.F. Zannoni, I. Stanafo, M. Mosca, C. Ferlini, E. Mantuano, and G. Scambia, Soy phytochemical decrease non-small cell lung growth in female athymic mice, *J Nutr* **138**(7): 1360–1364 (2008).
62. Hess, D. and R.A. Igal, Genistein downregulates *de novo* lipid synthesis and impairs cell proliferation in human lung cancer cells, *Exp Biol Med (Maywood)* **236**(6): 707–713 (2011).
63. Wu, T.C., Y.C. Yang, P.R. Huang, Y.D. Wen, and S.L. Yeh, Genistein enhances the effect of trichostatin A on inhibition of A549 cell growth by increasing expression of TNF receptor-1, *Toxicol Appl Pharmacol* **262**(3): 247–254 (2012).
64. Li, X., X. Wang, H. Ye, A. Peng, and L. Chen, Barbigerone, an isoflavone, inhibits tumor angiogenesis and human non-small-cell lung cancer xenografts growth through VEGFR2 signaling pathways, *Cancer Chemother Pharmacol* **70**(3): 425–437 (2012).
65. Peng, B., J. Cao, S. Yi, C. Wang, G. Zheng, and Z. He, Inhibition of proliferation and induction of G1-phase cell-cycle arrest by dFMGEN, a novel genistein derivative, in lung carcinoma A549 cells, *Drug Chem Toxicol* **36**(2): 196–204 (2013).
66. Matthew, B., L. Hernandez, X. Wu, P.C. Pillow, and R. Margaret, Dietary phytoestrogens and lung cancer risk, *JAMA* **294**(12): 1493–1504 (2005).
67. Yang, G., X.O. Shu, W.H. Chow, X. Zhang, H.L. Li, B.T. Ji, H. Cai, S. Wu, Y.T Gao, and W. Zheng, Soy food intake and risk of lung cancer: Evidence from the Shanghai Women's Health Study and a meta-analysis, *Am J Epidemiol* **176**(10): 846–855 (2012).
68. Shimazu, T., M. Inoue, S. Sasazuki, M. Iwasaki, N. Sawada, T. Yamaji, and S. Tsugane, JPHC Study Group, Plasma isoflavones and the risk of lung cancer in women: A nested case-control study in Japan, *Cancer Epidemiol Biomarkers Prev* **20**(3): 419–427 (2011).
69. Shimazu, T., M. Inoue, S. Sasazuki, M. Iwasaki, N. Sawada, T. Yamaji, and S. Tsugane, Japan Public Health Center-based Prospective Study Group, Isoflavone intake and risk of lung cancer: A prospective cohort study in Japan, *Am J Clin Nutr* **91**(3): 722–728 (2010).

70. Wu, X., Y. Zhu, H. Yan, B. Liu, H. Li, Q. Zhou, and K. Xu, Isothiocyanates induce oxidative stress and suppress the metastasis potential of human non-small cell lung cancer cells, *BMC Cancer* **10**: 269 (2010).
71. Priya, D.K., R. Gayathri, G.R. Gunassekaran, S. Murugan, and D. Sakthisekaran, Chemopreventive role of sulforaphane by upholding the GSH redox cycle in pre- and post-initiation phases of experimental lung carcinogenesis, *Asian Pacific J Cancer Prev* **12**: 103–110 (2011).
72. Hecht, S.S., F. Kassie, and D.K. Hatsukami, Chemoprevention of lung carcinogenesis in addicted smokers and ex-smokers, *Nat Rev Cancer* **9**(7): 476–488 (2009).
73. Rao, A.V., M.R. Ray, and L.G. Rao, Lycopene, *Adv Food Nutr Res* **51**: 99–164 (2006).
74. Santos, S.M., S.N. Meydani, L. Leka, W.U. Dayong, N. Fotouhi, M. Meydani, C.H. Hennekens, and J.M. Gaziano, Natural killer cell activity in elderly men is enhanced by β-carotene supplementation, *Am J Clin Nutr* **64**(5): 772–777 (1996).
75. Bendich, A. and S.S. Shapiro, Effect of beta-carotene and canthaxanthin on immune response of the rat, *J Nutr* **116**(11): 2254–2262 (1986).
76. Talalay, P., J.W. Fahey, W.D. Holtzclaw, T. Prestera, and Y. Zhang, Chemoprotection against cancer by phase 2 enzyme induction, *Toxicol Lett* **82**: 173–179 (1995).
77. Yu, H. and T. Rohan, Role of the insulin-like growth factor family in cancer development and progression, *J Natl Cancer Inst* **92**: 1472–1489 (2000).
78. Liu, C., F. Lian, D.E. Smith, R.M. Russell, and X.D. Wang, Lycopene supplementation inhibits lung squamous metaplasia and induces apoptosis via up-regulating insulin-like growth factor-binding protein 3 in cigarette smoke exposed ferrets, *Cancer Res* **63**(12): 3138–3144 (2003).
79. Kim, Y., N. Chongviriyaphan, C. Liu, R.M. Russell, and X.D. Wang, Combined antioxidant (β-carotene, α-tocopherol and ascorbic acid) supplementation increases the levels of lung retinoic acid and inhibits the activation of mitogen-activated protein kinase in the ferret lung cancer model, *Carcinogenesis* **27**(7): 1410–1419 (2006).
80. Sarkar, F.H., Y. Li, Z. Wang, and D. Kong, Cellular signaling perturbation by natural products, *Cell Signal* **21**(11): 1541–1547 (2009).
81. Park, C.H., J.Y. Chang, E.R. Hahm, S. Park, H.K. Kim, and C.H. Yang, Quercetin, a potent inhibitor against ß-catenin/Tcf signaling in SW480 colon cancer cells, *Biochem Biophys Res Commun* **328**(1): 227–234 (2005).
82. Kawahara, T., N. Kawaguchi-Ihara, Y. Okuhashi, M. Itoh, N. Nara, and S. Tohda, Cyclopamine and quercetin suppress the growth of leukemia and lymphoma cells, *Anticancer Res* **29**(11): 4629–4632 (2009).

83. Lam, W.K., Lung cancer in Asian women — the environment and genes, *Respirology* **10**(4): 408–417 (2005).
84. Curado, M.P., B. Edwards, H.R. Shin, H. Storm, J. Ferlay, M. Heanue, and P. Boyle (Eds.), *Cancer Incidence in Five Continents, Vol. IX*, IARC Scientific Publications, Lyon (2007).
85. Arts, C.W., A review of the epidemiological evidence on tea, flavonoids, and lung cancer, *J Nutr* **138**(8): 1561–1566 (2008).
86. Lagiou, P., E. Samoli, A. Lagiou, K. Katsouyanni, J. Peterson, J. Dwyer, and D. Trichopoulos, Flavonoid intake in relation to lung cancer risk: Casecontrol study among women in Greece, *Nutr Cancer* **49**(2): 139–143 (2004).
87. Gallicchio, L., K Boyd, G. Matanoski, X.G. Tao, L. Chen, T.K. Lam, M. Shiels, E. Hammond, K.A. Robinson, L.E. Caulfield, J.E. Herman, E. Guallar, and A.J. Alberg, Carotenoids and the risk of developing lung cancer: A systematic Review, *Am J Clin Nutr* **88**(2): 372–383 (2008).
88. Linseisen, J., S. Rohrmann, A.B. Miller, H.B. Bueno-de-Mesquita, F.L. Büchner, P. Vineis, A. Agudo, I.T. Gram, L. Janson, V. Krogh, K. Overvad, T. Rasmuson, M. Schulz, T. Pischon, R. Kaaks, A. Nieters, N.E. Allen, T.J. Key, S. Bingham, K.T. Khaw, P. Amiano, A. Barricarte, C. Martinez, C. Navarro, R. Quirós, F. Clavel-Chapelon, M.C. Boutron-Ruault, M. Touvier, P.H. Peeters, G. Berglund, G. Hallmans, E. Lund, D. Palli, S. Panico, R. Tumino, A. Tjønneland, A. Olsen, A. Trichopoulou, D. Trichopoulos, P. Autier, P. Boffetta, N. Slimani, and E. Riboli, Fruit and vegetable consumption and lung cancer risk: Updated information from the European Prospective Investigation into Cancer and Nutrition (EPIC), *Int J Cancer* **121**(5): 1103–1114 (2007).

9

Prostate Cancer: How Helpful are Natural Agents for Prevention?

Manoj K. Pandey, Ajaikumar B. Kunnumakkara and Shantu G. Amin*

INTRODUCTION

Prostate cancer (PCa) is the most common non-skin cancer in men in the world and second-leading cancer in American men with approximately 220,000 new cases and 32,000 deaths of PCa in 2012 (www.cancer.org). Out of the three well-known and indisputable risk factors, i.e., increasing age, ethnic origin, and hereditary/familial factors, age is the most significant risk factor for the development of prostate cancer, with a prevalence of approximately 35% in 60–69-year-old and 46% in 70–81-year-old men.[1,2] Growths in the prostate can be benign (non-cancerous) or malignant (cancerous) (Fig. 9.1).The PCa cells can spread by breaking away from a prostate tumor. These cells travel through blood vessels or lymph vessels, spread to other regions of the body, and grow to form new tumors that may damage those tissues. When PCa spreads from its original site to another part of the body, the new tumor has the same kind of abnormal cells as the primary tumor and is referred to as a secondary tumor. For example, if PCa spreads to the bones, the cancer cells in the bones are actually PCa cells. The disease is called metastatic prostate cancer, not bone cancer. How initiation

*Corresponding author: Manoj K. Pandey, Ph.D., Assistant Professor, Department of Pharmacology-CH72, Penn State College of Medicine, 500 University Drive, Hershey, PA 17033, USA. Tel: (+1) 717-531-0003 (ext. 284001), Fax: (+1) 717-531-5013, Email: mkp13@psu.edu.

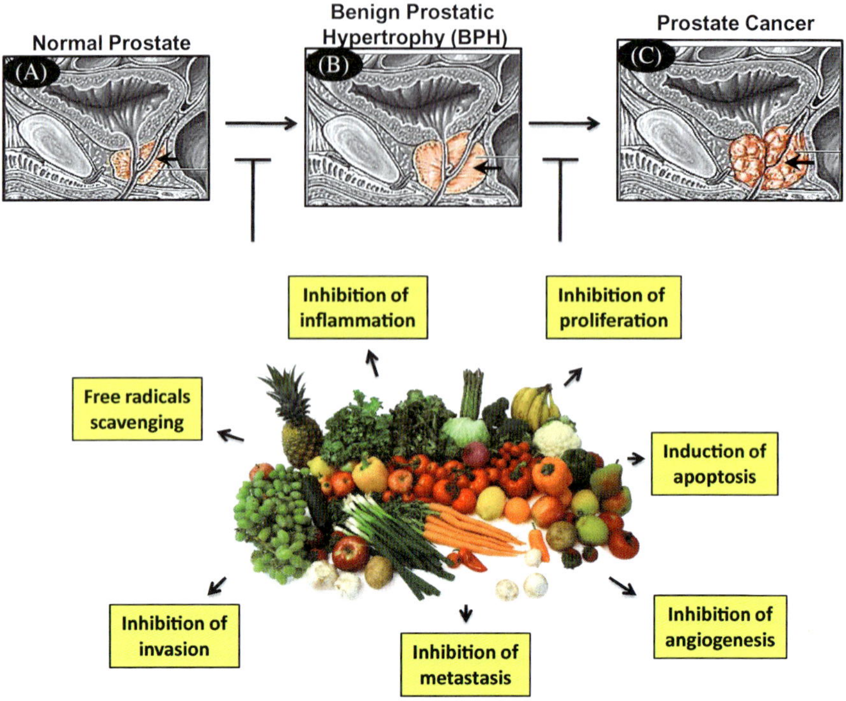

Figure 9.1: Fruits and vegetables prevent the initiation, promotion, and progression of prostate cancer (PCa) by different mechanisms.

and progression of PCa takes place is beyond the scope of the present chapter (see Ref. 3 for more details). This chapter will instead cover the markers of PCa, critical signaling pathways, and importance of diets (mainly fruits- and vegetables-based) for PCa prevention.

MARKERS OF PROSTATE CANCER

A number of markers associated with the prostate gland have been identified to date including prostate-specific antigen (PSA),[4] prostate carcinoma-associated glycoprotein complex (PAC),[5] prostatic acid phosphatase (PAP), prostate mucin antigen (PMA),[6] and prostate-specific membrane antigen (PSMA).[7] However, only a subset of these markers is elevated in or specifically associated with PCa.

GENETICS AND THE ROLE OF SIGNALING PATHWAYS IN THE DEVELOPMENT OF PROSTATE CANCER

PCa can be divided epidemiologically into hereditary and sporadic forms, with the latter being the most common. Although candidate-inherited prostate cancer susceptibility genes have been identified, such as *ELAC2*, *RNASEL*, *MSR1*, *NSB1*, and *CHEK2*, the proportion of cases of hereditary PCa attributable to germline mutations in these loci is small, and only occasional mutations in these candidate genes have been identified in sporadic PCa.[8–14]

The most common genetic irregularities in PCa are amplification of *c-MYC* and the androgen receptor (AR), mutation of *p53*, hemizygous deletion at 8p21 thought to target *NKX3.1*, and loss or mutation of *RB1*.[14] In 1997, the tumor suppressor gene *PTEN* was cloned from the 10q23 region, a region frequently targeted by loss of heterozygosity (LOH) in advanced cancers including PCa.[14–16] Thus, somatic inactivation of *PTEN* is common in PCa and it has become clear that the loss of *PTEN* and consequent activation of Akt is a critical event in the development of this disease, which presents a pathway for rationally targeted molecular therapeutics for the management of this disease.[14]

Somatic Mutation of *PTEN* or PI3K Pathway Genes in Human PCa

Inactivating mutations in PTEN

The discovery of somatic alterations in the PI3K pathway in PCa began with observations of LOH in the region of 10q (mainly 10q22–q24 and 10q25), which occurs at a high frequency of 30–60%,[14,17,18] which implies the presence of putative tumor suppressor genes at these loci.[14,18] Interest in genetic alterations in *PTEN* in PCa started with the observation that two of the three most commonly used PCa cell lines, PC-3 and LNCaP, harbor either a deletion (PC-3) or a point mutation in *PTEN* (LNCaP).[15] Somatic *PTEN* alterations have been reported for both localized and metastatic PCas (more common), and these include homozygous deletions, LOH, and inactivating missense and nonsense mutations.[19–23] These studies suggest that the prevalence of *PTEN* mutation increases in the metastatic PCa.

Alterations in IGFI in human PCa

An association between plasma levels of IGF-1 and the risk of death from prostate cancer has been observed in prospective population-based cohort studies.[14,24] These studies suggest that men who are in the top quintile of IGF1 levels have an increased risk of death from PCa. However, recent studies have failed to find this association.[14]

Akt, a Regulator of mTOR and Its Role in PCa

Loss-of-function mutations in *PTEN* lead to the activation of mammalian target of rapamycin (mTOR) pathway by either Akt-dependent inactivation of tuberous sclerosis (TSC)-2 or phosphoinositide-dependent kinase (PDK)-1-dependent activation of p70S6K. In either case, cells lacking *PTEN* or harboring activated alleles of Akt show high levels of mTOR activity which affects the regulation of cell size, organ size, and cell growth controls.[14] mTOR phosphorylates substrates critical for protein synthesis such as ribosomal subunit S6 kinase (S6K) and eukaryotic initiation factor 4E binding protein-1 (4E-BP1).[25] How mTOR activation leads to cellular transformation is still poorly understood in PCa.[14] However, it is now well established that activation of the Akt/mTOR pathway is common in PCa and induces in tumor promotion, progression, and resistance to chemotherapeutic agents.

NF-κB Signaling in Human PCa

The nuclear factor-kappaB (NF-κB) transcription factor is an important regulator of innate and adaptive immune responses, inflammation, and developmental processes.[26] Recent studies have shown that NF-κB plays a critical role in tumor initiation and progression. In resting cells, nearly every combination of the NF-κB family members (RelA, RelB, c-Rel, NF-κB1/p50, and NF-κB2/p52) forms a complex with IκB proteins in the cytoplasm.[26] Upon stimulation with bacterial or viral components, surface receptors, irradiation, or chemotherapeutic agents, the IκB proteins become phosphorylated and subsequently degraded, resulting in the translocation of NF-κB into the nucleus. Upon entering the nucleus, it binds to promoter and enhancer sites of its target genes and initiate the transcription of genes that are involved in PCa cell proliferation, survival (survivin), invasion, metastases, angiogenesis, chemoresistance, and radiation therapy resistance (Bcl-2, Bcl-x_L, cIAP1, survivin, cyclin D1, cyclin D2, VEGF, IL-6, IL-8, MMP-9, etc.).[26–28] It has been shown that androgen-independent PCa cell lines (PC-3 or DU145) express constitive NF-κB activation for their growth and inhibition of NF-κB either by pharmacological inhibitors or by the overexpression of a dominant negative mutant of IκBα (IκBα DN) caused apoptosis in these cell lines.[29] These studies show that chronic NF-κB activation replace AR to ensure cell survival and proliferation in an androgen-deprived environment, and the inhibition of NF-κB activation could be an effective therapy for the treatment of castration-resistant (CR) PCa. Increasing lines of evidence suggest that the inhibitor of NF-κB kinase subunit alpha (IKK-α, also known as IKK1) mediates the p52-dependent increase in nuclear AR, epigenetic regulation of MASPIN expression, and the mTOR pathway in PCa, and pharmacological inhibitors especially derived from natural agents such as butein[30] and gambogic acid[31] specific for IKK1 could be of use for the treatment of CR-PCa.[32]

PROSTATE CANCER PREVENTION: IS IT POSSIBLE?

Originally proposed by Sporn *et al.* in 1976, the classical definition of cancer chemoprevention is the use of natural, synthetic, or biological chemical agents to reverse, suppress, or prevent either the initial phase of carcinogenesis or the progression of neoplastic cells to cancer.[33,34] Research over the past several years revealed that carcinogenesis is a multi-step process which involves initiation, promotion, progression, tissue invasion, metastasis, and angiogenesis. During the process of carcinogenesis, many molecular changes take place inside the cell, such as genetic and epigenetic alterations, inactivation of tumor suppressor genes, activation of oncogenes, and modulation of different signaling pathways.[35] Identifying molecular mechanisms involved in carcinogenesis provides strong rationales for developing strategies for cancer treatment and prevention. Some of the molecularly targeted drugs that have been evaluated in cancer prevention trials include inhibitors of 5α-reductase (prostate cancer), COX2 (colon cancer), and selective estrogen receptor modulators (SERMs) (breast cancer).[36–38] The development of these drugs provides the rationale that molecular targeted compounds have high potential in the chemoprevention of this disease.

Many studies have shown that prostate cancer is an ideal candidate for chemoprevention because: (1) endocrine and hormonal dependency makes it susceptible to pharmacological manipulations; (2) prostate cancer progression is very slow (prostatic intraepithelial neoplasia (PIN) take about 10 years to develop into early invasive tumor) with a long latency period; and (3) PSA is a good serum marker for monitoring the progression of the disease.[39]

Herbal Compounds and Derivatives in the Prevention of PCa

Prostate cancer is an ideal candidate for chemoprevention by natural products because it is typically diagnosed in men over 50 years of age, and so a delay in disease progression achieved through nutritional intervention

Table 9.1: Clinical trials on prostate cancer (PCa) by compounds derived from dietary agents.

Compounds	Source	Aim of study	Results	Stage	Ref.
Soy products	Soy beans	Treatment of advanced PCa	No PCa response; no toxicity	Phase I	53
		Treatment of HSPC and HRPC	No PCa response; no toxicity	Phase II	53
Lycopenes	Fruits and vegetables, mainly tomatoes	Treatment of localized PRCA	Reduction in prostate oxidative damage (28%) and PSA (17.5%)	Neoadjuvants	101
			Reduction in positive margins, tumor volume and PIN diffusion	Neoadjuvants	102
β-carotenes	Fruits and vegetables	Prevention of cancer	No influence on overall PRCA incidence	Phase III	101
			PRCA increase	Phase III	103

could significantly impact a patient's quality of life.[40] Asian diets and Chinese medical therapies incorporate an extensive array of plant-derived foods, herbs, and herbal extracts that contain numerous polyphenolic components. These compounds are characterized by their diaryl nucleus and can be classified into flavones, flavonoids, isoflavones, and tannins. To date, more than 20,000 polyphenols have been isolated from Mother Nature and some of these compounds have been shown to possess cancer chemopreventive and therapeutic properties in preclinical and clinical settings. For example, polyphenols isolated from green tea, *Scutellaria baicalensis*, soy, and tomato have been shown to prevent PCa in rodent models and in humans. Keeping in view the focus of the chapter on fruits and vegetables, we will not discuss the importance of green tea, fats, meats, and dairy products in the prevention of PCa; however, numerous works have been performed on these dietary components (see detailed reviews in Refs. 34, 41, 42). Tables 9.1 and 9.2 describe the important studies of fruits and vegetables in the prevention and treatment of PCa.

Soy Isoflavones

Interest in soy phytoestrogens and isoflavones stem mainly from epidemiological findings that a lower incidence of PCa occurs in Far Eastern countries where the consumption of soy products is typically high. Food sources rich in isoflavones include soybean, tofu, kidney beans, chick peas, lentils, and peanuts. The principal isoflavones in soy include genistein and daidzeinandbiochanin A, which occur naturally as glucosidic conjugates and are metabolized to their active forms in the gut. Soy isoflavones have broad range of mechanisms for their cancer chemopreventive and therapeutic properties against PCa. They have been shown to alter the expression of numerous genes associated with PCa and to inhibit 5α-reductase (the enzyme that converts testosterone to the more potent androgen dihydrotestosterone), DNA topoisomerases, and various tyrosine kinases. They work mainly through their estrogenic effect. These compounds bind to estrogen receptors and this binding suppress cell proliferation and promote differentiation of cancer cells (reviewed in Ref. 43). It has been shown that these compounds inhibit the proliferation of different prostate cancer cells in laboratory conditions and in animal models.

Table 9.2: Studies of fruits and vegetables in prostate cancer chemoprevention.

Natural agents	Model	Mode of action	Ref.
Tomatoes and Lycopenes			
Lycopenes	*In vitro*	DNA strand breakage Mitotic arrest Apoptosis Inhibition of Akt and GSK3	61, 104–107
Lycopenes	*In vivo*	Increased necrosis	108
Lycopenes	*In vivo* (transgenic mouse model)	No reduction in PCa	109
Tomato paste and products	Patients with BPH	Reduction is PSA	110
	Prospective cohort	Increased PCa risk	55
	Open Phase II pilot study	No clinical benefits	111
Crucifer Vegetables			
Sulforaphane	*In vitro*	Cell death, caspase activation Increased ROS Inhibition of NF-κB and AP-1 Inhibition of HDAC Decreased AR expression	65, 112–115
Sulforaphane	*In vivo*	Tumor reduction Activation of phase II enzymes	116
Broccoli sprouts	*In vivo (xenografts)*	Retardation of tumor growth	113
Broccoli sprouts	*In vivo* (TRAMP mice)	Inhibition of tumor growth Increased apoptosis AKT inhibition	117
Broccoli	Prospective studies	Reduced cancer risk	118

The effect of soy isoflavones on the prevention of spontaneous prostate cancer has also been evaluated by many researchers. They found that these compounds prevent prostatic adenocarcinoma and increases the survival of TRAMP (transgenic mice with prostate cancer) mice by altering growth factor signaling and inhibiting the Akt/GSK-3 pathway.[44–47]

Recent studies have shown that genistein inhibits invasive potential of TRAMP-C2 cells by inducing the expression of a metastatic suppressor gene *kangai-1* (*KAI1*).[48]

The anticancer potential of soy isoflavones have also been evaluated in patients with prostate cancer. These studies suggest that soy isoflavones modulated the expression of many biomarkers of PCa prediction and progression including PSA, Bcl-2, etc. without any deleterious effects.[49–52] In addition, several randomized studies of soy isoflavones as chemopreventive agents are ongoing and the results are eagerly awaited (reviewed in Ref. 43).

Tomatoes and Lycopenes

Tomatoes or tomato products ingested daily seem to reduce the risk of PCa (Table 9.2). This fruit contain various chemopreventive and antineoplastic compounds such as carotenoids, polyphenols, and vitamins. Tomatoes also contain high levels of lycopene, a lipophilic carotenoid that gives red fruits their characteristic pigment. Lycopene is a linear hydrocarbon containing a series of conjugated and unconjugated double bonds; this structure renders it capable of limiting oxidative damage and confers high affinity for quenching singlet oxygen molecules.[53] While oxidative stress results in lipid peroxidation and DNA damage, culturing PCa cells with lycopene inhibits DNA strand breaks. Many epidemiological studies have shown that intake of two or more servings of raw or cooked tomato products decrease the risk of PCa.[53–57] Furthermore, lycopene and tomato paste extracts inhibit cell proliferation and induce cell cycle arrest and apoptosis in prostate cancer cells *in vitro* and *in vivo* by modulating the expression of different proteins including insulin-like growth factor I receptor (IGF-IR), cyclins D1 and E, cyclin-dependent kinase (Cdk)-4, peroxisome proliferator-activated receptor gamma (PPARγ), liver X receptor alpha (LXRα), ATP-binding cassette transporter 1 (ABCA1), and pRb phosphorylation.[58–62] Moreover, studies have also shown that lycopene enhanced the effect of docetaxel in CR PCa cells by modulating IGF-1R levels.[63] In addition to these *in vitro* and *in vivo* studies, others conducted in humans also revealed the potential of tomato and lycopene intake in the prevention of prostate cancer. Chen *et al.* carried out a meta-analysis to determine the effect of lycopene and tomatoes on the prevention of PCa. They have identified and analyzed 11 cohort studies and six nested case-control studies by searching international journal databases and reference lists of relevant publications, and suggest that that tomato intake play a modest role in the prevention of prostate cancer.[64]

Cruciferous Vegetables

Crucifers, or the family Brassicaceae, include vegetables such as horseradish, bok choy, wasabi, broccoli, cabbage, cauliflower, Brussels sprouts, Chinese cabbage, and turnips. Cruciferous vegetables contain anticancer phytochemicals such as phenethyl isothiocyanate, sulforaphane, indole-3-carbinol (I3C), and glucosinolates, which are converted into isothiocyanate metabolites in the body by the enzymatic action of plant-specific myrosinase or gut microflora. Evidence for the protective effect of crucifers against PCa comes from epidemiological studies of dietary intake in the United States (Table 9.2). In particular, a diet rich in broccoli has been shown to reduce PCa risk in men.

Sulforaphane (4-methyl sulfinylbutyl isothiocyanate) is a naturally occurring isothiocyanate, which was first isolated and identified as a major inducer of quinine reductase in broccoli. This compound has been shown to exhibit anti-proliferative and anti-metaststic properties, and has also been demonstrated to protect carcinogen-induced different types of tumors in animals. Its chemopreventive effects include inhibition of cytochrome P450 (CYP450) and modulation of the NF-κB and AP-1signaling pathways. Studies in TRAMP mice have evaluated the pharmacodynamics action of broccoli against prostate tumorigenesis. Administration of mice with 240 mg broccoli sprouts per day has been shown to inhibit prostate tumor growth, alongside increased expression of cleaved caspase-3, cleaved PARP, and apoptosis regulator Bax, and reduced levels of Bcl-x_L protein, and the phosphorylation and expression of Akt and PI3K, and mTOR, 4E-BP1, and cyclin D1. Sulforaphane also inhibits the action of histone deacetylase enzymes which are upregulated in PCa. One of these enzymes, histone deacetylase 6 (HDAC6), influences the acetylation state of a key AR chaperone, HSP90. Treatment with sulforaphane-hyperacetylated Hsp90 (heat shock protein 90), destabilized

AR and lowered AR protein and gene expression.[65] Other important isothiocynates present in cruciferous vegetables are erucin, phenylbutyl isothiocyanate (PBITC), phenylethyl isothiocyanate (PEITC), phenhexyl isothiocyanate (PHITC), and benzyl isothiocyanate (BITC). These isothiocyanates have been shown to alter DNA methylation patters, inhibit proliferation of PCa cells, and possess chemopreventive properties in PCa models *in vivo.*

I3C is another phytochemical derived from cruciferous vegetables, known to produce many oligomeric products in the acidic stomach. A major condensation product is diindolylmethane (DIM), formed from the dimerization of two molecules of I3C; DIM has been shown to inhibit PCa both *in vitro* and *in vivo.* Recent studies have demonstrated that I3C and DIM modulate androgen's effect on C–C chemokine ligand 2 (CCL2) and monocyte attraction to inhibit PCa cells.[66] These compounds have also been shown to suppress histone deacetylase and telomerase activity, and β-catenin expression in PCa cells.[67–69] In addition, DIM is able to prevent PCa development in TRAMP mice by reducing the expression of cyclin A, Cdk2, Cdk4, and Bcl-x_L, and increasing p27 and Bax expression. Finally, DIM has been shown to be safe in CR non-metastatic PCa patients at a dose of 225 mg orally twice daily.[70,71]

Garlic Compounds

Epidemiological studies suggest an inverse association between increased dietary intake of *Allium* vegetables, such as garlic, and PCa risk. Garlic contains many organosulfur compounds such as diallyl sulfide (DADS) and diallyl trisulfide (DATS) that are responsible for its anticancer effects. Recent studies have shown that these compounds inhibit the activation of the STAT3 and Akt pathways, and inhibit the expression of MMP-9, VEGF, and X-linked inhibitor of apoptosis (XIAP), thereby preventing PCa cell proliferation, survival, invasion, and metastasis.[72–75] Recent studies have also shown that DATS is more cytotoxic to PCa cells (PC-3) than to the non-cancerous epithelial cell line PNT1A, and suppresses the growth of PC-3 human PCa xenograft in animals.[76,77] In addition, the other compounds from garlic such as S-allylcysteine and S-allylmercaptocysteine have also been shown to inhibit PCa growth in animal models.[78,79]

Moreover, S-allylmercaptocysteine has been demonstrated to enhance the effects of docetaxel to induce apoptosis in hormone-refractory PCa cells.[80]

Recently, Zhou *et al.* carried out a literature search (up to May 2013) of the relation between *Allium* vegetables and reduced PCa risk.[81] The databases include PubMed, EMBASE, Scopus, the Web of Science, the Cochrane register, and the Chinese National Knowledge Infrastructure (CNKI). Thorough analysis of the studies published in these databases not only showed that the risk of PCa is significantly decreased through the consumption of garlic but also suggest through thte dietary intake of *Allium* vegetables.

Pomegranate: A "Superfruit"

Pomegranate (*Punica granatum*) is a fruit-bearing deciduous shrub that grows throughout the Mediterranean region and the United States. These fruits have a thick reddish skin that encapsulates hundreds of small red seeds, and when the seeds are crushed and dried, they produce a unique oil, 80% of which is puninic acid, a rare 18-carbon fatty acid. This oil also contains the isoflavone genistein and coumestrol, a phytoestrogen. As pomegranates possess high antioxidant properties, it termed a 'superfruit,' along with others such as blueberry and cranberry. The fruit is a rich source of anthocyanins, ellagic acid, and punicalagin, which account for the majority of the fruit's antioxidant activity. The polyphenols from this fruit has been shown to inhibit the proliferation and invasion of LNCaP, DU145, and PC-3 PCa cells in experimental conditions, e.g., cell growth is suppressed and apoptosis is induced in a dose-dependent manner in androgen-sensitive PC-3 cells via modulation of Cdk. They are known also to induce Bax and Bak, and inhibit Bcl-x_L, Bcl-2, cyclins D1, D2, and E, and Cdk2, 4, and 6.

Recent studies showed that ellagic acid at non-toxic concentrations significantly inhibited the motility and invasion of androgen-independent human (PC-3) and rat (PLS10) PCa cell lines by downregulating the expression of MMP-2,[40,82] and this compound in combination with urolithin A, synergistically inhibit androgen-independent PCa cell growth via inducing cell cycle arrest in the S phase and decreasing cyclin B1 and cyclin D1 levels.[83] The effect of luteolin, ellagic acid, and punicic acid has also been investigated in hormone-dependent and hormone-refractory PCa cells. The results suggest that these compounds inhibit the growth of such cells, and inhibit their migration and their chemotaxis toward stromal cell-derived factor 1α (SDF1α) — a chemokine that is important in PCa metastasis to the bone. These compounds also increased the expression of cell-adhesion genes and decrease the expression of genes involved in cell cycle control and cell migration.[84]

The role of the pomegranate and its components has also been explored in animal models of this disease. It has been shown that oral consumption of pomegranate fruit extract (PFE) inhibited PCa development in TRAMP mice and PCa cell growth and metastases in nude mice by downregulating the IGF-I/Akt/mTOR and NF-κB pathways in the prostate tissues and tumors.[85–87] Many studies have also shown that the administration of pomegranate juice increases PSA doubling time (PSADT) in PCa patients.[88,89] These studies suggest that the pomegranate has high potential in PCa prevention and treatment.

In addition to the above-mentioned agents, many other fruits and vegetables and their active ingredients have also been shown to possess cancer chemopreventive and therapeutic properties against PCa. These compounds include polyphenols from mangosteens (*Garcinia mangostana*), citrus peel flavonoids, polar biophenolics from sweet potatoes, American cranberries, gallic acid, ursolic acid, and resveratrol. However, more studies are required to evaluate these findings in humans.[90–99] Because of the potential of fruits and vegetables in the prevention of PCa, the American Cancer Society suggests the following guidelines for the prevention of this disease:[100]

(1) Maintain a healthy diet with a focus on fruit and vegetables;
(2) Try to maintain a healthy weight;
(3) Perform regular physical exercise; and
(4) Reduce alcohol intake.

To adopt a healthy diet with a focus on fruit and vegetables:

(1) Eat different fruits and vegetables every day;
(2) Eat whole wheat rather than refined wheat products; and
(3) Eat only small quantities of meat products and red meat.

CONCLUSION

PCa is one of the most common cancers in men, affecting and killing numerous people worldwide. However, recent studies have shown that the compounds present in fruits and vegetables have great potential in the prevention and treatment of this disease, and dietary intake of more fruits and vegetables have been associated with a reduced risk of this cancer. These studies suggest that leading a healthy lifestyle is the best way to prevent malignancies such as PCa, and this would avoid many health issues in the late stage of life. Therefore, it is encouraged to cultivate the habit of eating a diet rich in fruits and vegetables, which would to prevent many diseases including PCa.

REFERENCES

1. Heidenreich, A., G. Aus, M. Bolla, S. Joniau, V.B. Matveev, H.P. Schmid, and F. Zattoni, EAU guidelines on prostate cancer, *Eur Urol* **53**(1): 68–80 (2008).
2. Yin, M., S. Bastacky, U. Chandran, M.J. Becich, and R. Dhir, Prevalence of incidental prostate cancer in the general population: A study of healthy organ donors, *J Urol* **179**(3): 892–895 (2008).
3. Knudsen, B.S. and V. Vasioukhin, Mechanisms of prostate cancer initiation and progression, *Adv Cancer Res* **109**: 1–50 (2010).
4. Lundwall, A. and H. Lilja, Molecular cloning of human prostate specific antigen cDNA, *FEBS Lett* **214**(2): 317–322 (1987).
5. Wright Jr., G.L., M.L. Beckett, G.B. Lipford, C.L. Haley, and P.F. Schellhammer, A novel prostate carcinoma-associated glycoprotein complex (PAC) recognized by monoclonal antibody TURP-27, *Int J Cancer* **47**(5): 717–725 (1991).
6. Beckett, M.L. and G.L. Wright Jr., Characterization of a prostate carcinoma mucin-like antigen (PMA), *Int J Cancer* **62**(6): 703–710 (1995).
7. Israeli, R.S., C.T. Powell, W.R. Fair, and W.D. Heston, Molecular cloning of a complementary DNA encoding a prostate-specific membrane antigen, *Cancer Res* **53**(2): 227–230 (1993).
8. Hsieh, C.L., I. Oakley-Girvan, R.R. Balise, J. Halpern, R.P. Gallagher, A.H. Wu, L.N. Kolonel, L.E. O'Brien, I.G. Lin, D.J. Van Den Berg, C.Z. Teh, D.W. West, and A.S. Whittemore, A genome screen of families with multiple cases of prostate cancer: Evidence of genetic heterogeneity, *Am J Hum Genet* **69**(1): 148–158 (2001).
9. Xu, J., S.L. Zheng, J.D. Carpten, N.N. Nupponen, C.M. Robbins, J. Mestre, T.Y. Moses, D.A. Faith, B.D. Kelly, S.D. Isaacs, K.E. Wiley, C.M. Ewing,

P. Bujnovszky, B. Chang, J. Bailey-Wilson, E.R. Bleecker, P.C. Walsh, D.A. Trent, D.A. Meyers, and W.B. Isaacs, Evaluation of linkage and association of HPC2/ELAC2 in patients with familial or sporadic prostate cancer, *Am J Hum Genet* **68**(4): 901–911 (2001).

10. Casey, G., P.J. Neville, S.J. Plummer, Y. Xiang, L.M. Krumroy, E.A. Klein, W.J. Catalona, N. Nupponen, J.D. Carpten, J.M. Trent, and R.H. Silverman, and J.S. Witte, RNASEL Arg462Gln variant is implicated in up to 13% of prostate cancer cases, *Nat Genet* **32**(4): 581–583 (2002).
11. Rennert, H., D. Bercovich, A. Hubert, D. Abeliovich, U. Rozovsky, A. Bar-Shira, S. Soloviov, L. Schreiber, H. Matzkin, G. Rennert, L. Kadouri, T. Peretz, Y. Yaron, and A. Orr-Urtreger, A novel founder mutation in the *RNASEL* gene, 471delAAAG, is associated with prostate cancer in Ashkenazi Jews, *Am J Hum Genet* **71**(4): 981–984 (2002).
12. Rokman, A., T. Ikonen, E.H. Seppala, N. Nupponen, V. Autio, N. Mononen, J. Bailey-Wilson, J. Trent, J. Carpten, M.P. Matikainen, P.A. Koivisto, T.L. Tammela, O.P. Kallioniemi, and J. Schleutker, Germline alterations of the *RNASEL* gene, a candidate HPC1 gene at 1q25, in patients and families with prostate cancer, *Am J Hum Genet* **70**(5): 1299–1304 (2002).
13. Xu, J., S.L. Zheng, A. Komiya, J.C. Mychaleckyj, S.D. Isaacs, J.J. Hu, D. Sterling, E.M. Lange, G.A. Hawkins, A. Turner, C.M. Ewing, D.A. Faith, J.R. Johnson, H. Suzuki, P. Bujnovszky, K.E. Wiley, A.M. DeMarzo, G.S. Bova, B. Chang, M.C. Hall, D.L. McCullough, A.W. Partin, V.S. Kassabian, J.D. Carpten, J.E. Bailey-Wilson, J.M. Trent, J. Ohar, E.R. Bleecker, P.C.Walsh, W.B. Isaacs, and D.A. Meyers, Germline mutations and sequence variants of the macrophage scavenger receptor 1 gene are associated with prostate cancer risk, *Nat Genet* **32**: 321–325 (2002).
14. Majumder, P.K. and W.R. Sellers, Akt-regulated pathways in prostate cancer, *Oncogene* **24**(50): 7465–7474 (2005).
15. Li, J., C. Yen, D. Liaw, K. Podsypanina, S. Bose, S.I. Wang, J. Puc, C. Miliaresis, L. Rodgers, R. McCombie, S.H. Bigner, B.C. Giovanella, M. Ittmann, B. Tycko, H. Hibshoosh, M.H. Wigler, and R. Parsons, *PTEN*, a putative protein tyrosine phosphatase gene mutated in human brain, breast, and prostate cancer, *Science* **275**(5308): 1943–1947 (1997).
16. Steck, P.A., M.A. Pershouse, S.A. Jasser, W.K. Yung, H. Lin, A.H. Ligon, L.A. Langford, M.L. Baumgard, T. Hattier, T. Davis, C. Frye, R. Hu, B. Swedlund, D.H. Teng, and S.V. Tavtigian, Identification of a candidate tumour suppressor gene, *MMAC1*, at chromosome 10q23.3 that is mutated in multiple advanced cancers, *Nat Genet* **15**(4): 356–362 (1997).

17. Gray, I.C., S.M. Phillips, S.J. Lee, J.P. Neoptolemos, J. Weissenbach, and N.K. Spurr, Loss of the chromosomal region 10q23–25 in prostate cancer, *Cancer Res* **55**(21): 4800–4803 (1995).
18. Komiya, A., H. Suzuki, T. Ueda, R. Yatani, M. Emi, H. Ito, and J. Shimazaki, Allelic losses at loci on chromosome 10 are associated with metastasis and progression of human prostate cancer, *Genes Chromosomes Cancer* **17**(4): 245–253 (1996).
19. Dong, J.T., T.W. Sipe, E.R. Hyytinen, C.L. Li, C. Heise, D.E. McClintock, C.D. Grant, L.W. Chung, and H.F. Frierson Jr., *PTEN/MMAC1* is infrequently mutated in pT2 and pT3 carcinomas of the prostate, *Oncogene* **17**(15): 1979–1982 (1998).
20. Gray, I.C., L.M. Stewart, S.M. Phillips, J.A. Hamilton, N.E. Gray, G.J. Watson, N.K. Spurr, and D. Snary, Mutation and expression analysis of the putative prostate tumour-suppressor gene *PTEN*, *Br J Cancer* **78**(10): 1296–1300 (1998).
21. Wang, S.I., R. Parsons, and M. Ittmann, Homozygous deletion of the *PTEN* tumor suppressor gene in a subset of prostate adenocarcinomas, *Clin Cancer Res* **4**(3): 811–815 (1998).
22. Suzuki, H., D. Freije, D.R. Nusskern, K. Okami, P. Cairns, D. Sidransky, W.B. Isaacs, and G.S. Bova, Interfocal heterogeneity of *PTEN/MMAC1* gene alterations in multiple metastatic prostate cancer tissues, *Cancer Res* **58**(2): 204–209 (1998).
23. Vlietstra, R.J., D.C. van Alewijk, K.G. Hermans, G.J. van Steenbrugge, and J. Trapman, Frequent inactivation of *PTEN* in prostate cancer cell lines and xenografts, *Cancer Res* **58**(13): 2720–2723 (1998).
24. Chan, J.M., M.J. Stampfer, E. Giovannucci, P.H. Gann, J. Ma, P. Wilkinson, C.H. Hennekens, and M. Pollak, Plasma insulin-like growth factor-I and prostate cancer risk: A prospective study, *Science* **279**(5350): 563–566 (1998).
25. Schmelzle, T. and M.N. Hall, TOR, a central controller of cell growth, *Cell* **103**(2): 253–262 (2000).
26. Aggarwal, B.B., Nuclear factor-kappaB: The enemy within, *Cancer Cell* **6**(3): 203–208 (2004).
27. Deeb, D., X. Gao, H. Jiang, A.S. Arbab, S.A. Dulchavsky, and S.C. Gautam, Growth inhibitory and apoptosis-inducing effects of xanthohumol, a prenylated chalone present in hops, in human prostate cancer cells, *Anticancer Res* **30**(9): 3333–3339 (2010).
28. Ben Jemaa, A., Y. Bouraoui, S. Sallami, A. Banasr, N. Ben Rais, L. Ouertani, Y. Nouira, A. Horchani, and R. Oueslati, Co-expression and impact of prostate

specific membrane antigen and prostate specific antigen in prostatic pathologies, *J Exp Clin Cancer Res* **29**(1): 171 (2010).

29. Suh, J., F. Payvandi, L.C. Edelstein, P.S. Amenta, W.X. Zong, C. Gelinas, and A.B. Rabson, Mechanisms of constitutive NF-kappaB activation in human prostate cancer cells, *Prostate* **52**(3): 183–200 (2002).
30. Pandey, M.K., S.K. Sandur, B. Sung, G. Sethi, A.B. Kunnumakkara, and B.B. Aggarwal, Butein, a tetrahydroxychalcone, inhibits nuclear factor (NF)-kappaB and NF-kappaB-regulated gene expression through direct inhibition of IkappaBalpha kinase beta on cysteine 179 residue, *J Biol Chem* **282**(24): 17340–17350 (2007).
31. Pandey, M.K., B. Sung, K.S. Ahn, A.B. Kunnumakkara, M.M. Chaturvedi, and B.B. Aggarwal, Gambogic acid, a novel ligand for transferrin receptor, potentiates TNF-induced apoptosis through modulation of the nuclear factor-kappaB signaling pathway, *Blood* **110**(10): 3517–3525 (2007).
32. Jain, G., M.V. Cronauer, M. Schrader, P. Moller, and R.B. Marienfeld, NF-kappaB signaling in prostate cancer: A promising therapeutic target?, *World J Urol* **30**(3): 303–310 (2012).
33. Sporn, M.B., N.M. Dunlop, D.L. Newton, and J.M. Smith, Prevention of chemical carcinogenesis by vitamin A and its synthetic analogs (retinoids), *Fed Proc* **35**(6): 1332–1338 (1976).
34. William, W.N., Jr., J.V. Heymach, E.S. Kim, and S.M. Lippman, Molecular targets for cancer chemoprevention, *Nat Rev Drug Discov* **8**(3): 213–225 (2009).
35. Lippman, S.M. and W.K. Hong, Cancer prevention science and practice, *Cancer Res* **62**(18): 5119–5125 (2002).
36. Thompson, I.M., P.J. Goodman, C.M. Tangen, M.S. Lucia, G.J. Miller, L.G. Ford, M.M. Lieber, R.D. Cespedes, J.N. Atkins, S.M. Lippman, S.M. Carlin, A. Ryan, C.M. Szczepanek, J.J. Crowley, and C.A. Coltman Jr., The influence of finasteride on the development of prostate cancer, *N Engl J Med* **349**(3): 215–224 (2003).
37. Arber, N., C.J. Eagle, J. Spicak, I. Racz, P. Dite, J. Hajer, M. Zavoral, M.J. Lechuga, P. Gerletti, J. Tang, R.B. Rosenstein, K. Macdonald, P. Bhadra, R. Fowler, J. Wittes, A.G. Zauber, S.D. Solomon, and B. Levin, Celecoxib for the prevention of colorectal adenomatous polyps, *N Engl J Med* **355**(9): 885–895 (2006).
38. Fisher, B., J.P. Costantino, D.L. Wickerham, D.L. Redmond, M. Kavanah, W.M. Cronin, V. Vogel, A. Robidoux, N. Dimitrov, J. Atkins, M. Daly, S. Wieand, E. Tan-Chiu, L. Ford, and N. Wolmark, Tamoxifen for prevention of breast cancer: Report of the National Surgical Adjuvant Breast and Bowel Project P-1 Study, *J Natl Cancer Inst* **90**(18): 1371–1388 (1998).

39. Schmid, H.P., J.E. McNeal, and T.A. Stamey, Clinical observations on the doubling time of prostate cancer, *Eur Urol* **23**(Suppl. 2): 60–63 (1993).
40. Bell, C. and S. Hawthorne, Ellagic acid, pomegranate and prostate cancer — a mini review, *J Pharm Pharmacol.* **60**(2): 139–144 (2008).
41. Schmid, H.P., C. Fischer, D.S. Engeler, M.L. Bendhack, and B.J. Schmitz-Drager, Nutritional aspects of primary prostate cancer prevention, *Recent Results Cancer Res* **188**: 101–107 (2011).
42. Venkateswaran, V. and L.H. Klotz, Diet and prostate cancer: Mechanisms of action and implications for chemoprevention, *Nat Rev Urol* **7**(8): 442–453 (2010).
43. Hori, S., E. Butler, and J. McLoughlin, Prostate cancer and diet: Food for thought?, *BJU Int* **107**(9): 1348–1359 (2011).
44. Mentor-Marcel, R., C.A. Lamartiniere, I.E. Eltoum, N.M. Greenberg, and A. Elgavish, Genistein in the diet reduces the incidence of poorly differentiated prostatic adenocarcinoma in transgenic mice (TRAMP), *Cancer Res* **61**(18): 6777–6782 (2005).
45. Mentor-Marcel, R., C.A. Lamartiniere, I.A. Eltoum, N.M. Greenberg, and A. Elgavish, Dietary genistein improves survival and reduces expression of osteopontin in the prostate of transgenic mice with prostatic adenocarcinoma (TRAMP), *J Nutr* **135**(5): 989–995 (2005).
46. Wang, J., I.E. Eltoum, and C.A. Lamartiniere, Genistein alters growth factor signaling in transgenic prostate model (TRAMP), *Mol Cell Endocrinol.* **219**(1–2): 171–180 (2004).
47. El Touny, L.H. and P.P. Banerjee, Akt GSK-3 pathway as a target in genistein-induced inhibition of TRAMP prostate cancer progression toward a poorly differentiated phenotype, *Carcinogenesis* **28**(8): 1710–1717 (2007).
48. El Touny, L.H. and P.P. Banerjee, Genistein induces the metastasis suppressor kangai-1 which mediates its anti-invasive effects in TRAMP cancer cells, *Biochem Biophys Res Commun* **361**(1): 169–175 (2007).
49. Pendleton, J.M., W.W. Tan, S. Anai, M. Chang, W. Hou, K.T. Shiverick, and C.J. Rosser, Phase II trial of isoflavone in prostate-specific antigen recurrent prostate cancer after previous local therapy, *BMC Cancer* **8**: 132 (2008).
50. Swami, S., A.V. Krishnan, J. Moreno, R.S. Bhattacharyya, C. Gardner, J.D. Brooks, D.M. Peehl, and D. Feldman, Inhibition of prostaglandin synthesis and actions by genistein in human prostate cancer cells and by soy isoflavones in prostate cancer patients, *Int J Cancer* **124**(9): 2050–2059 (2009).
51. Lazarevic, B., G. Boezelijn, L.M. Diep, K.K. Vernrod, O. Ogren, H. Ramberg, A. Moen, N. Wessel, R.E. Berg, W. Egge-Jacobsen, C. Hammarstrom, A. Svindland, O. Kucuk, F. Saatcioglu, K.A. Taskèn, and S.J. Karlsen, Efficacy

and safety of short-term genistein intervention in patients with localized prostate cancer prior to radical prostatectomy: A randomized, placebo-controlled, double-blind Phase 2 clinical trial, *Nutr Cancer* **63**(6): 889–898 (2011).
52. Lazarevic, B., C. Hammarström, J. Yang, H. Ramberg, L.M. Diep, S.J. Karlsen, O. Kucuk, F. Saatcioglu, K.A. Taskèn, and A. Svindland, The effects of short-term genistein intervention on prostate biomarker expression in patients with localised prostate cancer before radical prostatectomy, *Br J Nutr* **108**(12): 2138–2147 (2012).
53. Nelson, P.S. and B. Montgomery, Unconventional therapy for prostate cancer: Good, bad or questionable?, *Nat Rev Cancer* **3**(11): 845–858 (2003).
54. Mills, P.K., W.L. Beeson, R.L. Phillips, and G.E. Fraser, Cohort study of diet, lifestyle, and prostate cancer in Adventist men, *Cancer* **64**: 598–604 (1989).
55. Giovannucci, E., E.B. Rimm, Y. Liu, M.J. Stampfer, and W.C. Willett, A prospective study of tomato products, lycopene, and prostate cancer risk, *J Natl Cancer Inst* **94**(5): 391–398 (2002).
56. Ambrosini, G.L., N.H. de Klerk, L. Fritschi, D. Mackerras, and B. Musk, Fruit, vegetable, vitamin A intakes, and prostate cancer risk, *Prostate Cancer Prostatic Dis* **11**(1): 61–66 (2008).
57. Tan, H.L., J.M. Thomas-Ahner, E.M. Grainger, L. Wan, D.M. Francis, S.J. Schwartz, J.W. Erdman Jr., and S.K. Clinton, Tomato-based food products for prostate cancer prevention: What have we learned?, *Cancer Metastasis Rev* **29**(3): 553–568 (2010).
58. Yang, C.M., I.H. Lu, H.Y. Chen, and M.L. Hu, Lycopene inhibits the proliferation of androgen-dependent human prostate tumor cells through activation of PPARγ-LXRα-ABCA1 pathway, *J Nutr Biochem* **23**(1): 8–17(2012).
59. Yang, C.M., Y.T. Yen, C.S. Huang, and C.S. Hux, Growth inhibitory efficacy of lycopene and β-carotene against androgen-independent prostate tumor cells xenografted in nude mice, *Mol Nutr Food Res* **55**(4): 606–612 (2011).
60. Kanagaraj, P., M.R. Vijayababu, B. Ravisankar, J. Anbalagan, M.M. Aruldhas, and J. Arunakaran, Effect of lycopene on insulin-like growth factor-I, IGF binding protein-3 and IGF type-I receptor in prostate cancer cells, *J Cancer Res Clin Oncol* **133**(6): 351–359 (2007).
61. Ivanov, N.I., S.P. Cowell, P. Brown, P.S. Rennie, E.S. Guns, and M.E. Cox, Lycopene differentially induces quiescence and apoptosis in androgen-responsive and -independent prostate cancer cell lines, *Clin Nutr* **26**(2): 252–263 (2007).
62. Soares, N.D., A.J. Teodoro, F.L. Oliveira, C.A. Santos, C.M. Takiya, O.S. Junior, M. Bianco, A.P. Junior, L.E. Nasciutti, L.B. Ferreira, E.R. Gimba, and R. Borojevic, Influence of lycopene on cell viability, cell cycle, and apoptosis of human prostate cancer and benign hyperplastic cells, *Nutr Cancer* **65**(7): 1076–1085 (2013).

63. Tang, Y., B. Parmakhtiar, A.R. Simoneau, J. Xie, J. Fruehauf, M. Lilly, and X. Zi, Lycopene enhances docetaxel's effect in castration-resistant prostate cancer associated with insulin-like growth factor I receptor levels, *Neoplasia* **13**(2): 108–119 (2011).
64. Chen, J., Y. Song, and L. Zhang, Lycopene/tomato consumption and the risk of prostate cancer: A systematic review and meta-analysis of prospective studies, *J Nutr Sci Vitaminol (Tokyo)* **59**(3): 213–223 (2013).
65. Gibbs, A., J. Schwartzman, V. Deng, and J. Alumkal, Sulforaphane destabilizes the androgen receptor in prostate cancer cells by inactivating histone deacetylase 6, *Proc Natl Acad Sci USA* **106**(39): 16663–16668 (2009).
66. Kim, E.K., J.A. Kim Milner, and T.T. Wang, Indole-3-carbinol and 3′,3′-diindolylmethane modulate androgen's effect on C–C chemokine ligand 2 and monocyte attraction to prostate cancer cells, *Cancer Prev Res (Phila)* **6**(6): 519–529 (2013).
67. Beaver, L.M., T.W. Yu, E.I. Sokolowski, D.E. Williams, R.H. Dashwood, and E. Ho, 3,3′-diindolylmethane, but not indole-3-carbinol, inhibits histone deacetylase activity in prostate cancer cells, *Toxicol Appl Pharmacol* **263**(3): 345–351 (2012).
68. Adler, S., G. Rashid, and A. Klein, Indole-3-carbinol inhibits telomerase activity and gene expression in prostate cancer cell lines, *Anticancer Res* **31**(11): 3733–3737 (2011).
69. Jeong, Y.M., H. Li, S.Y. Kim, H.Y. Yun, K.J. Baek, N.S. Kwon, S.C. Myung, and D.S. Kim, Indole-3-carbinol inhibits prostate cancer cell migration via degradation of beta-catenin, *Oncol Res* **19**(5): 237–243 (2011).
70. Cho, H.J., S.Y. Park, E.J. Kim, J.K. Kim, and J.H. Park, 3,3′-diindolylmethane inhibits prostate cancer development in the transgenic adenocarcinoma mouse prostate model, *Mol Carcinog* **50**(2): 100–112 (2011).
71. Heath, E.I., L.K. Heilbrun, J. Li, U. Vaishampayan, F. Harper, P. Pemberton, and F.H. Sarkar, A phase I dose-escalation study of oral BR-DIM (BioResponse 3,3′-diindolylmethane) in castrate-resistant, non-metastatic prostate cancer, *Am J Transl Res* **2**(4): 402–411 (2010).
72. Chandra-Kuntal, K. and S.V. Singh, Diallyl trisulfide inhibits activation of signal transducer and activator of transcription 3 in prostate cancer cells in culture and *in vivo*, *Cancer Prev Res (Phila)* **3**(11): 1473–1483 (2010).
73. Xiao, D., M. Li, A. Herman-Antosiewicz, J. Antosiewicz, H. Xiao, K.L. Lew, Y. Zeng, S.W. Marynowski, and S.V. Singh, Diallyl trisulfide inhibits angiogenic features of human umbilical vein endothelial cells by causing Akt inactivation and down-regulation of VEGF and VEGF-R2, *Nutr Cancer* **55**(1): 94–107 (2006).

74. Kim, S.H., A. Bommareddy, and S.V. Singh, Garlic constituent diallyl trisulfide suppresses x-linked inhibitor of apoptosis protein in prostate cancer cells in culture and *in vivo*, *Cancer Prev Res (Phila)* **4**(6): 897–906 (2011).
75. Shin, D.Y., G.Y. Kim, J.I. Kim, M.K. Yoon, T.K. Kwon, S.J. Lee, Y.W. Choi, H.S. Kang, Y.H. Yoo, and Y.H. Choi, Anti-invasive activity of diallyl disulfide through tightening of tight junctions and inhibition of matrix metalloproteinase activities in LNCaP prostate cancer cells, *Toxicol In Vitro* **24**(6): 1569–1576 (2010).
76. Borkowska, A., N. Knap, and J. Antosiewicz, Diallyl trisulfide is more cytotoxic to prostate cancer cells PC-3 than to noncancerous epithelial cell line PNT1A: A possible role of p66Shc signaling axis, *Nutr Cancer* **65**(5): 711–717 (2013).
77. Xiao, D., K.L. Lew, Y.A. Kim, Y. Zeng, E.R. Hahm, R. Dhir, and S.V. Singh, Diallyl trisulfide suppresses growth of PC-3 human prostate cancer xenograft *in vivo* in association with Bax and Bak induction, *Clin Cancer Res* **12**(22): 6836–6843 (2006).
78. Chu, Q., D.T. Lee, S.W. Tsao, X. Wang, and Y.C. Wong, S-allylcysteine, a water-soluble garlic derivative, suppresses the growth of a human androgen-independent prostate cancer xenograft, CWR22R, under *in vivo* conditions, *BJU Int* **99**(4): 925–932 (2007).
79. Howard, E.W., M.T. Ling, C.W. Chua, H.W. Cheung, X. Wang, and Y.C. Wong, Garlic-derived S-allylmercaptocysteine is a novel *in vivo* antimetastatic agent for androgen-independent prostate cancer, *Clin Cancer Res* **13**(6): 1847–1856 (2007).
80. Howard, E.W., D.T. Lee, Y.T. Chiu, C.W. Chua, X. Wang, and Y.C. Wong, Evidence of a novel docetaxel sensitizer, garlic-derived S-allylmercaptocysteine, as a treatment option for hormone refractory prostate cancer, *Int J Cancer* **122**(9): 1941–1948 (2008).
81. Zhou, X.F., Z.S. Ding, and N.B. Liu, Allium vegetables and risk of prostate cancer: Evidence from 132,192 subjects, *Asian Pac J Cancer Prev* **14**(7): 4131–4134 (2013).
82. Pitchakarn, P., T. Chewonarin, K. Ogawa, S. Suzuki, M. Asamoto, S. Takahashi, T. Shirai, and P. Limtrakul, Ellagic Acid inhibits migration and invasion by prostate cancer cell lines, *Asian Pac J Cancer Prev* **14**(5): 2859–2863 (2013).
83. Vicinanza, R., Y. Zhang, S.M. Henning, and D. Heber, Pomegranate juice metabolites, ellagic acid and urolithin A, synergistically inhibit androgen-independent prostate cancer cell growth via distinct effects on cell cycle control and apoptosis, *Evid Based Complement Alternat Med* 247504 doi: 10.1155/2013/247504 (2013).

84. Wang, L., J. Ho, C. Glackin, and M. Martins-Green, Specific pomegranate juice components as potential inhibitors of prostate cancer metastasis, *Transl Oncol* **5**(5): 344–355 (2012).
85. Paller, C.J., X. Ye, P.J. Wozniak, B.K. Gillespie, P.R. Sieber, R.H. Greengold, B.R. Stockton, B.L. Hertzman, M.D. Efros, R.P. Roper, H.R. Liker, and M.A. Carducci, A randomized phase II study of pomegranate extract for men with rising PSA following initial therapy for localized prostate cancer, *Prostate Cancer Prostatic Dis* **16**(1): 50–55 (2013).
86. Adhami, V.M., I.A. Siddiqui, D.N. Syed, R.K. Lall, and H. Mukhtar, Oral infusion of pomegranate fruit extract inhibits prostate carcinogenesis in the TRAMP model, *Carcinogenesis* **33**(3): 644–651 (2012).
87. Rettig, M.B., D. Heber, J. An, N.P. Seeram, J.Y. Rao, H. Liu, T. Klatte, A. Belldegrun, A. Moro, S.M. Henning, D. Mo, W.J. Aronson, and A. Pantuck, Pomegranate extract inhibits androgen-independent prostate cancer growth through a nuclear factor-kappaB-dependent mechanism, *Mol Cancer Ther* **7**(9): 2662–2671 (2008).
88. Seeram, N.P., W.J. Aronson, Y. Zhang, S.M. Henning, A. Moro, R.P. Lee, M. Sartippour, D.M. Harris, M. Rettig, M.A. Suchard, A.J. Pantuck, A. Belldegrun, and D. Heber, Pomegranate ellagitannin-derived metabolites inhibit prostate cancer growth and localize to the mouse prostate gland, *J Agric Food Chem* **55**(19): 7732–7737 (2007).
89. Pantuck, A.J., J.T. Leppert, N. Zomorodian, W. Aronson, J. Hong, R.J. Barnard, N. Seeram, H. Liker, H. Wang, R. Elashoff, D. Heber, M. Aviram, L. Ignarro, and A. Belldegrun, Phase II study of pomegranate juice for men with rising prostate-specific antigen following surgery or radiation for prostate cancer, *Clin Cancer Res* **12**(13): 4018–4026 (2006).
90. Li, G., S. Thomas, and J.J. Johnson, Polyphenols from the mangosteen (*Garcinia mangostana*) fruit for breast and prostate cancer, *Front Pharmacol* **4**: 80 (2013).
91. Lai, C.S., S. Li, Y. Miyauchi, M. Suzawa, C.T Ho, and M.H. Pan, Potent anticancer effects of citrus peel flavonoids in human prostate xenograft tumors, *Food Funct* **4**(6): 944–949 (2013).
92. Gundala, S.R., C. Yang, N. Lakshminarayana, G. Asif, M.V. Gupta, S. Shamsi, and R. Aneja, Polar biophenolics in sweet potato greens extract synergize to inhibit prostate cancer cell proliferation and *in vivo* tumor growth, *Carcinogenesis* **34**(9): 2039–2049 (2013).
93. Déziel, B., J. MacPhee, K. Patel, A. Catalli, M. Kulka, C. Neto, K. Gottschall-Pass, and R. Hurta, American cranberry (*Vaccinium macrocarpon*) extract affects human prostate cancer cell growth via cell cycle arrest by modulating expression of cell cycle regulators, *Food Funct* **3**(5): 556–564 (2012).

94. Johnson, J.J., S.M. Petiwala, D.N. Syed, J.T. Rasmussen, V.M. Adhami, I.A. Siddiqui, A.M. Kohl, and H. Mukhtar, α-Mangostin, a xanthone from mangosteen fruit, promotes cell cycle arrest in prostate cancer and decreases xenograft tumor growth, *Carcinogenesis* **33**(2): 413–419 (2012).
95. Liu, K.C., A.C. Huang, P.P. Wu, H.Y. Lin, F.S. Chueh, J.S. Yang, C.C. Lu, J.H. Chiang, M. Meng, and J.G. Chung, Gallic acid suppresses the migration and invasion of PC-3 human prostate cancer cells via inhibition of matrix metalloproteinase-2 and -9 signaling pathways, *Oncol Rep* **26**(1): 177–184 (2011).
96. Kondo, M., S.L. MacKinnon, C.C. Craft, M.D. Matchett, R.A. Hurta, and C.C. Neto, Ursolic acid and its esters: Occurrence in cranberries and other *Vaccinium* fruit and effects on matrix metalloproteinase activity in DU145 prostate tumor cells, *J Sci Food Agric* **91**(5): 789–796 (2011).
97. MacLean, M.A., B.E. Scott, B.A. Deziel, M.C. Nunnelley, A.M. Liberty, K.T. Gottschall-Pass, C.C. Neto, and R.A. Hurta, North American cranberry (*Vaccinium macrocarpon*) stimulates apoptotic pathways in DU145 human prostate cancer cells *in vitro*, *Nutr Cancer* **63**(1): 109–120 (2011).
98. Li, G., P. Rivas, R. Bedolla, D. Thapa, R.L. Reddick, R. Ghosh, and A.P. Kumar, Dietary resveratrol prevents development of high-grade prostatic intraepithelial neoplastic lesions: Involvement of SIRT1/S6K axis, *Cancer Prev Res (Phila)* **6**(1): 27–39 (2013).
99. Osmond, G.W., E.M. Masko, D.S. Tyler, S.J. Freedland, and S. Pizzo, *In vitro* and *in vivo* evaluation of resveratrol and 3,5-dihydroxy-4′-acetoxy-trans-stilbene in the treatment of human prostate carcinoma and melanoma, *J Surg Res* **179**(1): e141–e148 (2013).
100. Kushi, L.H., T. Byers, C. Doyle, E.V. Bandera, M. McCullough, A. McTiernan, T. Gansler, K.S. Andrews, and M.J. Thun, American Cancer Society Guidelines on Nutrition and Physical Activity for cancer prevention: Reducing the risk of cancer with healthy food choices and physical activity, *CA Cancer J Clin* **56**(5): 254–281 (2006).
101. Chen, L., M. Stacewicz-Sapuntzakis, C. Duncan, R. Sharifi, L. Ghosh, R. van Breemen, D. Ashton, and P.E. Bowen, Oxidative DNA damage in prostate cancer patients consuming tomato sauce-based entrees as a whole-food intervention, *J Natl Cancer Inst* **93**(24): 1872–1879 (2001).
102. Kucuk, O., F.H. Sarkar, W. Sakr, Z. Djuric, M.N. Pollak, F. Khachik, Y.W. Li, M. Banerjee, D. Grignon, J.S. Bertram, J.D. Crissman, E.J. Pontes, and D.P. Wood, Jr., Phase II randomized clinical trial of lycopene supplementation before radical prostatectomy, *Cancer Epidemiol Biomarkers Prev* **10**(8): 861–868 (2001).
103. Heinonen, O.P., D. Albanes, J. Virtamo, P.R. Taylor, J.K. Huttunen, A.M. Hartman, J. Haapakoski, N. Malila, M. Rautalahti, S. Ripatti, H. Maenpaa,

L. Teerenhovi, L. Koss, M. Virolainen, and B.K. Edwards, Prostate cancer and supplementation with alpha-tocopherol and beta-carotene: Incidence and mortality in a controlled trial, *J Natl Cancer Inst* **90**(6): 440–446 (1998).
104. Muzandu, K., K. El Bohi, Z. Shaban, M. Ishizuka, A. Kazusaka, and S. Fujita, Lycopene and beta-carotene ameliorate catechol estrogen-mediated DNA damage, *Jpn J Vet Res* **52**(4): 173–184 (2005).
105. Muzandu, K., M. Ishizuka, K.Q. Sakamoto, Z. Shaban, K. El Bohi, A. Kazusaka, and S. Fujita, Effect of lycopene and beta-carotene on peroxynitrite-mediated cellular modifications, *Toxicol Appl Pharmacol* **215**(3): 330–340 (2006).
106. Hantz, H.L., L.F. Young, and K.R. Martin, Physiologically attainable concentrations of lycopene induce mitochondrial apoptosis in LNCaP human prostate cancer cells, *Exp Biol Med (Maywood)* **230**(3): 171–179 (2005).
107. Liu, X., J.D. Allen, J.T. Arnold, and M.R. Blackman, Lycopene inhibits IGF-I signal transduction and growth in normal prostate epithelial cells by decreasing DHT-modulated IGF-I production in co-cultured reactive stromal cells, *Carcinogenesis* **29**(4): 816–823 (2008).
108. Siler, U., A. Herzog, V. Spitzer, N. Seifert, A. Denelavas, P.B. Hunziker, L. Barella, W. Hunziker, M. Lein, R. Goralczyk, and K. Wertz, Lycopene effects on rat normal prostate and prostate tumor tissue, *J Nutr* **135**(8): 2050S–2052S (2005).
109. Venkateswaran, V., L.H. Klotz, M. Ramani, L.M. Sugar, L.E. Jacob, R.K. Nam, and N.E. Fleshner, A combination of micronutrients is beneficial in reducing the incidence of prostate cancer and increasing survival in the Lady transgenic model, *Cancer Prev Res (Phila)* **2**(5): 473–483 (2009).
110. Edinger, M.S. and W.J. Koff, Effect of the consumption of tomato paste on plasma prostate-specific antigen levels in patients with benign prostate hyperplasia, *Braz J Med Biol Res* **39**(8): 1115–1119 (2006).
111. Schwenke, C., B. Ubrig, P. Thurmann, C. Eggersmann, and S. Roth, Lycopene for advanced hormone refractory prostate cancer: A prospective, open phase II pilot study, *J Urol* **181**(3): 1098–1103 (2009).
112. Singh, S.V., S.K. Srivastava, S. Choi, K.L. Lew, J. Antosiewicz, D. Xiao, Y. Zeng, S.C. Watkins, C.S. Johnson, D.L. Trump, Y.J. Lee, H. Xiao, and A. Herman-Antosiewicz, Sulforaphane-induced cell death in human prostate cancer cells is initiated by reactive oxygen species, *J Biol Chem* **280**(20): 19911–19924 (2005).
113. Singh, A.V., D. Xiao, K.L. Lew, R. Dhir, and S.V. Singh, Sulforaphane induces caspase-mediated apoptosis in cultured PC-3 human prostate cancer cells and retards growth of PC-3 xenografts *in vivo*, *Carcinogenesis* **25**(1): 83–90 (2004).
114. Jakubikova, J., J. Sedlak, J. Bod'o, and Y. Bao, Effect of isothiocyanates on nuclear accumulation of NF-kappaB, Nrf2, and thioredoxin in caco-2 cells, *J Agric Food Chem* **54**(5): 1656–1662 (2006).

115. Myzak, M.C., K. Hardin, R. Wang, R.H. Dashwood, and E. Ho, Sulforaphane inhibits histone deacetylase activity in BPH-1, LnCaP and PC-3 prostate epithelial cells, *Carcinogenesis* **27**(4): 811–819 (2006).
116. Jones, S.B. and J.D. Brooks, Modest induction of phase 2 enzyme activity in the F-344 rat prostate, *BMC Cancer* **6**: 62 (2006).
117. Keum, Y.S., T.O. Khor, W. Lin, G. Shen, K.H. Kwon, A. Barve, W. Li, and A.N. Kong, Pharmacokinetics and pharmacodynamics of broccoli sprouts on the suppression of prostate cancer in transgenic adenocarcinoma of mouse prostate (TRAMP) mice: Implication of induction of Nrf2, HO-1 and apoptosis and the suppression of Akt-dependent kinase pathway, *Pharm Res* **26**(10): 2324–2331 (2009).
118. Erba, D., P. Riso, A. Bordoni, P. Foti, P.L. Biagi, and G. Testolin, Effectiveness of moderate green tea consumption on antioxidative status and plasma lipid profile in humans, *J Nutr Biochem* **16**(3): 144–149 (2005).

10

Phytochemicals from Fruits and Vegetables as Potential Anticancer Agents: Special Reference to Skin Cancer

*Jayesh Antony**, *Minakshi Saikia** *and Ruby John Anto*[†]

INTRODUCTION

Fruits and vegetables contain active ingredients that have both therapeutic as well as preventive properties against most diseases including cancer. Epidemiological studies have consistently shown that a high dietary intake of fruits and vegetables is strongly associated with reduced risk of developing chronic diseases, such as cancer and cardiovascular disease, which are the top two causes of death in the United States and in most industrialized countries.[1] In 1982, the National Academy of Sciences of the United States included guidelines in their report on diet and cancer, emphasizing the importance of fruits and vegetables. The value of adding citrus fruits, cruciferous vegetables, and carotene-rich fruits and vegetables to the diet for reducing the risk of cancer was specifically highlighted and subsequently

---

*Both authors contributed equally to the work.
[†]Corresponding author: Ruby John Anto, Ph.D., Scientist E-II, Cancer Research Program, Division of Cancer Research, Rajiv Gandhi Centre for Biotechnology, Thiruvananthapuram, Kerala-695014, India. Tel: (+91) 471-252-9473, Fax: (+91) 471-234-8096, Email: rjanto@rgcb.res.in.

in 1989; it was recommended to consume five or more servings of fruits and vegetables daily for reducing the risk of both cancer and heart disease, in a report on diet and health.[2]

SKIN CANCER

Skin is the first line of defense that protects us from harmful genotoxic environmental carcinogens, such as ultraviolet (UV) solar radiations, which may lead to development of skin cancer. Skin cancer is the most common type of cancer in fair-skinned populations around the world. The common cutaneous malignancies are basal cell carcinoma (BCC), squamous cell carcinoma (SCC), and malignant melanoma, among which, malignant melanoma has a much higher mortality rate than non-melanoma skin cancer (NMSC) that includes BCC and SCC. Together, malignant melanoma and NMSC comprise the vast majority of skin cancers. Some rare malignancies such as Merkel cell carcinoma, atypical fibroxanthoma, malignant fibrohistiocytoma, dermatofibrosarcoma protuberans, and eccrine and sebaceous carcinomas also come under skin cancer.

Melanoma is a rare but deadly form of skin cancer. The number of new cases of melanoma has steadily increased for the last 30 years.[3] According to the American Cancer Society's "Cancer Facts and Figures" in 2012, an estimated 76,250 new cases of melanoma will occur in the United States in 2012, which is a significant rise of 6,020 cases from 2011 figures. The number of melanoma-related deaths rose as well, by almost 400 cases from 8,790 deaths in 2011 to a predicted 9,180 deaths in 2012. In fact, since 2004, incidence rates among Caucasians have been increasing by almost 3% per year in both men and women. Melanoma is currently the fifth most common cancer among men in the United States, with 44,250 expected to be diagnosed in 2012, and the sixth most common cancer among women, with 32,000 new cases anticipated in 2012. The lifetime risk of developing the disease is one in 36 for men, and one in 55 for women.

Most melanomas develop in the skin, which includes nail beds, soles of the hands or feet, and the scalp, but it can also occur in the eye, or on mucosal surfaces such as the anal canal, rectum, and vagina. Because most cutaneous melanomas are visible, it is a cancer that is extremely amenable to early detection. The survival rates are high if melanoma is diagnosed early when it is confined within the skin and is not associated with ulceration.

Signs and Symptoms

Signs and symptoms of skin cancer include a new skin lesion or open sores that bleed, ooze, or crust and fail to heal in an expected time frame. Enlargement of an existing skin lesion, change in color, size, shape, or texture of a mole, a reddish patch frequently occurring on the chest, shoulders, arms, or legs, or a shiny bump that is pearly or translucent may also indicate development of skin cancer.[4]

Causative Factors

Skin cancer can be caused by UV exposure, diet, and chemical carcinogens such as arsenic pesticides, ionizing radiation, viruses, bacteria, and parasites. Organ transplant recipients and AIDS patients have an increased incidence of skin cancer. Some treatment modalities including radiation therapy, phototherapy, psoralen and long-wave ultraviolet radiation (PUVA), as well as all immunosuppressive treatments can also predispose to skin cancer.

Mechanisms of action

Example of mechanisms of action are as follows: aberrant activation of hedgehog signaling by mutations in *PTCH* and *SMOH* genes; UVB-initiating effects including chromosomal alterations and mutations as well as promotion and progression effects including altered gene expression; cell membrane damage, apoptosis, and a compromised immune system; UVB-mediated activation of phosphatidylinositol-3-kinase (PI3K) and p38 mitogen-activated protein kinase, resulting in increased transcription of the *c-FOS* and *COX-2* (cyclooxygenase-2) genes; and mutation of the *p53* tumor suppressor gene. Other factors such as cell cycle inhibitor *p16INK4* mutation, *Ras* oncogenes mutation, telomere dysfunction, and *c-myc* oncogenes-induced genomic instability are also involved in skin cancer development.

Diagnosis

Skin cancer can be diagnosis via biopsy, which can determine the type of tumor and rate of tumor growth, along with X-ray, CT, MRI, or ultrasound scans that can determine how far the cancer has spread. Karyotyping, study of loss of heterozygosity or allelic imbalance, and comparative genomic hybridization can be used for genomic DNA analyses, while Northern blots, RT-PCR, nuclease protection assays, *in-situ* hybridization, etc. can be used for RNA analyses.

Treatment

Treatment for skin cancer includes surgery, as well as non-surgical treatments such as radiotherapy, photodynamic therapy (laser), and immunotherapy. If the cancer has spread, the patient may be given chemotherapy, while NMSCs can also be destroyed by freezing them with liquid nitrogen (cryotherapy). Therapies using complementary and alternative medicines (CAMs) can involve therapeutic diets, herbs and herbal combinations, homeopathy, acupuncture, etc.; these are used for preventing rather than treating skin cancer and to reduce the side effects of conventional treatments.

ANTICANCER PROPERTIES OF FRUITS AND VEGETABLES

Fruits and vegetables represent an untapped reservoir of various nutritive and non-nutritive phytochemicals with potential cancer chemopreventive activity. Taking cue from the epidemiological data indicating that dietary habits influence cancer risk, considerable scientific interest has been generated in developing various preventive measures based on diet, especially those involving fruits and vegetables,[5,6] which represent a vast source of phytochemicals having potential anticancer or chemopreventive efficacy.[7] As such, interventions based on fruits and vegetables are more natural, since they lower the cancer risk without posing any side effects and help to maintain good general health as they are major sources of vitamins, and fiber.[8] Numerous dietary agents have been demonstrated to block malignancy by interfering with the various stages in the multi-step events of cancer development (Table 10.1).

Table 10.1: Molecular mechanisms of the phytochemicals regulating their anticancer activities.

No	Phytochemical/ Extract	Biological activity	Mode of action/ Target molecules	References
1	Apigenin	Anticancer	⊥ ODC, PKC activity and nuclear oncogene expression	44–48
2	Asperulosidic acid	Anticancer	⊥ AP-1 transactivation and c-Jun phosphorylation	20
3	Auraptene	Antitumor	Suppression of leukocyte activation	16
4	Betanin	Chemo-preventive; anti-cancer	Protect against Epstein–Barr early antigen activation	51, 52
5	Canthaxanthin	Antitumor; antioxidant	—	53
6	α-carotene	Antitumor	—	54
7	β-carotene	Antitumor; antioxidant	Quenching free radicals	53, 54
8	Chebulagic acid	Cytotoxic	—	34
9	Chebulinic acid	Cytotoxic	—	34
10	β-Cryptoxanthin	Antitumor	—	55
11	Delphinidin	Anticancer; photochemo-preventive	COX-2, MAPKK4, PI3K, AP-1, and NF-κB transactivation; JNKs, p38, and Akt phosphorylation; lipid peroxidation; 8-OHdG formation; decrease in PCNA and Bcl-2; increase in PARP cleavage and Bax; caspases activation ↑ Bid and Bak and ↓ Bcl-x_L	41–43
12	Diallyl sulfide	Antioxidant; antitumor	↑ GSH activity	46
13	Ethyl gallate	Cytotoxic	—	36
14	Gallic acid	Cytotoxic	—	34
15	Garlic oil	Antitumor	—	57

(*Continued*)

Table 10.1: (*Continued*)

No	Phytochemical/ Extract	Biological activity	Mode of action/ Target molecules	References
16	Genistein	Antioxidant; anticancer	⊥ Bulky DNA adduct formation; H_2O_2; inflammatory responses; tyrosine protein kinase (TPK) activity; *c-fos* and *c-jun* expression ↓ EGFR phosphorylation ↑ Catalase, superoxide dismutase, glutathione peroxidase, and glutathione	46, 58, 59
17	Ginger extract	Antitumor	⊥ Epidermal edema, hyperplasia, ODC, COX, and lipoxygenase activities	60
18	[6]-gingerol	Antioxidant; chemopreventive; antitumor	⊥ AP-1 activation, ODC activity and inflammation	61, 62
19	Grape seed extract/grape seed polyphenol (GSP)	Antioxidant; antitumor	Inhibition of lipid peroxidation Reduction in activities of ornithine decarboxylase (ODC) and myeloperoxidase (MPO) enzymes ↓ MAPK and ↓ NF-κB	8, 17, 18
20	Lupeol	Antitumor; anti-inflammatory; antioxidant; antimutagenic; chemopreventive; chemotherapeutic	⊥ Protein kinases, DNA topoisomerase II, antioxidant enzymes, prostaglandin (PGE2), and cytokine production Reduction in ODC, COX-2, NO synthase, lipid peroxidation, and hydrogen peroxide generation ⊥ Activation of PI3K, NF-κB, and IKKα, and phosphorylation of Akt and IκBα	21–24, 64
21	Lutein	Antitumor	—	55
22	Luteolin	Cytotoxic; antitumor; antimutagenic; chemopreventive	⊥ COX-2 , AP-1, and NF-κB activity; MAPK and Akt phosphorylation; PKCε and Src kinase activity ↓ TNFα, and PCNA	37, 63

(*Continued*)

Table 10.1: (*Continued*)

No	Phytochemical/ Extract	Biological activity	Mode of action/ Target molecules	References
23	Lycopene	Antioxidant; anti-cancer	Quench free radical reactions	39, 40
24	*Momordica charantia*	Antitumor; chemopreventive	—	9–11
25	Nobiletin	Anti-inflammatory; antioxidant; antitumor	↓ COX-2 ⊥ Induction of nitric oxide (NO) synthase proteins Release of prostaglandin E2 (PGE2)	15
26	Onion oil	Antitumor	⊥ ODC	46
27	[6]-paradol	Antioxidant; chemopreventive	Induction of apoptosis	61
28	Pomegranate fruit extract (PFE)	Antioxidant; anti-inflammatory; antitumor	⊥ ODC, COX-2, PCNA, p21, p53, and Ki-67 ⊥ ERK1/2, JNK1/2, p38, and IκBα phosphorylation ⊥ NF-κB and IKKα, STAT3, AKT, and mTOR activation ↑ Bax and Bad ↓ Bcl-x_L	30–34
29	Quercetin	Antioxidant	Protects glutathione peroxidase, glutathione reductase, catalase, and superoxide dismutase activities ⊥ Peroxidation in liposomal membranes, suppression of contact hypersensitivity, and reduction of CD8-positive cells	65–67
30	Resveratrol	Antiproliferative; cell cycle arrest; anticancer	↓ Cyclins D1, D2, and E, Cdk 2, 4, and 6, PCNA, hyperphosphorylated pRb proteins, ERK1/2, and AP-1 signaling ↑ p21WAF1/CIP1 ⊥ Survivin, COX-2, and ODC	19
31	Silibinin	Antioxidant; anti-cancer	Reduction in thymine dimer positive cells ↑ p53-p21/Cip1 and CHOP	26–29

(*Continued*)

Table 10.1. (*Continued*)

No	Phytochemical/ Extract	Biological activity	Mode of action/ Target molecules	References
32	Silymarin	Antioxidant; antitumor; anti-inflammatory, chemopreventive; chemotherapeutic; cell cycle inhibition	⊥ Lipid peroxidation, COX and ODC activity, malondialdehyde formation, TNFα and IL-1α mRNA expression, EGFR kinase and its receptor tyrosine kinase activity, ERK1/2 activation, and depletion of catalase activity Scavenging free radicals and reactive oxygen species Decreases PCNA positive cells Inhibition of DNA synthesis ⊥ Depletion of SOD, catalase, and GPx activities and increase in myeloperoxidase and lipoxygenase activity Activation of JNK signaling ⊥ Cyclin A, B, D1, and E, and CDK1, 2, and 6 ↑ $p21^{Cip1}$and $p27^{Kip1}$	16, 25
33	*Terminalia arjuna* extract	Anticancer; Antimutagenic	—	36–38

Some of the commonly available fruits and vegetables with their anticancer properties pertaining to the prevention of skin malignancies are discussed below.

Bitter gourd

The bitter gourd (*Momordica charantia*) is a fruit belonging to the Cucurbitaceae family, which along with its peel, pulp, and seed have been reported to inhibit dimethylbenz[a]anthracene (DMBA)-induced mouse skin papillomas.[9] Extracts of *Momordica* peel, pulp, seed, and whole fruit have been shown to result in an appreciable decrease in the tumor burden, the cumulative numbers of papillomas, and the incidence of skin papillomas.[10] A report indicates the chemopreventive activity of *Momordia charantia* fruit and leaves on DMBA and croton oil induced skin papilliomagenesis in mice model. A significant reduction in tumor burden, tumor incidence, and cumulative number of papillomas has also been reported in *Momordica* extract-treated animals as compared to animals treated with single topical application of DMBA alone and croton oil.[11]

Citrus

Citrus is one of the major world fruit crops and is consumed mostly fresh or as juices because of its nutritional value and unqiue flavor. An Indian citrus species, *C. aurantifolia*, is reported to have significant antioxidant activity due to its high hesperidin content.[12] Hesperidin is known to act as anticancer agent through prostaglandin[13] and inhibition of chemical carcinogenesis.[14]

Nobiletin, a polymethoxyflavonoid isolated from the species *C. unshiu*, which is extremely popular in Japan, is reported to have anti-inflammatory, antioxidative, and antitumor activity in murine skin.[15] This compound inhibits skin inflammation induced by 12-O-tetradecanoylphorbol-13-acetate (TPA) by suppressing the expression of COX-2, inducing production of nitric oxide (NO) synthase proteins, and release of prostaglandin E2.[15] The chemopreventive efficacy of nobiletin has also been documented by a DMBA/TPA-induced mouse skin tumor model.[15]

A coumarin-related compound, auraptene, has also been isolated from the cold-pressed oil of *Citrus natsudaidai* Hayata, commonly known as *natsumikan*, which was shown to reduce tumor incidence and tumor number as assessed by a two-stage carcinogenesis model, possibly through the suppression of leukocyte activation, which inhibits tumor promotion.[16] This compound has been also reported in *hassaku* orange (*C. hassaku*) and grapefruit (*C. paradisi*).

Grape

In 1999, it was reported for the first time that grape seed polyphenols (GSPs) possess antitumor-promoting activities, due to the strong antioxidant effect of procynidins present in them,[17] in a dose-dependent manner, by reducing tumor incidence, multiplicity, and volume. The same study has also reported the isolation and identification of five polyphenols from the extract, namely, catechin, procyanidin B2, procyanidin B5, procyanidin C1, and procyanidin B5-3′-gallate. All these compounds have been shown to have significant antioxidant capabilities as assessed by their epidermal lipid peroxidation inhibition activity. They have also conducted a structure-activity relationship study and the result showed that the activity increases with increase in polymerization in polyphenol structure and position of linkage between inter-flavan units. A sharp increase in the activity was noticed when a gallate group was linked at the 3′-hydroxyl position of a procyanidin dimer. Overall, the study put forward GSPs, especially procyanidin B5-3′-gallate, as promising candidate molecules for the development of a chemopreventive or anticarcinogenic agent. GSPs are also reported to have antitumor-promoting activities in murine skin epidermis[18] through the reduction in the activities of both ornithine decarboxylase (ODC) and myeloperoxidase (MPO) enzymes, which are treated as two markers of tumor promotion in murine skin.

In a UVB radiation-induced mouse skin carcinogenesis model, dietary feeding of GSPs was effective in preventing photocarcinogenesis at both the initiation and promotion stages and in malignant transformation of skin papillomas to carcinomas. The mechanism for this anticarcinogenic effect has been attributed to the antioxidant property, reduction in MAPK and NF-κB expression, and inhibition of lipid peroxidation by GSPs.[8]

Another important compound isolated from the skin and seed of grapes and several other plants of grape vine species is resveratrol (3,5,4′-trihydroxy-trans-stilbene), which is a stilbenoid, a type of phenol. Many studies have shown that the topical application of resveratrol inhibits the development of several cutaneous disorders, including skin cancer and phototoxicity.[19] Resveratrol induces its anti-proliferative effect by modulating cell cycle regulatory proteins and has been shown to downregulate the expression of cyclins D1 and D2, Cdk 2, 4, and 6, and proliferating cell nuclear antigen (PCNA), and upregulate the expression of p21WAF1/CIP1. Moreover, the expression of anti-apoptotic proteins such as survivin and markers of tumor promotion, COX-2 and ODC, are found to be inhibited by resveratrol. Ninety-eight percent reduction in skin tumors and 60% reduction in papillomas have been reported with the topical application of resveratrol, which could be related to its cytotoxic and free radical scavenging activities. Orally administered resveratrol was also shown to inhibit DMBA/croton oil-induced murine skin papillomas, correlating with prolonging the latent period of tumor occurrence and inhibiting croton oil-induced enhancement of epidermal ODC activities.

Resveratrol induces G1-phase cell cycle arrest, accompanied by p21WAF1/CIP1 induction in human squamous cell carcinoma cells; it decreases the cell cycle regulators, cyclins D1/D2/E and Cdks, hyperphosphorylated pRb proteins, ERK1/2, and AP-1 signaling.[19] It also potentiates generation of 8-oxo-7 and 8-dihydro-2′-deoxyguanosine (8-OHdG), an oxidative damage which can lead to DNA strand breaks, and finally cell death in UVA-irradiated immortalized human keratinocyte cells.[19]

In vitro studies have proven the cytotoxic effect of resveratrol in melanoma cells through induction of apoptosis. An *in vivo* study conducted to evaluate this effect report that, though oral administration of resveratrol did not inhibit the growth of melanoma cells inoculated into the footpads of mice, it decreased the hepatic metastatic invasion of cells inoculated intrasplenically.[19] Moreover, the intraperitoneal administration of resveratrol has been shown to result in a dose-dependent delay of tumor growth, without toxicity. Altogether, the *in vivo* studies indicate that resveratrol is not an effective chemotherapeutic agent in inhibiting melanoma growth in animals, although more preclinical studies would be required for confirmation.[19]

Great morinda

Morinda citrifolia, commonly known as great morinda or Indian mulberry (locally called 'noni'), is a plant originally grown in the Hawaiian and Tahitian islands and is used traditionally to treat a broad range of diseases including cancer. Two novel glycosides, 6-O-(b-D-glucopyranosyl)-1-O-octanoyl-b-D-glucopyranose and asperulosidic acid, extracted from the juice of noni fruits, were found to inhibit TPA and epidermal growth factor (EGF)-induced AP-1 transactivation and cell transformation in murine epidermal cells by inhibiting the phosphorylation of c-Jun, but not extracellular signal-regulated kinases or p38 kinases, indicating that c-Jun N-terminal kinases regulate TPA or EGF-induced AP-1 activity and subsequent cell transformation.[20]

Mango

The mango (*Mangifera indica*), also known as the Ayurvedic king of fruits, contains a vast number of phenolic compounds such as quercetin, isoquercitrin, astragalin, fisetin, gallic acid, and methylgallate, all of which possess chemopreventive properties. Lupeol [lup-20(29)-en-3β-ol] is a naturally occurring triterpene found in various fruits and vegetables and many medicinal plants. A significant quantity of this compound is present in mangoes along with olives, strawberries, and figs, and is reported to possess several important biological properties which can be correlated to the mango's antitumor-promoting effect. It has been shown to possess strong anti-inflammatory and antimutagenic activity in both *in vitro* and *in vivo* systems, possibly through inhibiting protein kinases and DNA topoisomerase II, a target for anticancer chemotherapy. Studies have also been reported that lupeol induces differentiation and inhibits the cell growth of melanoma cells.[21,22] The anti-inflammatory, antimutagenic, and antioxidative activities as well as its inhibitory potential against prostaglandin (PGE2) and cytokine production suggests the antitumor-promoting effect of lupeol.

Lupeol prevents oxidative stress during the early stages of tumor promotion and it is reported to reverse benzoyl peroxide (BPO)-mediated inhibition of the activities of several antioxidant enzymes such as catalase, glutathione peroxidase, glucose 6-phosphate dehydrogenase, glutathione reductase, and glutathione S transferase, along with the amelioration of BPO-induced lipid peroxidation, increased generation of hydrogen peroxide, and depleted levels of glutathione.[23] Lupeol is found to be able to intercept free radicals and protect cellular macromolecules and effectively inhibits ODC activity which plays a major role in tumor promotion.[23] Topical application of lupeol prior to TPA application onto the skin of mice was found to induce significant inhibition of skin edema and hyperplasia as assessed by a reduction in ODC, COX-2, and NO synthase, which may be correlated to the inhibition of TPA-induced activation of PI3K, phosphorylation of Akt, activation of NF-κB and IKKα, and degradation and phosphorylation of IκB. Animals pretreated with lupeol were found to significantly reduce tumor incidence, lower tumor body burden, and a significant delay in the latency period for tumor appearance.[24]

Milk thistle plant

Milk thistle, *Silybum marianum* (*L.*) Gaertn, belongs to the Asteraceae family. The ripe seed of the plant is used in herbal remedies and contain the antioxidant silymarin which is a flavanolignan complex, present in the black shiny seeds (fruit) of milk thistle plant and exhibits potential anticancer activity against skin cancer as assessed by both *in vitro* and *in vivo* studies. Silibinin is the most active and abundant constituent present in silymarin.

Silibinin is found to inhibit skin inflammation, DNA damage, epithelial cell proliferation and sunburn, alter mitogenic, apoptotic, and survival signals, activate p53, induce cell cycle arrest, and enhance repair of DNA damage. Studies report that silymarin inhibit lipid peroxidation and provide significant protection against UVB-induced depletion of catalase activity. Therefore, silymarin can effectively terminate the harmful biochemical reactions by scavenging free radicals and reactive oxygen species (ROS) and by strengthening the cellular antioxidant status. It also inhibits UVB-caused induction of COX and ODC activity, which provides an insight into the molecular mechanisms of the protective effect of silymarin against UV-induced skin carcinogenesis.

Several other studies have reported the chemopreventive as well as chemotherapeutic activities of silymarin in various carcinogenesis models. It is also reported to show complete protection against okadaic acid-triggered tumor promotion in DMBA-initiated skin cancer and led to the complete inhibition of TPA-caused skin edema and induction of epidermal hyperplasia in mice. Silymarin decreases PCNA positive cells in TPA-induced epidermal proliferation in mouse skin and inhibits [methyl-3H]thymidine incorporation (DNA synthesis) in human epidermoid carcinoma cells.[25] The inhibitory effect of silymarin on malondialdehyde formation in epidermal microsome and TPA-caused lipid peroxidation in murine skin epidermis, supports its strong *in vivo* antioxidant activity.[25]

It has also been shown that silymarin strongly inhibits TPA-caused depletion of epidermal enzyme activities of superoxide dismutase, catalase, and glutathione peroxidase and TPA-caused increase in myeloperoxidase activity, that is closely associated with neutrophil infiltration, which is a characteristic feature of TPA and UV radiation-caused skin inflammation. Silymarin is also shown to inhibit the TPA-caused increase in lipoxygenase activity in terms of 8-HETE formation in murine skin and inhibits both TPA caused COX-2 expression, and COX activity in terms of PGE2, PGF2α, and PGD2 formation in murine epidermis. Inhibition of TPA-induced COX-2 expression by silymarin is found to be selective as it does not alter COX-1 (constitutive COX) expression, suggesting that it can be targeted toward COX-2 modulation in epithelial cancers.

Silymarin inhibits TPA- and okadaic acid-induced expression of TNFα mRNA, which is a cytokine that has been shown to be associated with skin inflammation and tumor promotion, in a dose-dependent manner in mouse skin. Consistent with inhibition of skin inflammation and tumor promotion, silymarin strongly inhibits the TPA-caused increase in IL-1α mRNA expression and corresponding IL-1α protein level in murine skin.

In vitro studies by another group showed that silymarin inhibits both the ligand activation of receptor tyrosine kinase EGFR and its intrinsic kinase activity, and subsequently inhibits the activation of an immediate downstream target Shc, an adaptor protein containing src homology-2 (SH-2) domain. Silymarin also inhibits the EGF-induced activation of ERK1/2 in starved skin cancer cells at lower doses while it does not show any effect on ERK1/2 activation at higher doses though it is activating JNK signaling as an apoptotic effect of the compound. In cell growth studies, silymarin has shown dose and time-dependent death accompanied by growth inhibition in cancer cells of epidermoid and epithelial origin.

Silymarin is also shown to inhibit the expression of cell cycle proteins such as cyclin A, B, D1, and E and Cdk1, 2, and 6, and decreases the kinase activity associated with Cdk1, 2, and 6 and cyclin D1 and E in human epidermoid carcinoma cells. Increase in the protein expression of p21Cip1and p27Kip1 and their binding with Cdk1, 2, and 6 was also documented along with the report of accumulation of the cells in the G2/M phase at lesser treatment time while, longer treatment (24 h) with silymarin shows both G0/G1 and G2/M arrest at the expense of the S-phase cell population.[25]

Silibinin is the major bioactive flavanone present in milk thistle seeds having very strong antioxidant activity by which it is capable of scavenging both free radicals and ROS, hence enhancing cellular antioxidant defense mechanisms.[26] A study has reported that the topical application of silibinin prior to or immediately after UV irradiation resulted in strong protective effect toward the radiation-induced skin damages by reduction in thymine dimer positive cells as well as an upregulation of p53-p21/Cip1 in the murine epidermis.[27] Dietary feeding of silibinin to mice indicated that silibinin affords strong protection in skin epidermis by either preventing DNA damage or enhancing repair, reducing UVB-induced hyperproliferative response, and inhibiting UVB-caused apoptosis and sunburn, possibly through the upregulation of p53 and p21/cip1 as major UVB-damage control sensors.[28] A recent study has proven that silibinin is acting as a potent sensitizer of UVA radiation-induced oxidative stress and enhances endoplasmic reticulum (ER) stress-mediated apoptosis in human keratinocyte cells by increasing the expression of CHOP protein.[29]

Pomegranate

The pomegranate (*Punica granatum*), native to Persia, is an edible fruit cultivated in Mediterranean countries, Afghanistan, India, China, Japan, Russia, and the United States. Edible parts of pomegranate fruit comprise 80% juice and 20% seed. Pomegranate fruit extract (PFE) is a rich source of two types of polyphenolic compounds, namely, anthocyanins and hydrolysable tannins. PFE possesses strong antioxidant and antiinflammatory properties.

Afaq *et al.* reported the inhibition of TPA-induced tumor promotion and epidermal ODC activity and COX-2 expression by PFE for the first time.[30] They also found that the topical application of PFE inhibits TPA-induced phosphorylation of ERK1/2, p38 and JNK1/2, as well as activation of NF-κB and IKKα and phosphorylation and degradation of IκBα. Later, they also demonstrated that mice pre-treated with PFE showed substantially reduced tumor incidence and multiplicity as assessed by a DMBA/TPA-induced skin carcinogenesis model.

The same group has also reported that pre-treatment of normal human epidermal keratinocytes (NHEKs) with PFE for 24 h before UVB exposure inhibited UVB-mediated activation of several survival signals such as MAPKs and NF-κB.[31] They have evaluated the effect *in vivo*[32] and have demonstrated that oral feeding of PFE to mice resulted in the inhibition of UVB-induced increase in skin edema, hyperplasia, infiltration of leukocytes, generation of hydrogen peroxide, DNA damage, and UVB-induced PCNA, ODC, and COX-2 protein expression, and the induction of UVB mediated increase in p21 and p53 protein expression.[33]

It was also shown that pre-treatment of NHEKs with PFE for 24 h before UVA exposure inhibited the activation of STAT3, AKT, ERK1/2, and mTOR, and overexpression of Ki-67 and PCNA, which led to cell cycle arrest in the G1 phase, with an enhancement in the expression of Bax and Bad (pro-apoptotic proteins) and the downregulation of Bcl-x_L (anti-apoptotic protein).[34]

Terminalia species

Terminalia chebula is a medicinal plant found in tropical regions of the world and is commonly used in Ayurvedic preparations as a traditional medicine due to the wide spectrum of pharmacological activities associated with the biologically active constituents present in the plant. The methanolic extract of *T. chebula* as well as its isolated compounds, gallic acid, 1,2,3,4,6-penta-O-galloyl-b-D-gulcopyranose, chebulagic acid, and chebulinic acid are reported to have moderate *in vitro* cytotoxicity against human melanoma cells.[35] Another species of the genus, *T. arjuna* (Roxb.) Wight and Arn., has numerous medicinal uses in India including treatment of cancer.[36] The bark of the plant is rich in polyphenols including flavones, flavonols, phenylpropanoids, and tannins which contribute to its various medicinal properties. A group has reported the isolation of anticancer compounds gallic acid, ethyl gallate, and luteolin from *T. arjuna* with strong inhibition of growth of different cancer cell lines including melanoma cells.[37] Another study has identified the antimutagenic effect of different organic extracts from *T. arjuna.*[38] The active extracts showed to inhibit the S9-dependent mutagens more effectively than the direct-acting mutagens in the TA98 frameshift mutagen tester strain of *Salmonella typhimurium.*

Tomato

The tomato is a storehouse of the antioxidant lycopene and also contains vitamins A, C, and E, which are all enemies of cancer-friendly free radicals. Lycopene is an acyclic hydrocarbon carotenoid also present in other fruits such as the watermelon, pink grapefruit, guava and papaya. Skin lycopene is also reported to have the ability to interact with the reactive species formed in the skin upon UV exposure and to quench free radical reactions.[39] Because carotenoids are consumed in the process of quenching free radicals, when skin is subjected to UV light stress, skin lycopene is destroyed, suggesting a role of lycopene in mitigating oxidative damage in tissues, which may be an important defense mechanism against adverse effects of UV irradiation on the skin.

A dose-dependent inhibition of UVB-induced ODC and myeloperoxidase and significant reduction in bifold skin thickness upon the application of lycopene has been reported. The topical application of lycopene was also reported to show significant reversal of UVB-induced PCNA inhibition, and normal PCNA staining was found to be restored in the carotenoid-treated skin.[40]

Fruits and vegetables contain ample compounds that have chemopreventive as well as chemotherapeutic properties against various cancers including the cancer of skin. We have conducted a detailed survey of the major compounds, which might have potential therapeutic efficacy against skin cancer.

Anthocyanins

Anthocyanins are abundant natural polyphenolic compounds that generally are responsible for conferring the bright-red, blue, and purple color to fruits and vegetables. Vegetables such as the purple cabbage, red onion, red radish, red lettuce, and corn contain anthocyanins. They influence various factors that control skin tumor development.[41]

Delphinidin, the aglycon form of anthocyanin, has the most potent anticarcinogenic properties. It is reported to exert a stronger inhibitory potency against cancer cell migration and cell transformation. A study has shown that delphinidin suppresses UVB-induced COX-2 expression by acting as a potent inhibitor of MAPKK4 and PI3K, and also inhibits UVB-induced transactivation of AP-1 and NF-κB and phosphorylation of JNKs, p38, and Akt in murine epidermal cells.[42] Afaq *et al.* found that pre-treatment of HaCaT cells with delphinidin inhibited UVB-mediated increase in lipid peroxidation, formed 8-OHdG, decreased PCNA expression, increased PARP cleavage, activated caspases, increased Bax, decreased Bcl-2, upregulated Bid and Bak, and downregulated Bcl-x_L.[43] The photochemopreventive effect of delphinidin was also shown *in vivo* by the same group on UVB-induced biomarkers of skin cancer development. The topical application of delphinidin to murine skin inhibited apoptosis and markers of DNA damage such as cyclobutane pyrimidine dimers and 8-OHdG, and it is suggested that delphinidin protects the cells from UVB-induced apoptosis by inhibiting UVB-mediated oxidative stress and reducing DNA damage.[41]

Apigenin

Apigenin (5,7,4′-trihydroxyflavone) is a plant flavonoid found in vegetables such as beans, broccoli, Chinese cabbage, celeries, leeks, onions, garlics, barley, and parsley, and has been reported to be effective in the prevention of UVA-/B-induced skin carcinogenesis in mice.[44] Studies have shown that it inhibits epidermal ODC induction by TPA and the incidence and numbers of carcinoma in mice, and decreases the tendency of conversion of papillomas to carcinomas. It has also been shown to suppress PKC activity and nuclear oncogene expression in TPA-induced tumor promotion that might contribute to the molecular mechanisms of skin cancer inhibition.[45] The mechanism underlying apigenin action in human diploid fibroblasts has also been investigated and was found to be G1 cell cycle arrest by inhibiting Cdk2 kinase activity, phosphorylation of retinoblastoma protein, induction of the Cdk inhibitor p21/WAF1, and stabilization of tumor suppressor gene *p53*. The photoprotective action of apigenin may be the p53-p21/waf1 response pathway. In another *in-vivo* study, apigenin treatment to murine skin was found to result in inhibition of UV-mediated induction of ODC activity and reduction in tumor incidence and an increase in tumor free survival in the mice. These studies suggest that apigenin may be an effective agent against photocarcinogenesis.[46]

It has been established that the topical application of apigenin suppresses the UVB-induced increase in COX-2 expression in murine and human keratinocyte cells.[47,48] One study has evaluated the combined effect of quercetin and apigenin, and demonstrated that *in vivo* administration of both together was effective in inhibiting melanoma lung tumor metastasis in a murine melanoma metastasis model, which was postulated to be due to the impairment of endothelial interactions in malignant cells.[49] Another study has shown that apigenin markedly induces the expression of death receptor 5 (DR5) and synergistically acts with exogenous soluble recombinant human tumor necrosis factor-related apoptosis-inducing ligand (TRAIL) to induce apoptosis in malignant tumor cells.[50]

Betanin

The root of the plant *Beta vulgaris L.* (Chenopodiaceae), commonly called beetroot, contains betanin, a potent chemopreventive agent. Studies have shown that betanin inhibits DMBA/UVB promoted and (±)-(E)-4-methyl-2-[(E)-hydroxyamino]-5-nitro-6-methoxy-3-hexanamide (NOR-1)-induced TPA promoted skin carcinogenesis. The spleen in the DMBA/UVB-treated mice bioassay showed that the experimental group treated with DMBA/UVB alone had enlarged spleens (splenomegaly), whereas mice that received DMBA/UVB along with betanin in drinking water had normal-sized spleens. Betanin, therefore, offers significant protection against UVB-induced tumors as well as against splenomegaly. It is orally active in preventing skin carcinogenesis[51] and has been shown to protect against TPA induced Epstein–Barr early antigen activation (EBV-EA), which correlates with the promotion stage of carcinogenesis.[52] Hence, betanin inhibits both initiation and promotion steps of chemical carcinogenesis.

Carotenoids

Vegetables such as green leaves, carrots, pumpkin, kale, spinach, and winter squash are rich sources of carotenoids. Cells exposed to mutagenic agents such as nucleophilic agents, X-rays, and ROS are prevented by carotenoids against nuclear damage. Carotenoids have been implicated as chemoprotective and chemopreventive agents in many cancers including cancer of the skin. Various *in vivo* experiments have been performed to validate its cancer protective roles. Studies have shown that injection of β-carotene slowed the skin tumor progression in mice exposed to UV light (UVA, UVB), and feeding of β-carotene, canthaxanthin, or polyenes delays and reduces skin tumor development in mice exposed to UVB. Carotenoids are found to prevent oxidative stress to the cells by quenching free radicals capable of causing cellular damage.[53] Murakoshi *et al.* have proven that α-carotene is more potent in suppressing the promoting activity of TPA in DMBA-induced mice model than β-carotene.[54] Other carotenoids such as lutein, lycopene, β-cryptoxanthin are also found to have a chemoprotective role in skin tumorigenesis.[55]

Diallyl sulphide

Diallyl sulfide is a natural compound present in *Allium* vegetables such as garlics and onions and is known to possess strong antioxidant potential. One group has shown that diallyl sulfide completely abolishes the prolonged inhibitory effect of TPA on glutathione (GSH) peroxidase and increases the enzyme activity in isolated epidermal cells incubated in the presence or absence of TPA. Garlic oil is also reported to inhibit TPA-induced ODC activity significantly.[56] Another study has demonstrated that the topical application of garlic oil decreases the number of tumor-bearing mice and the mean number of tumors per mouse in benzo[a]-pyrene-induced skin tumor formation in mice. Onion oil is also reported to produce the same effect on murine skin. It has been demonstrated that the topical application of diallyl sulfide and diallyl disulfide inhibit benzoyl peroxide-mediated tumor promotion in DMBA-initiated murine skin.[46]

Genistein

Genistein is a soy bean-derived isoflavone (4′,5,7-trihydroxyisoflavone), which exhibits antioxidant and anticarcinogenic effects in the skin. The topical application of genistein has been shown to reduce tumor incidence and multiplicity. Studies indicate that genistein exerts its anti-initiational and anti-promotional effects on skin carcinogenesis, probably through the inhibition of oxidative and inflammatory events *in vivo*, and inhibits DMBA-induced bulky DNA adduct formation and TPA-stimulated H_2O_2 and inflammatory responses in murine skin.[57] Dietary administration of genistein has shown to substantially enhance the activities of antioxidant enzymes in murine skin and trigger the inhibition of the tyrosine protein kinase (TPK) activity and downregulation of EGF receptor (EGFR) phosphorylation, which ultimately inhibits UVB-induced expression of the proto-oncogenes, *c-fos* and *c-jun* in murine skin.[58] Dietary feeding of genistein is also found to significantly increase the activities of catalase, superoxide dismutase, glutathione peroxidase, and glutathione reductase in the skin. Suppression of UVB-induced proto-oncogene expression in murine skin suggests that genistein may serve as a potential preventive agent against photodamage and photocarcinogenesis.[46]

Ginger compounds

Ginger rhizome (*Zingiber officinale*) is consumed as a spice and a flavoring agent. An ethanolic extract of ginger is reported to mediate antitumor-promoting effects and has been shown to inhibit TPA-caused epidermal edema and hyperplasia in a murine skin tumorigenesis model.[9] Various studies revealed that the application of this extract on murine skin inhibits TPA-caused induction of epidermal ODC, COX, and lipoxygenase activities.[59]

The antioxidant potential of its constituents is responsible for the cancer chemopreventive properties of ginger. Reports have demonstrated that two structurally related compounds of the ginger family, [6]-gingerol and [6]-paradol, block EGF-induced cell transformation in mouse epidermal cell lines and, although closely related structurally, both of them act through different mechanisms. While [6]-gingerol acts through inhibition of AP-1 activation, [6]-paradol appear to act through the induction of apoptosis.[60] A study evaluated the antitumor promotional activity of [6]-gingerol, in a two-stage murine skin carcinogenesis model and observed significant inhibition of skin papilloma formation as well as TPA-induced epidermal ODC activity and inflammation.[61]

Luteolin

Luteolin is a flavonoid present in various vegetables, including onions and broccoli, and has been reported to possess anticarcinogenic effects. A study on the chemopreventive effect and associated mechanisms of luteolin indicates that it suppresses UVB-induced COX-2 expression and activation of AP-1 and NF-κB in mice. Luteolin is reported to attenuate protein kinase Cε (PKCε) and Src kinase activities that subsequently inhibit UVB-induced phosphorylation of the MAPK and Akt signaling pathways.[62] It suppresses tumor incidence, multiplicity, and overall size of the tumor size in mice and produces a substantial reduction in the levels of COX-2, TNF-α, and PCNA against groups treated with only UVB, as assessed by immunohistochemistry and immunoblotting. Hence, luteolin exerts potent chemopreventive activity against UVB-induced skin cancer mainly by targeting PKCε and Src.[62]

Lupeol

Lupeol, is found in vegetables such as white cabbage, pepper, cucumbers, soy beans, and carrots, and also present in a good amount in mangoes. It is a non-toxic but highly potent chemopreventive and chemotherapeutic agent which has been proven to be beneficial against skin tumorigenesis by various *in vivo* studies.[63] A detailed account of the anticancer activity of this compound has already been discussed in the section above on 'Fruits and Treatment of Skin Cancer.'

Quercetin

Quercetin (3,5,7,3′,4′-pentahydroxyflavon) is one of the most abundant natural flavonoids, which is present in various common vegetables such as onions, lettuce, broccoli, kales, and cotton-seed. It is a powerful antioxidant and metal ion chelator. Reports show that quercetin protects skin antioxidant systems, namely, glutathione peroxidase, glutathione reductase, catalase, and superoxide dismutase activities, against UVA-irradiating damage in rats to a considerable degree.[64] Oral intake of quercetin was reported to reduce development of tumors after UVB exposure by protecting the immune system against UVB-induced immunosuppression. Studies indicate that it prevents the UV-induced suppression of the contact hypersensitivity (CHS) and the reduction of the percentage of CD8-positive cells in the spleen and lymph nodes.[65] *In vitro*, quercetin and its semisynthetic derivatives (quercetin 3-O-acetate, quercetin 3-O-propionate, and quercetin 3-O-palmitate) were found to inhibit UVC radiation-induced peroxidation in liposomal membranes.[66]

CLINICAL TRIALS

Very few clinical trials have been conducted using phytochemicals reported from fruits and vegetables in skin cancer, and in most cases, the results are not published. A 12-year randomized primary prevention trial of β-carotene supplementation for NMSC has been conducted and the results showed that there was no effect for β-carotene on the incidence of both BCC and SCC.[67] A Phase II study on the placebo-controlled intervention trial of oral N-acetylcysteine (NAC) for the protection of human nevi against UV-induced oxidative stress/damage is ongoing in the Huntsman Cancer Institute in the United States. Tomato and pomegranate juices are two of the best natural sources of NAC. The available details regarding the clinical trials of the different compounds mentioned in the chapter is given in the Table 10.2.

CONCLUSION

Ozone layer depletion has led to increased UV infiltration, which is expected to raise skin cancer incidences. This warrants more chemotherapeutic and chemopreventive approaches against skin cancer. In this chapter, we have conducted a detailed review of various compounds which have been reported to show significant anticancer potential in preventing skin carcinogenesis. Mechanistic evaluation of the regulatory pathways followed by these compounds has also been addressed as much as possible (Fig. 10.1). It is evident from the above citations that phytochemicals from fruits and vegetables can modulate the molecules that interplay and result in development of cancer, and hence can be used to control the disease. These phytochemicals are safe and have no side effects, unlike other synthetic compounds. However, the bioavailability may pose a problem in their administration and therefore demands further studies in this area. Though the mechanisms of the beneficial aspects of these compounds have already been illustrated, this information has not been translated into practical use. More clinical trials and epidemiological studies should be encouraged to prove the effectiveness of these natural phytocompounds that hold great potential in saving humans from this deadly disease.

Table 10.2: Clinical trials evaluating the potential of various compounds isolated from fruits and vegetables in inhibiting skin tumor development.

No	Phytochemical	Status	Phase	No of patients	Reference/ Identification no	Lead organization	Outcome/Result
1	Catechin	Completed	—	95	NCT01032031	Royal NHS Foundation Trust, Manchester, UK	Not reported
		Completed	1	30	NCT01490008	CardioSec Clinical Research GmbH, Erfurt, Germany	Not reported
		Completed	4	43	NCT01082302	Charite Research Organization, Berlin, Germany	Not reported
2	Carotene	Completed	—	81	(67) NCT00836342	Clinical Unit for Research Trials in Skin-MGH, Boston, Massachusettes, USA	12 years supplementation of β-carotene in healthy men does not affect the development of both BCC and SCC
3	Garlic oil	Completed	2	60	NCT01748669	Bangabandhu Sheikh Mujib Medical University, Dhaka, Bengladesh	Not reported
4	Genistein	Ongoing	0	15	NCT00276835	Robert H. Lurie Comprehensive Cancer Centre at Northwestern University, Chicago, Illinois, USA	Not reported
5	N-acetylcysteine	Ongoing	2	218	NCT01612221	Huntsman Cancer Institute, Salt Lake City, Utah, USA	Not reported
6	Resveratrol	Completed	1	42	NCT00721877	Arizona Cancer Centre at University of Arizona Health Science Centre, Tucson, Arizona, USA	Not reported

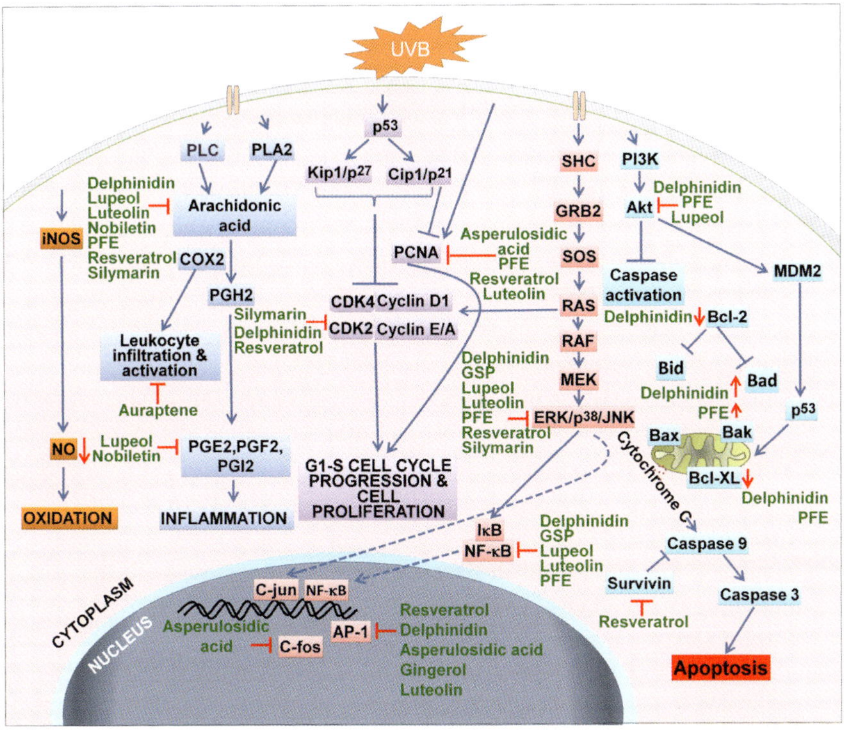

Figure 10.1: Molecular targets of UV-induced multiple signaling pathways leading to skin carcinogenesis, regulated by phytochemicals isolated from fruits and vegetables.

ACKNOWLEDGMENT

The authors acknowledge Abdul Rahim C.S. and Shanid Mohiyuddin, K.V.M. College of Engineering and IT, Cherthala for their technical help.

REFERENCES

1. Willett, W.C., Balancing life-style and genomics research for disease prevention, *Science* **296**(5568): 695–698 (2002).
2. Liu, R.H., Potential synergy of phytochemicals in cancer prevention: Mechanism of action, *J Nutr* **134**(12 Suppl.): 3479S–3485S (2004).
3. McGettigan, S., Have questions about your melanoma diagnosis?, from askanurse@melanoma.org, The Abramson Cancer Center of the University of Pennsylvania (2008).

4. Ehrlich, S.D., Skin cancer, from http://averaorg.adam.com/content.aspx?productId=107&pid=33&gid=000029, VeriMed Healthcare Network (2006).
5. Wu, H., Q. Dai, M.J. Shrubsole, R.M. Ness, D. Schlundt, W.E. Smalley, H. Chen, M. Li, Y. Shyr, and W. Zheng, Fruit and vegetable intakes are associated with lower risk of colorectal adenomas, *J Nutr* **139**(2): 340–344 (2009).
6. Kurahashi, N., M. Inoue, M. Iwasaki, Y. Tanaka, M. Mizokami, and S. Tsugane, Vegetable, fruit and antioxidant nutrient consumption and subsequent risk of hepatocellular carcinoma: A prospective cohort study in Japan, *Br J Cancer* **100**(1): 181–184 (2009).
7. Ramos, S., Cancer chemoprevention and chemotherapy: Dietary polyphenols and signalling pathways, *Mol Nutr Food Res* **52**(5): 507–526 (2008).
8. Kaur, M., C. Agarwal, and R. Agarwal, Anticancer and cancer chemopreventive potential of grape seed extract and other grape-based products, *J Nutr* **139**(9): 1806S–1812S (2009).
9. Park, E.J. and J.M. Pezzuto, Botanicals in cancer chemoprevention, *Cancer Metastasis Rev* **21**(3–4): 231–255 (2002).
10. Singh, A., S.P. Singh, and R. Bamezai, *Momordica charantia* (bitter gourd) peel, pulp, seed and whole fruit extract inhibits mouse skin papillomagenesis, *Toxicol Lett* **94**(1): 37–46 (1998).
11. Agrawal, R.C. and T. Beohar, Chemopreventive and anticarcinogenic effects of *Momordica charantia* extract, *Asian Pac J Cancer Prev* **11**(2): 371–375 (2010).
12. Abd Ghafar, M.F., K.N. Prasad, K. K. Weng, and A. Ismail, Flavonoid, hesperidine, total phenolic contents and antioxidant activities from *Citrus* species, *Afr J Biotechnol* **9**(3): 326–330 (2010).
13. Miller, E.G., A.P. Gonzales-Sanders, A.M. Couvillon, J.M. Wright, S. Hasegawa, L.K.T. Lam, and G.I. Sunahara, Inhibition of oral carcinogenesis by green coffee beans and limoinoid glucosides, M.-T. Huang, T. Osawa, C.-T. Ho, and R.T. Rosen (Eds.), in *Food Phytochemicals for Cancer Prevention*, American Chemical Society: Washington, D.C., *ACS Symp* **546**: 220–229 (1994).
14. Kupfer, D. and W.H. Bulger, Metabolic activation of pesticides with proestrogenic activity, *Fed Proc* **46**(5): 1864–1869 (1987).
15. Murakami, A., Y. Nakamura, K. Torikai, T. Tanaka, T. Koshiba, K. Koshimizu, S. Kuwahara, Y. Takahashi, K. Ogawa, M. Yano, H. Tokuda, H. Nishino, Y. Mimaki, Y. Sashida, S. Kitanaka, and H. Ohigashi, Inhibitory effect of citrus nobiletin on phorbol ester-induced skin inflammation, oxidative stress, and tumor promotion in mice, *Cancer Res* **60**(18): 5059–5066 (2000).
16. Murakami, A., W. Kuki, Y. Takahashi, H. Yonei, Y. Nakamura, Y. Ohto, H. Ohigashi, and K. Koshimizu, Auraptene, a citrus coumarin, inhibits 12-O-tetradecanoylphorbol-13-acetate-induced tumor promotion in ICR mouse

skin, possibly through suppression of superoxide generation in leukocytes, *Jpn J Cancer Res* **88**(5): 443–452 (1997).
17. Zhao, J., J. Wang, Y. Chen, and R. Agarwal, Anti-tumor-promoting activity of a polyphenolic fraction isolated from grape seeds in the mouse skin two-stage initiation-promotion protocol and identification of procyanidin B5-3′-gallate as the most effective antioxidant constituent, *Carcinogenesis* **20**(9): 1737–1745 (1999).
18. Bomser, J.A., K.W. Singletary, M.A. Wallig, and M.A. Smith, Inhibition of TPA-induced tumor promotion in CD-1 mouse epidermis by a polyphenolic fraction from grape seeds, *Cancer Lett* **135**(2): 151–157 (1999).
19. Athar, M., J.H. Back, X. Tang, K.H. Kim, L. Kopelovich, D.R. Bickers, and A.L. Kim, Resveratrol: A review of preclinical studies for human cancer prevention, *Toxicol Appl Pharmacol* **61**(15): 5749–5756 (2007).
20. Liu, G., A. Bode, W.Y. Ma, S. Sang, C.T. Ho, and Z. Dong, Two novel glycosides from the fruits of *Morinda citrifolia* (noni) inhibit AP-1 transactivation and cell transformation in the mouse epidermal JB6 cell line, *Cancer Res* **61**(15): 5749–5756 (2001).
21. Hata, K., K. Hori, and S. Takahashi, Differentiation- and apoptosis-inducing activities by pentacyclic triterpenes on a mouse melanoma cell line, *J Nat Prod* **65**(5):645–648 (2002).
22. Hata, K., K. Hori, and S. Takahashi, Role of p38 MAPK in lupeol-induced B16 2F2 mouse melanoma cell differentiation, *J Biochem* **134**(3): 441–445 (2003).
23. Saleem, M., A. Alam, S. Arifin, M.S. Shah, B. Ahmed, and S. Sultana, Lupeol, a triterpene, inhibits early responses of tumor promotion induced by benzoyl peroxide in murine skin, *Pharmacol Res* **43**(2): 127–134 (2001).
24. Saleem, M., F. Afaq, V.M. Adhami, and H. Mukhtar, Lupeol modulates NF-κB and PI3K/Akt pathways and inhibits skin cancer in CD-1 mice, *Oncogene* **23**(30): 5203–5214 (2004).
25. Singh, R.P. and R. Agarwal, Flavonoid antioxidant silymarin and skin cancer, *Antioxid Redox Signal* **4**(4): 655–663 (2002).
26. Singh, R.P. and R. Agarwal, Mechanisms and preclinical efficacy of silibinin in preventing skin cancer, *Eur J Cancer* **41**(13): 1969–1979 (2005).
27. Dhanalakshmi, S., G.U. Mallikarjuna, R.P. Singh, and R. Agarwal, Silibinin prevents ultraviolet radiation-caused skin damages in SKH-1 hairless mice via a decrease in thymine dimer positive cells and an up-regulation of p53-p21/Cip1 in epidermis, *Carcinogenesis* **25**(8): 1459–1465 (2004).
28. Gu, M., S. Dhanalakshmi, R.P. Singh, and R. Agarwal, Dietary feeding of silibinin prevents early biomarkers of UVB radiation-induced carcinogenesis in SKH-1 hairless mouse epidermis, *Cancer Epidemiol Biomarkers Prev* **14**(5): 1344–1349 (2005).

29. Narayanapillai, S., C. Agarwal, C. Tilley, and R. Agarwal, Silibinin is a potent sensitizer of UVA radiation-induced oxidative stress and apoptosis in human keratinocyte HaCaT cells, *Photochem Photobiol* **88**(5): 1135–1140 (2012).
30. Afaq, F., M. Saleem, C.G. Krueger, J.D. Reed, and H. Mukhtar, Anthocyanin- and hydrolyzable tannin-rich pomegranate fruit extract modulates MAPK and NF-κB pathways and inhibits skin tumorigenesis in CD-1 mice, *Int J Cancer* **113**(3): 423–433 (2005).
31. Afaq, F., A. Malik, D. Syed, D. Maes, M.S. Matsui, and H. Mukhtar, Pomegranate fruit extract modulates UVB-mediated phosphorylation of mitogen-activated protein kinases and activation of nuclear factor kappa B in normal human epidermal keratinocytes paragraph sign, *Photochem Photobiol* **81**(1): 38–45 (2005).
32. Afaq, F. and H. Mukhtar, Botanical antioxidants in the prevention of photocarcinogenesis and photoaging, *Exp Dermatol* **15**(9): 678–684 (2006).
33. Syed, D.N., F. Afaq, and H. Mukhtar, Pomegranate derived products for cancer chemoprevention, *Semin Cancer Biol* **17**(5): 377–385 (2007).
34. Syed, D.N., A. Malik, N. Hadi, S. Sarfaraz, F. Afaq, and H. Mukhtar, Photochemopreventive effect of pomegranate fruit extract on UVA-mediated activation of cellular pathways in normal human epidermal keratinocytes, *Photochem Photobiol* **82**(2): 398–405 (2006).
35. Saleem, A., M. Husheem, P. Harkonen, and K. Pihlaja, Inhibition of cancer cell growth by crude extract and the phenolics of *Terminalia chebula* Retz. fruit, *J Ethnopharmacol* **81**(3): 327–336 (2002).
36. Hartwell, J.L., *Plants Used Against Cancer*, Quarterman Publications, Lawrence: MA (1982).
37. Pettit, G.R., M.S. Hoard, D.L. Doubek, J.M. Schmidt, R.K. Pettit, L.P. Tackett, and J.C. Chapuis, Antineoplastic agents 338. The cancer cell growth inhibitory. Constituents of *Terminalia arjuna* (Combretaceae), *J Ethnopharmacol* **53**(2): 57–63 (1996).
38. Kaur, K., S. Arora, S. Kumar, and A. Nagpal, Antimutagenic activities of acetone and methanol fractions of *Terminalia arjuna*, *Food Chem Toxicol* **40**(10): 1475–1482 (2002).
39. Ribaya-Mercado, J.D., M. Garmyn, B.A. Gilchrest, and R.M. Russell, Skin lycopene is destroyed preferentially over beta-carotene during ultraviolet irradiation in humans, *J Nutr* **125**(7): 1854–1859 (1995).
40. Fazekas, Z., D. Gao, R.N. Saladi, Y. Lu, M. Lebwohl, and H. Wei, Protective effects of lycopene against ultraviolet B-induced photodamage, *Nutr Cancer* **47**(2): 181–187 (2003).

41. Wang, L.S. and G.D. Stoner, Anthocyanins and their role in cancer prevention, *Cancer Lett* **269**(2): 281–290 (2008).
42. Kwon, J.Y., K.W. Lee, J.E. Kim, S.K. Jung, N.J. Kang, M.K. Hwang, Y.S. Heo, A.M. Bode, Z. Dong, and H.J. Lee, Delphinidin suppresses ultraviolet B-induced cyclooxygenases-2 expression through inhibition of MAPKK4 and PI-3 kinase, *Carcinogenesis* **30**(11): 1932–1940 (2009).
43. Afaq, F., D.N. Syed, A. Malik, N. Hadi, S. Sarfaraz, M.H. Kweon, N. Khan, M.A. Zaid, and H. Mukhtar, Delphinidin, an anthocyanidin in pigmented fruits and vegetables, protects human HaCaT keratinocytes and mouse skin against UVB-mediated oxidative stress and apoptosis, *J Invest Dermatol* **127**(1): 222–232 (2007).
44. Svobodova, A., P. Psotova, and D. Walterova, Natural phenolics in the prevention of UV-induced skin damage. A review, *Biomed Pap Med Fac Univ Palacky Olomouc Czech Repub* **147**(2): 137–145 (2003).
45. Lin, J.K., Y.C. Chen, Y.T. Huang, and S.Y. Lin-Shiau, Suppression of protein kinase C and nuclear oncogene expression as possible molecular mechanisms of cancer chemoprevention by apigenin and curcumin, *J Cell Biochem Suppl* **28–29**: 39–48 (1997).
46. Gupta, S. and H. Mukhtar, Chemoprevention of skin cancer: Current status and future prospects, *Cancer Metastasis Rev* **21**(3–4): 363–380 (2002).
47. Tong, X., R.T. Van Dross, A. Abu-Yousif, A.R. Morrison, and J.C. Pelling, Apigenin prevents UVB-induced cyclooxygenase 2 expression: Coupled mRNA stabilization and translational inhibition, *Mol Cell Biol* **27**(1): 283–296 (2007).
48. Van Dross, R. T., X. Hong, S. Essengue, S.M. Fischer, and J.C. Pelling, Modulation of UVB-induced and basal cyclooxygenase-2 (COX-2) expression by apigenin in mouse keratinocytes: Role of USF transcription factors, *Mol Carcinog* **46**(4): 303–314 (2007).
49. Shukla, S. and S. Gupta, Apigenin: A promising molecule for cancer prevention, *Pharm Res* **27**(6): 962–978 (2010).
50. Horinaka, M., T. Yoshida, T. Shiraishi, S. Nakata, M. Wakada, and T. Sakai, The dietary flavonoid apigenin sensitizes malignant tumor cells to tumor necrosis factor-related apoptosis-inducing ligand, *Mol Cancer Ther* **5**(4): 945–951 (2006).
51. Kapadia, G.J., M.A. Azuine, R. Sridhar, Y. Okuda, A. Tsuruta, E. Ichiishi, T. Mukainake, M. Takasaki, T. Konoshima, H. Nishino, and H. Tokuda, Chemoprevention of DMBA-induced UVB promoted, NOR-1-induced TPA promoted skin carcinogenesis, and DEN-induced phenobarbital promoted liver tumors in mice by extract of beetroot, *Pharmacol Res* **47**(2): 141–148 (2003).

52. Kapadia, G.J., H. Tokuda, T. Konoshima, and H. Nishino, Chemoprevention of lung and skin cancer by *Beta vulgaris* (beet) root extract, *Cancer Lett* **100**(1–2): 211–214 (1996).
53. Bendich, A. and J.A. Olson, Biological actions of carotenoids, *FASEB J* **3**(8): 1927–1932 (1989).
54. Murakoshi, M., H. Nishino, Y. Satomi, J. Takayasu, T. Hasegawa, H. Tokuda, A. Iwashima, J. Okuzumi, H. Okabe, and H. Kitano, Potent preventive action of alpha-carotene against carcinogenesis: Spontaneous liver carcinogenesis and promoting stage of lung and skin carcinogenesis in mice are suppressed more effectively by alpha-carotene than by beta-carotene, *Cancer Res* **52**(23): 6583–6587 (1992).
55. Nishino, H., M. Murakosh, T. Ii, M. Takemura, M. Kuchide, M. Kanazawa, X.Y. Mou, S. Wada, M. Masuda, Y. Ohsaka, S. Yogosawa, Y. Satomi, and K. Jinno, Carotenoids in cancer chemoprevention, *Cancer Metastasis Rev* **21**(3–4): 257–264 (2002).
56. Athar, M., H. Raza, D.R. Bickers, and H. Mukhtar, Inhibition of benzoyl peroxide-mediated tumor promotion in 7,12-dimethylbenz(a)anthracene-initiated skin of Sencar mice by antioxidants nordihydroguaiaretic acid and diallyl sulfide, *J Invest Dermatol* **94**(2): 162–165 (1990).
57. Wei, H., R. Bowen, X. Zhang, and M. Lebwohl, Isoflavone genistein inhibits the initiation and promotion of two-stage skin carcinogenesis in mice, *Carcinogenesis* **19**(8): 1509–1514 (1998).
58. Wang, Y., X. Zhang, M. Lebwohl, V. DeLeo, and H. Wei, Inhibition of ultraviolet B (UVB)-induced c-fos and c-jun expression *in vivo* by a tyrosine kinase inhibitor genistein, *Carcinogenesis* **19**(4): 649–654 (1998).
59. Katiyar, S.K., R. Agarwal, and H. Mukhtar, Inhibition of tumor promotion in SENCAR mouse skin by ethanol extract of *Zingiber officinale* rhizome, *Cancer Res* **56**(5): 1023–1030 (1996).
60. Bode, A.M., W.Y. Ma, Y.J. Surh, and Z. Dong, Inhibition of epidermal growth factor-induced cell transformation and activator protein 1 activation by [6]-gingerol, *Cancer Res* **61**(3): 850–853 (2001).
61. Park, K.K., K.S. Chun, J.M. Lee, S.S. Lee, and Y.J. Surh, Inhibitory effects of [6]-gingerol, a major pungent principle of ginger, on phorbol ester-induced inflammation, epidermal ornithine decarboxylase activity and skin tumor promotion in ICR mice, *Cancer Lett* **129**(2): 139–144 (1998).
62. Byun, S., K.W. Lee, S.K. Jung, E.J. Lee, M.K. Hwang, S.H. Lim, A.M. Bode, H.J. Lee, and Z. Dong, Luteolin inhibits protein kinase C(epsilon) and c-Src activities and UVB-induced skin cancer, *Cancer Res* **70**(6): 2415–2423 (2010).
63. Saleem, M., Lupeol, a novel anti-inflammatory and anti-cancer dietary triterpene, *Cancer Lett* **285**(2): 109–115 (2009).

64. Erden Inal, M., A. Kahraman, and T. Koken, Beneficial effects of quercetin on oxidative stress induced by ultraviolet A, *Clin Exp Dermatol* **26**(6): 536–539 (2001).
65. Steerenberg, P.A., J. Garssen, P.M. Dortant, H. van der Vliet, E. Geerse, A.P. Verlaan, W.G. Goettsch, Y. Sontag, H.B. Bueno-de-Mesquita, and H. Van Loveren, The effect of oral quercetin on UVB-induced tumor growth and local immunosuppression in SKH-1, *Cancer Lett* **114**(1–2): 187–189 (1997).
66. Saija, A., A. Tomaino, D. Trombetta, M.L. Pellegrino, B. Tita, C. Messina, F.P. Bonina, C. Rocco, G. Nicolosi, and F. Castelli, "*In-vitro*" antioxidant and photoprotective properties and interaction with model membranes of three new quercetin esters, *Eur J Pharm Biopharm* **56**(2): 167–174 (2003).
67. Frieling, U.M., D.A. Schaumberg, T.S. Kupper, J. Muntwyler, and C.H. Hennekens, A randomized, 12-year primary-prevention trial of beta carotene supplementation for nonmelanoma skin cancer in the physician's health study, *Arch Dermatol* **136**(2): 179–184 (2000).

11

Anticancer Effects of Agents Derived from Fruits and Vegetables Against Stomach Cancer

*Sakshi Sikka and Gautam Sethi**

INTRODUCTION

Gastric (stomach) cancer is the second most common cancer worldwide and the second most common cause of cancer-related deaths. Despite complete resection of gastric cancer and lymph node dissection, as well as improvements in chemotherapy and radiotherapy, there are still 700,000 gastric cancer-related deaths per year globally, and more than 80% of patients with advanced gastric cancer die of the disease or recurrent disease within one year after diagnosis. The overall five-year relative survival rate for gastric cancer is about 28%.[1] The bacterium *Helicobacter pylorus* is the primary known risk factor for gastric carcinogenesis.[2,3] A multistage sequence in the development of intestinal-type gastric carcinoma has been identified, beginning with chronic gastritis, proceeding to mucosal atrophy, and then further into intestinal metaplasia.[4] The latter stage involves the development of a cellular phenotype similar to that of the

*Corresponding author: Gautam Sethi, Ph.D., Assistant Professor, Department of Pharmacology, Yong Loo Lin School of Medicine and Cancer Science Institute of Singapore, National University of Singapore, Singapore 117597. Tel: (+65) 6516-3267, Fax: (+65) 6873-7690, Email: phcgs@nus.edu.sg.

intestine, which is associated with the ectopic expression of the protein CDX2, a transcription factor normally expressed by intestinal epithelial cells.[5] The final stage of malignant transformation leads to the appearance of a discreet tumor with glandular histology. The development of effective therapy for advanced gastric cancer is rather slow and no globally acceptable standard regimen has been established yet.[6] Moreover, therapies such as surgical operation or radiotherapy at later stages[7] incur a poor prognosis with an overall five-year survival rates of less than 25%.

Lately, the treatment for gastric cancer has shifted to genetic engineering that inhibits the proliferation and differentiation of cancer cells.[8] Cancer is now believed to be a disease that can be prevented. It is known that the inheritance of mutated genes and somatic mutations causes 5–10% of all cancers, whereas the remaining 90–95% has been associated with lifestyle factors and environmental agents.[9,10] Almost 30% of all cancers have been attributed to tobacco smoke, 35% to diet, 14–20% to obesity, 18% to infectious agents, and 7% to radiation as well as environmental toxins and pollutants.[11,12] Epidemiology has revealed that certain cancers are more common among people of some cultures than others;[13,14] for instance, stomach cancer is most prevalent in Japan. Natural dietary agents including fruits, vegetables and spices have drawn a great deal of attention from both the scientific community and the general public owing to their demonstrated ability to suppress cancer.[15] Naturally occurring dietary compounds have received increasing attention in cancer chemoprevention.[16] Since diet has an important role in the aetiology of gastric cancer, dietary chemoprevention has received great attention for their prevention. However, identification of an agent with chemopreventive potential requires *in vitro* studies and efficacy and toxicity studies in animal models before embarking on human clinical trials. An ideal chemopreventive agent should have little or no toxicity, high efficacy in multiple sites, capability of oral consumption, known mechanisms of action, low cost and human acceptance.[17] A number of other important transcription factors (AP-1, STAT3, PPARγ, Wnt/β-catenin), pro-apoptotic proteins (e.g., caspases, PARP, Bax), cell adhesion molecules (ICAM, VCAM, ELAM), and metastatic proteins (COX-2, 5-LOX, MMP-9, VEGF) have also been found to be modulated by dietary agents (Fig. 11.1). The chemical diversity, structural complexity, affordability, lack of

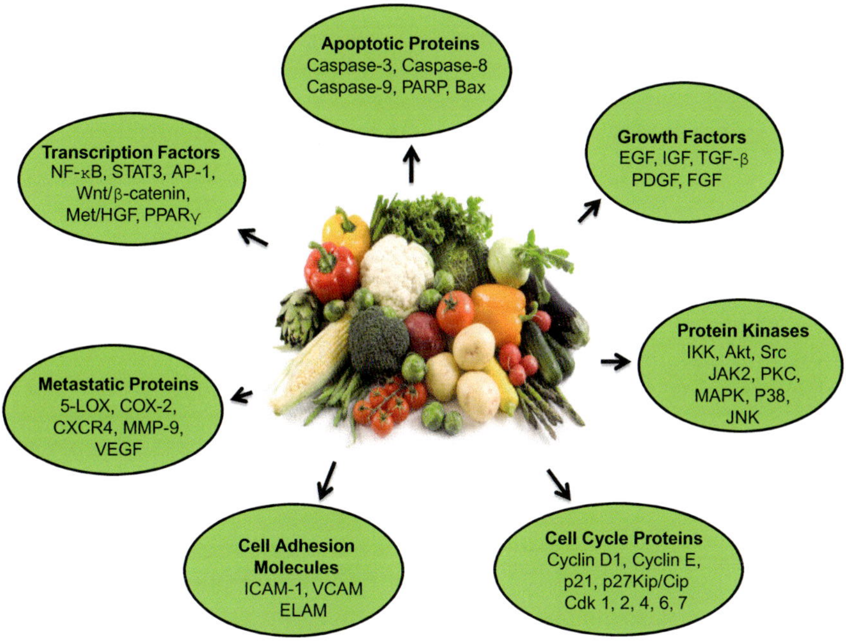

Figure 11.1: Diverse molecular targets modulated by dietary agents in gastric cancer.

substantial toxic effects and inherent biologic activity of natural products makes them ideal candidates for new therapeutics. Natural products not only disrupt aberrant signalling pathways leading to cancer, but also synergize with chemotherapy and radiotherapy.[18] This chapter will focus on the mechanisms of action of key natural products derived from fruits and vegetables as well as promising preclinical data on their efficacy as anticancer agents against gastric cancer.

IMPORTANT ONCOGENIC PATHWAYS TARGETED BY DIETARY AGENTS IN GASTRIC CANCER

Cancer is a hyperproliferative disorder that involves the transformation and dysregulation of apoptosis, proliferation, invasion, angiogenesis, and metastasis. Dietary agents used for both cancer prevention and treatment generally target multiple cell signalling molecules, including growth factor receptors (EGF, FGF); inflammatory transcription factors (HIF-1α, NF-κB);

protein kinases (PI3K/Akt, MAPKs, PKC, IKK); cell cycle regulators (cyclin D1 and cyclin E); and anti-apoptotic proteins (Bcl-2, Bcl-X_L, XIAP, survivin, FLIP). This section briefly describes few important signal transduction pathways involved in both gastric cancer initiation and progression.

Growth Factor Signalling Pathway

Growth factors are proteins that bind to receptors on the cell surface, with the primary result of activating cellular proliferation and/or differentiation. Some of the growth factors implicated in carcinogenesis are EGF, platelet-derived growth factor (PDGF), FGFs, transforming growth factors (TGF), erythropoietin (Epo), and insulin-like growth factor (IGF). The potent cell proliferation signals generated by various growth factor receptors such as the EGF receptor, IGF-1 receptor, and vascular endothelial growth factor (VEGF) receptor networks constitute the basis for receptor-driven tumorigenicity in the progression of several cancers.[19] Abnormal growth factor signalling pathways lead to increased cell proliferation, suppression of apoptotic signals, and invasion contributing to metastasis. IGF-1 is also shown to mediate the activation of NF-κB, induce the phosphorylation of FKHR (forkhead) transcription factor, and upregulate a series of intracellular anti-apoptotic proteins (including FLIP, survivin, cIAP-2, A1/Bfl-1 and XIAP).[20,21] Transforming growth factor-beta (TGF-β) is a growth factor that controls proliferation, cellular growth and differentiation, and embryonic development.[20] During tumorigenesis, the TGF-β signalling pathway becomes mutated and TGF-β no longer controls the cell cycle. The cancer cells along with the surrounding stromal cells (fibroblasts) proliferate unchecked. Both types of cells increase their production of TGF-β, which acts on the surrounding stromal, immune, endothelial and smooth muscle cells, increasing the invasiveness and motility of cancer.[20] Several chemopreventive phytochemicals including genistein, resveratrol and catechins have been shown to be potent inhibitors of several growth factor signalling pathways.

HIF-1α Pathway

Hypoxic areas are frequently found in human solid tumors as a result of morphologically and functionally inappropriate vascularization, irregular blood flow, anaemia and high oxygen consumption of rapidly proliferating cells.[22] A large body of clinical evidence suggests that intra-tumoral hypoxia correlates with the elevated aggressive behavior of cancer cells and their resistance to therapy, leading to poor patient prognosis.[23] Tumor cells must adapt to hypoxic stress through alterations of cellular metabolism and stimulation of neovascularization. A key regulator of the cellular response to oxygen deprivation is the transcription factor hypoxia-inducible factor 1 (HIF-1) whose accumulation results in the induction of a plethora of target genes that collectively confer cellular adaptation to hypoxia.[24] HIF-1 can directly upregulate a number of angiogenic factors, including VEGF, VEGF receptors, plasminogen activator inhibitor-1, angiopoietins (ANG-1 and -2), PDGF-B, TIE-2 receptor and matrix metalloproteinases (MMPs).[20] HIF-1 is comprised of a labile oxygen-regulated α-subunit mainly targeted for normoxia-dependent degradation by the proteasomal system, whereas its β-subunit is constitutively expressed in most cells.[24,25] Therefore, HIF-1 activity is dependent upon the limiting expression of α-subunit. Under hypoxia, HIF-1α is stabilized, enters the nucleus and heterodimerizes with HIF-1β. The heterodimer HIF-1 binds hypoxia-responsive elements to transactivate a variety of hypoxia-responsive genes, therefore contributing to the adaptive response to hypoxic conditions.[23] HIF-1α is overexpressed in many human cancers including gastric cancer and correlates with poor prognosis outcome.[26–28] In most of these cases, overexpression is due to the stabilisation of the HIF-1α protein by hypoxia. However, there is an increasing body of evidence demonstrating that a number of non-hypoxic stimuli such as genetic alterations that activate oncogenes and inactivate tumor suppressor genes or growth factor signalling are also highly capable of turning on this transcription factor.[25] Accordingly, HIF-1α represents an attractive, yet challenging, target for the development of pharmacological inhibitors.[29,30]

PI3K/Akt Pathway

Proliferation, survival, differentiation and motility of cancer cells are regulated by different intracellular signalling pathways. Among these, the role of the (1) MAPK [RAS/RAF/MAP kinase–ERK kinase (MEK)/extracellular signal-regulated kinase (ERK)] pathway and (2) the P13K/Akt [PI3K/protein kinase B (PKB/AKT)/mammalian target of rapamycin (mTOR)] pathway in the pathogenesis of human carcinoma have long been established.[31] Constitutive MAPK and PI3K/Akt pathways activation is a frequent event in different human cancers including gastric cancer, as a result of molecular alterations in genes encoding key components of the pathways or upstream activation mediated by mutations or amplification of cell-surface receptors.[31–33] Deregulated signalling due to constitutive activation of these pathways can lead to uncontrolled cell growth and survival, ultimately resulting in oncogenic transformation and progression.

PI3Ks belong to a conserved family of lipid kinases that phosphorylate the 3′-hydroxyl group of phosphoinositides.[34] There are three classes of PI3Ks grouped according to their substrate preference and sequence homology, but only the class IA PI3Ks are implicated in human cancer. Class IA PI3Ks are heterodimers comprised of a regulatory subunit (p85α, p55α, p50α, p85β, p55γ) and a catalytic subunit (p110α, p110β, p110δ).[35] PI3Ks are activated by growth factor stimulation through receptor tyrosine kinases (RTKs). In particular, the p85 regulatory subunit binds to phosphotyrosine residues on activated RTKs or adaptor molecules, such as insulin receptor substrate-1 (IRS-1), via its SH2 domains. This binding relieves the inhibition of the p110 catalytic subunit by p85 and recruits PI3K heterodimer to the plasma membrane where its substrate PIP_2 is located. PI3K can also been stimulated by activated Ras, which directly binds p110.[34] PI3K phosphorylates PIP_2 on the 3′-OH position to produce PIP_3. The tumor suppressor phosphatase and tensin homolog deleted on chromosome ten (*PTEN*) negatively regulates the PI3K pathway by dephosphorylating PIP_3 to PIP_2. PIP_3 acts by localizing several signalling proteins with pleckstrin homology (PH) domains to the membrane, where they become activated and propagate the intracellular signalling.[35] Among the PH domain-containing proteins, the Akt protein is recruited to the plasma membrane and activated by 3-phosphoinositide-dependent kinase 1 (PDK1). Akt promotes cellular survival through the phosphorylation and inactivation of the pro-apoptotic protein B cell leukemia 2 antagonist of cell death (Bad).[36] In addition, Akt induces the activation of NF-κB and inhibitor of NF-κB (IκB) kinase α (IKKα).[37] Akt also promotes the phosphorylation of mouse double minute 2 (Mdm2) that antagonizes p53-mediated apoptosis. The constitutive activation of Akt in human tumors may be due, in addition to the activation of PI3K, to loss or mutation of *PTEN*. *PTEN* is frequently mutated or downregulated in a broad range of human cancers.[38,39]

ANTICANCER EFFECTS OF DIETARY AGENTS AGAINST GASTRIC CANCER

In the past several decades, many studies have been performed to evaluate cancer preventive and therapeutic effects of fruits and vegetables against stomach cancer. The following section describes the detailed effects of diverse dietary agents on the prevention and treatment of gastric cancer.

Resveratrol

Resveratrol has been shown to suppress the proliferation of gastric cancer cells in experimental conditions.[40] Atten *et al.* reported that resveratrol inhibited proliferation of nitrosamine-stimulated human gastric adenocarcinoma KATO-III and RF-1 cells.[41] It arrested KATO-III cells in the G0/G1 phase of the cell cycle and eventually induced apoptotic cell death by utilizing a protein kinase C (PKC)-mediated mechanism to deactivate these gastric adenocarcinoma cells. Resveratrol can exhibit anti-inflammatory, cell growth modulatory and anticarcinogenic effects by suppressing NF-κB, a nuclear transcription factor that regulates the expression of various genes involved in inflammation, cytoprotection and carcinogenesis.[42] Bertilli *et al.* studied the plasma kinetics and tissue bioavailability of resveratol after oral administration in rats, which showed significant cardiac bioavailability and a strong affinity for the liver and kidneys.[43] Andlauer *et al.* investigated the absorption and metabolism of resveratrol by using an isolated preparation of luminally and vascularly perfused rat small intestine, which showed a 20.5% vascular uptake of resveratrol.[44] These results demonstrate an ample uptake and metabolic conversion of resveratrol in experimental conditions. Zaidi *et al.*[45] evaluated the effect of resveratrol on the induction of IL-8 in *H. pylori*-infected gastric epithelial cells. The results showed that lower concentrations (non-toxic) of resveratrol did not show any inhibitory effect against *H. pylori* adhesion to gastric epithelial cells, whereas pre-incubation of the cells with resveratrol (75 and 100 μM) significantly suppressed the *H. pylori*-induced secretion of IL-8 and reactive oxygen species (ROS) and morphological changes. These results suggest the protective effect of resveratrol against various *H. pylori*-related gastric pathogenic ailments. In another study, Wang *et al.*[46] showed that treatment with resveratrol (50–200 μmol/L) significantly induced apoptosis and DNA damage in human gastric cancer SGC7901 cells due to the increased generation of ROS following resveratrol treatment, because incubation of cells with superoxide dismutase or catalase attenuated resveratrol-induced cellular apoptosis. These data provide evidence that resveratrol induces apoptosis via ROS in the human gastric cancer cell line SGC7901. In addition, several studies showed that resveratrol inhibits proliferation of human gastric adenocarcinoma cells both *in vitro* and *in vivo* conditions.[47–49]

Honokiol

Honokiol, a small molecular weight natural product, is a main active compound of *Magnolia officinalis*. *Magnolia* bark is widely known to ameliorate microbial infection, inflammation and gastrointestinal disorder in traditional Asian medicinal systems such as traditional Chinese medicine and Kampo medicine in Japan.[50] Honokiol markedly inhibited PPAR-γ and (cyclooxygenase-2) COX-2 expressions in gastric cancer cells and tumors of xenograft mice, and induced apoptosis and cell death.[51] It has been shown that honokiol inhibits gastric cancer cell proliferation by activation of 15-lipoxygenase-1 and inhibition of peroxisome proliferator-activated receptor-gamma (PPARγ) and COX-2-dependent signals in human gastric cancer cell lines AGS, MKN45, N87 and SCM-1 and cell line-induced tumor xenograft in mice.[52] Sheu *et al.*[53] explored the effects of honokiol on the regulation of glucose-regulated proteins (GRPs) and apoptosis in human gastric cancer cells and tumor growth. Treatment with honokiol induced GRP94 cleavage (but not GRP78), calpain activity, calpain-II protein level and inhibited MKN45-induced tumor growth in BALB/c nude mice. Moreover, Liu *et al.*[54] determined the effects of honokiol on angiogenic activity and peritoneal dissemination using *in vivo*, *ex vivo* and *in vitro* assay systems. Honokiol significantly inhibited peritoneal dissemination in a xenograft gastric tumor mouse model and attenuated angiogenesis in different angiogenesis assays such as the chick chorioallantoic membrane assay, mouse matrigel plug assay, rat aortic ring endothelial cell sprouting assay and endothelial cell tube formation assay. In addition, honokiol significantly inhibited STAT3 phosphorylation, inhibited STAT3 DNA binding activity and VEGF expression in human gastric cancer cells and HUVECs, which was correlated with the upregulation of the activity and protein expression of Src homology 2 (SH2)-containing tyrosine phosphatase-1 (SHP-1).[54] These studies suggest the potential of honokiol in gastric cancer therapy.

Quercetin

The flavone quercetin (3,3′,4′,5,7-pentahydroxyflavone), one of the major dietary flavonoids, is found in a broad range of fruits, vegetables and beverages such as tea and wine.[55] It is known to block NF-κB activation and has been approved in clinical trials for tyrosine kinase inhibition.[55–58] A Phase I clinical trial indicated that the molecule can be safely administered and that its plasma levels are sufficient to inhibit lymphocyte tyrosine kinase activity. Quercetin is a promising cancer chemopreventive agent that inhibits tumor promotion by inducing cell cycle arrest and promoting apoptotic cell death.[56] A study was carried out to examine the biological activities of quercetin against gastric cancer. The results demonstrated that exposure of gastric cancer cells AGS and MKN28 to quercetin resulted in pronounced pro-apoptotic activity through the activation of the mitochondria pathway, and this compound activated autophagy both *in vitro* and *in vivo* conditions.[56] Quercetin inhibited the phosphorylation of Akt and mTOR as well as p70 S6K and 4E-BP1 (two best-characterised targets of the mTOR1 complex) in gastric cancer cells, which revealed the importance of the involvement of Akt/mTOR signalling in quercetin-mediated protective autophagy in gastric cancer cells.[56] Wang *et al.*[59] investigated the effect of quercetin on apoptosis and morphology of gastric carcinoma BGC-823 cells, as well as its mechanism of action. Quercetin induced apoptosis in BGC-823 cells, changed apoptotic protein expression and decreased Bcl-2/Bax ratio with the increased expression of caspase 3, which provide evidence that quercetin-induced apoptosis may be mediated via the mitochondrial pathway. Furthermore, many studies have shown that quercetin induces apoptosis in different gastric cancer cell lines such as EPG85-257P, EPG85-257RDB (daunorubicin-resistant) and MGC803 by modulating different cell signalling pathways.[60–62] These studies show the potential of quercetin in the prevention and treatment of gastric cancer.

Sanguinarine

Sanguinarine is a benzophenanthridine alkaloid, derived from the root of *Sanguinaria canadensis* and other poppy *Fumaria* species, which is known to have antimicrobial, anti-inflammatory and antioxidant properties.[63] Choi *et al.*[63] showed that treatment with tumor necrosis factor-related apoptosis-inducing ligand (TRAIL) in combination with subtoxic concentrations of sanguinarine sensitized TRAIL-mediated apoptosis in AGS cells (TRAIL-resistant cells), effectively induced Bid cleavage and loss of mitochondrial membrane potential, leading to the activation of caspases, and cleavage of poly(ADP-ribose) polymerase (PARP) and β-catenin. In addition, the combination of TRAIL and sanguinarine markedly reduced Akt protein expression, suggesting that interactions of the synergistic effect were at least partially mediated through the Akt-dependent pathway. However, further studies are needed to evaluate the potential of this compound against gastric cancer.

Phenethyl Isothiocyanate

Phenethyl isothiocyanate (PEITC) is found in dietary cruciferous vegetables and has been proven to exhibit antitumor properties.[64] Plasma concentrations of PEITC in rats could reach 9.2 to 42.1 μM after oral doses of 10 and 100 μmol/kg of PEITC. Pharmacokinetic analysis of this molecule shows that micromolar concentrations of PEITC are easily achievable *in vivo*. In animal and cell culture models, micromolar concentrations of PEITC have been shown to prevent cancer.[65] Yang *et al.*[66] reported that in addition to its function as an anticancer agent, PEITC can inhibit migration and invasion through the suppression of ERK1/2, PKC and NF-κB signalling pathways in human gastric cells (AGS). In addition, studies have shown that PEITC inhibits ERK1/2, mitogen-activated protein kinase kinase 7 (MKK7), MAP kinase kinase kinase 3 (MEKK3), son of sevenless 1 (SOS1), PKC, Ras homolog gene family, member A (Rho A), urokinase-type plasminogen activator (uPA) and MMP-2 and -9. PEITC also inhibits Ras, growth factor receptor-bound protein 2 (GRB2), VEGF, focal adhesion kinase (FAK), inducible nitric oxide synthase (iNOS) and COX-2, which lead to the suppression of AGS cell proliferation. Moreover, studies have shown that treatment with this molecule reverses multi-drug resistance of human gastric cancer SGC7901/DDP cells.[67] These studies suggest that this agent has high potential in the prevention and treatment of gastric cancer.

Olives

Olives contain a range of phenolic compounds; these natural antioxidants may contribute to the prevention of chronic conditions including cancer.[68] Kountouri *et al.*[69] investigated the effect of a methanol extract of olives in AGS cell proliferation, induction of apoptosis and inhibition of inflammation. Olive extract significantly suppressed cell proliferation, induced apoptosis and decreased ICAM-1 and IL-8 expression, suggesting that the methanol extract from olives, rich in phenolic compounds, exhibits gastric cancer preventive activity by limiting cell proliferation, inducing cell death and suppressing inflammation in AGS cells.[69] However, more studies in animal models are needed to validate these findings.

Eugenol

Eugenol (4-allyl-2-methoxyphenol) is the active component of *Syzigium aromaticum* (cloves).[70] Aromatic plants like nutmeg, basil, cinnamon and bay leaves also contain eugenol. Eugenol has a wide range of applications like perfumeries, flavorings, essential oils and in medicine as a local antiseptic and anaesthetic. Eugenol possesses antioxidant, antimutagenic, antigenotoxic, anti-inflammatory and anticancer properties.[70] The molecular mechanism of eugenol-induced apoptosis in gastric cells has been well documented.[70] Manikandan *et al.*[71] evaluated the chemopreventive potential of this compound against N-methyl-N′-nitro-N-nitrosoguanidine (MNNG)-induced gastric carcinogenesis by analyzing markers of apoptosis, invasion and angiogenesis. The results suggest that the administration of eugenol induced apoptosis via the mitochondrial pathway by modulating the Bcl-2 family proteins, Apaf-1, cytochrome c and caspases and inhibiting invasion and angiogenesis as evidenced by changes in the activities of MMPs and the expression of MMP-2 and -9, VEGF, VEGF receptor 1,

TIMP-2 and RECK. Moreover the same group have shown that eugenol suppressed the incidence of MNNG-induced gastric tumors by suppressing NF-κB activation and modulating the expression of NF-κB target genes that regulate cell proliferation and cell survival.[72] However, further studies in humans are needed to evaluate these findings.

Nobiletin

Nobiletin, a compound isolated from citrus fruits, is a polymethoxylated flavone derivative shown to have anti-inflammatory, antitumor and neuro-protective properties.[73] A study conducted by Lee *et al.*[74] investigated the inhibitory effects of nobiletin on AGS cell adhesion, invasion and migration under non-cytotoxic concentrations. The results showed that nobiletin inhibited the activation of FAK and PI3K/Akt and messenger RNA levels of MMP-2 and -9, and expression of Ras, c-Raf, Rac-1, Cdc42 and RhoA. Nobiletin-treated AGS cells also showed tremendous decrease in the phosphorylation and degradation of inhibitor of kappaBα (IκBα), the nuclear level of NF-κB and the binding ability of NF-κB to NF-κB response element. Furthermore, nobiletin significantly reduced invasion and migration of AGS cells. Minagawa *et al.*[75] demonstrated the inhibitory effects of nobiletin on the proliferation of the cancer cell line, TMK-1, and its production of MMPs. In animals, nobiletin inhibited the formation of peritoneal dissemination nodules from TMK-1 and inhibited MMP-9 enzymatic activity, indicating that nobiletin may be a candidate anti-metastatic drug for prevention of peritoneal dissemination of gastric cancer.

Isorhamnetin

Isorhamnetin (IH), an immediate metabolite of quercetin, also called 3′-O-methylquercetin, has been gaining interest for its anti-inflammatory and antiproliferative properties in a number of cancers.[76,77] Prior studies have focused on quercetin as an anticancer agent, but recent research has shown that IH can induce higher cytotoxicity in tumor cells as compared to quercetin.[76] It is now well established that PPAR-γ is overexpressed in patients with gastric carcinoma.[78] The same study also suggested that PPAR-γ might be a molecular marker for the development of gastric cancer from chronic gastritis. Other studies have shown that PPAR-γ plays a protective role in gastric carcinogenesis and activation of the receptor has a chemopreventive effect.[79] Because of the critical role of PPAR-γ in gastric cancer proliferation, survival, invasion and metastasis, Ramachandran *et al.*[80] investigated whether IH can mediate its antiproliferative and pro-apoptotic effects in gastric cancer cells and xenograft models through the activation of the PPAR-γ signalling cascade. It was observed that this flavonoid increased PPAR-γ activity, modulated the expression of the PPAR-γ-regulated genes, decreased proliferation, induced apoptosis and also potentiated the apoptotic effects of chemotherapeutic drugs in gastric cancer cells. Moreover, the increase in PPAR-γ activity was reversed in the presence of a PPAR-γ pharmacological blocker and a mutated PPAR-γ dominant negative plasmid, thereby indicating that IH can act as a potential novel ligand of PPAR-γ. In addition, intraperitoneal injection of IH into nude mice bearing subcutaneous SNU-5 xenografts resulted in significant increase in the expression of PPAR-γ and the downregulation of Bcl-2 and CD31 in treated tumor tissues.[80] These studies suggest the anticancer properties of this compound against gastric cancer.

Isothiocyanate Sulforaphane

Isothiocyanate sulforaphane [SF; 1-isothiocyanato-4(R)-methylsulfinylbutane] is abundant in broccoli sprouts in the form of its glucosinolate precursor (glucoraphanin).[81] SF is powerful against *H. pylori* infections, which are strongly associated with the worldwide pandemic of gastric cancer. Studies showed that oral administration of SF-rich broccoli sprouts inhibited gastric bacterial colonization, attenuated mucosal expression of TNF-α and interleukin-1β, mitigated corpus inflammation and prevented expression of high salt-induced gastric corpus atrophy in *H. pylori*-infected mice.[81] This therapeutic effect was not observed in mice in which the Nrf2 gene was deleted, which implicates the important role of Nrf2-dependent antioxidant and anti-inflammatory proteins in SF-dependent protection.[81]

S-allylcysteine

S-allylcysteine (SAC) is a water-soluble garlic constituent shown to prevent different cancers. Studies have shown that this compound inhibits

MNNG-induced gastric cancer in animals.[82] Velmurugan *et al.*[83] investigated the apoptosis-inducing potential of a combination of SAC and lycopene, a tomato carotenoid during MNNG- and saturated sodium chloride (S-NaCl)-induced gastric carcinogenesis in rats using the apoptosis-associated proteins Bcl-2, Bax, Bim, caspase 8 and caspase 3 as markers. Results showed that SAC and lycopene, when used singly, significantly inhibited the development of gastric cancer; however, their combination was more effective in inhibiting MNNG-induced stomach tumors and modulating the expression of apoptosis-associated proteins. These results suggest that the combination of SAC and lycopene has a great potential in the chemoprevention of gastric cancer.[83]

Diallyl Disulfide

The effect of diallyl disulfide (DADS), a major component of an oil-soluble allylsulphide garlic (*Allium sativum*) derivative, on the correlation between anti-invasive activity and tightening of tight junctions (TJs), was investigated in human gastric adenocarcinoma AGS cells by Park *et al.*[84] Their data indicated that the inhibitory effects of DADS on cell motility and invasiveness were found to be associated with increased tightness of the TJs, which was demonstrated by an increase in transepithelial electrical resistance. DADS inhibited MMP-2 and -9 activities in AGS cells, and this was also correlated with a decrease in expression of their mRNA and proteins. These results suggest that DADS can act as a dietary source to decrease the risk of gastric cancer metastasis.[84] In addition, many studies have shown that this compound inhibits gastric cancer cell proliferation and inhibits gastric cancer cell-induced tumor xenografts by modulating the p38 MAPK, ERK and Wnt signalling pathways, and upregulating miR-200b and miR-22 expression.[85–88]

Thymoquinone

Thymoquinone (TQ), a component derived from the bioactive constituent of black seed (*Nigella sativa*), has been shown to exert biological activity on various types of human cancers including gastric cancer. Studies have shown that this compound inhibits benzo[a]pyrene-induced forestomach carcinogenesis in mice by preventing the generation of ROS.[89] Lei *et al.*[90] described the chemosensitizing effect of TQ and 5-fluorouracil (5-FU) on gastric cancer preclinical models. The results showed that pre-treatment with TQ significantly increased the apoptotic effects induced by 5-FU in gastric cancer cell lines *in vitro*, downregulated anti-apoptotic protein Bcl-2, upregulated pro-apoptotic protein Bax and activated caspases-3 and -9. Moreover, the combination of TQ and 5-FU significantly inhibited xenograft tumors than either agent alone. These results suggest that thymoquinone be used as chemosensitizing agent in gastric cancer.[90]

Green Tea Extract

The consumption of green tea is associated with a reduced risk for gastrointestinal cancers.[91,92] Inflammatory processes, such as the secretion of IL-8 from the gastric epithelium in response to chronic chemokine or antigen exposure, serve both as a chemoattractant for white blood cells and a prerequisite for gastric carcinogenesis. The gastric adenocarcinoma cell line AGS was used to investigate the effect of green tea extract, black tea extract and epigallocatechin gallate (EGCG) on cytokine-induced inflammation. The results showed that both green and black tea extracts significantly inhibited IL-1β-induced IL-8 production and secretion, and inhibited NF-κB activity.[93] Moreover, several studies have shown that EGCG, one of the components of green tea, inhibited cell proliferation and induced apoptosis in gastric cancer cells by modulating different cell signalling pathways.[94,95] These studies thus show that green tea holds promise in the prevention of gastric cancer.

Cranberry

Cranberry extract possesses potent antioxidant and anti-proliferative activities. Liu *et al.*[96] determined the effect of cranberry extract human gastric cancer SGC-7901 cell proliferation and human gastric cancer cells-induced tumor xenografts in animals. Treatment with cranberry extract at doses of 0, 5, 10, 20 and 40 mg/mL significantly inhibited proliferation of

SGC-7901 cells and decreased PCNA expression. In addition, the administration of cranberry extract significantly inhibited gastric tumor xenografts in animals.[97] Moreover, it has been shown that the administration of cranberry juice suppressed *H. pylori* infection in an endemically infected population at high risk for gastric cancer.[98] These results demonstrate fresh cranberries to be a potential chemopreventive reagent.

Tocotrienols

Recent research has revealed that tocotrienols, especially γ-tocotrienol, exhibit not only a similar antioxidant ability as tocopherols, but also a remarkable anticancer capacity in cancer cell lines. Several studies have demonstrated that tocotrienol inhibits proliferation and induces apoptosis in gastric cancer cells.[98–100] Liu *et al.*[101] explored the invasion and metastatic capacities of gastric adenocarcinoma SGC-7901 cells and the correlation with anti-metastasis mechanisms induced by γ-tocotrienol. The results showed γ-tocotrienol inhibited cell migration and invasion. Moreover, γ-tocotrienol significantly inhibited MMP-2 and -9 mRNA expression and upregulated tissue inhibitor of metalloproteinase-1 (TIMP-1) and -2 in SGC-7901 cells. Additionally, γ-tocotrienol induced the activation of caspase-3 and increased the cleavage of the downstream substrate PARP in gastric cancer cells.[102] Due to poor prognosis and development of resistance against chemotherapeutic drugs, the existing treatment modalities for gastric cancer are ineffective. Hence, novel agents that are safe and effective are urgently needed. Manu *et al.*[103] showed that γ-tocotrienol inhibited proliferation of various gastric cancer cell lines, potentiated the apoptotic effects of capecitabine, inhibited the constitutive activation of NF-κB and suppressed the NF-κB-regulated expression of COX-2, cyclin D1, Bcl-2, CXCR4, VEGF and MMP-9. Moreover, the administration of γ-tocotrienol alone (1 mg/kg body weight, intraperitoneally three times/week) and in combination with capecitabine significantly suppressed gastric cancer cells-induced xenograft tumors in animals by inhibiting activation of NF-κB and the expression of cyclin D1, COX-2, intercellular adhesion molecule-1 (ICAM-1), MMP-9, survivin, $Bcl\text{-}x_L$ and XIAP.[78] These results suggest that tocotrienols have high potential in the prevention and treatment of gastric cancer.

CONCLUSION

Together, the above summarized studies clearly and convincingly show that there is a vast range of phytochemicals isolated from various fruits and vegetables, which exert potent cell growth inhibitory, cell cycle arrest and apoptosis-inducing effects in a wide panel of human gastric cancer cell lines with varying degrees of genetic alterations by targeting various signal transduction pathways. Some of the most common mechanisms by which these phytochemicals inhibit survival of tumor cells are by activating caspases, inducing pro-apoptotic proteins and downregulating anti-apoptotic proteins. Induction of apoptosis and/or inhibition of cell proliferation are highly correlated with the activation of variety of intracellular signalling pathways leading to arrest of cell cycle in the G1, S or G2/M phases. The intake of 400–600 g/day of fruits and vegetables is associated with reduced incidence of many common forms of cancer, and diets rich in plant foods are also associated with a reduced risk of heart disease and numerous chronic inflammatory conditions. However, more human studies are needed to translate the enormous preclinical data that currently exists on the significant anticancer effects of various phytochemicals derived from various fruits and vegetables.

ABBREVIATIONS

ANG-1: angiopoietin-1; AOM: azoxymethane; AP-1: activator protein-1; BAD: Bcl-2-associated death promoter; Bcl-2: B-cell lymphoma 2; Bcl-x_L: B-cell lymphoma-extra large; COX-2: cyclooxygenase-2; CSF: colony-stimulating factor; ; CXCR4: C-X-C chemokine receptor type 4; EGCG: epigallocatechin gallate; EGF: epidermal growth factor; Epo: erythropoietin; ERK1/2: extracellular signal-regulated kinases; FAK: focal adhesion kinase; FLIP: FLICE-like inhibitory protein; ICAM-1: intracellular adhesion molecule-1; IGF: insulin growth factor; IKK: IκB kinase; IL-6: interleukin-6; HIF-1α: hypoxia-inducible factor 1-alpha; HUVEC: human umbilical vein endothelial cells; LOX: lipooxygenase; MAPK-ERK: mitogen-activated protein kinase-extracellular signal regulated kinase; MDM2: mouse double minute 2; MKK7: MAP kinase kinase 7; MMP: matrix metalloproteinase; NF-κB: nuclear factor-kappa B; Nrf2: nuclear factor (erythroid-derived 2)-like 2; PARP: poly(ADP-ribose) polymerase; PEITC: phenethylisothiocyanate; PI3K: phosphoinositide-3-kinase; PKC: protein kinase C; PPAR-γ: peroxisome proliferator activated receptor-gamma; PTEN: phosphatase and tensin homolog; ROS: reactive oxygen species; SCID: severe combined immunodeficiency; SHP-1: Src homology region 2 domain-containing phosphatase-1; SOS1: son of sevenless homolog 1; STAT3: signal transducer and activator of transcription; TGF-β: transforming growth factor-beta; TNF-α: tumor necrosis factor-alpha; TQ: thymoquinone; TRAIL: TNF-related apoptosis-inducing ligand; VEGF: vascular endothelial growth factor; XIAP: X-linked inhibitor of apoptosis protein

ACKNOWLEDGMENT

This work was supported by a grant from the NUS Academic Research Fund (Grant R-184-000-207-112] to Dr. Gautam Sethi.

CONFLICT OF INTEREST

None declared.

REFERENCES

1. Gomceli, I., B. Demiriz, and M. Tez, Gastric carcinogenesis, *World J Gastroenterol* **18**(37): 5164–5170 (2012).
2. Peek, R.M. Jr. and M.J. Blaser, *Helicobacter pylori* and gastrointestinal tract adenocarcinomas, *Nat Rev Cancer* **2**(1): 28–37 (2002).
3. Rocco, A., G. Nardone and H. Diet, *Pylori* infection and gastric cancer: Evidence and controversies, *World J Gastroenterol* **13**(21): 2901–2912 (2007).
4. Correa, P., Human gastric carcinogenesis: A multistep and multifactorial process — First American Cancer Society Award Lecture on Cancer Epidemiology and Prevention, *Cancer Res* **52**(24): 6735–6740 (1992).
5. Barros R., J.N. Freund, L. David, and R. Almeida, Gastric intestinal metaplasia revisited: Function and regulation of CDX2, *Trends Mol Med* **18**(9): 555–563 (2012).
6. Ohtsu, A., Chemotherapy for metastatic gastric cancer: Past, present, and future, *J Gastroenterol* **43**(4): 256–264 (2008).

7. Shih, P.H., C.T. Yeh, and G.C. Yen, Effects of anthocyanidin on the inhibition of proliferation and induction of apoptosis in human gastric adenocarcinoma cells, *Food Chem Toxicol* **43**(10): 1557–1566 (2005).
8. Cascinu, S., M. Scartozzi, R. Labianca, V. Catalano, R.R. Silva, S. Barni, A. Zaniboni, A. D'Angelo, S. Salvagni, G. Martignoni, G.D. Beretta, F. Graziano, R. Berardi and V. Franciosi, High curative resection rate with weekly cisplatin, 5-fluorouracil, epidoxorubicin, 6S-leucovorin, glutathione, and filgastrim in patients with locally advanced, unresectable gastric cancer: A report from the Italian Group for the Study of Digestive Tract Cancer (GISCAD), *Br J Cancer* **90**(8): 1521–1525 (2004).
9. Aggarwal, B.B., R.V. Vijayalekshmi and B. Sung, Targeting inflammatory pathways for prevention and therapy of cancer: Short-term friend, long-term foe, *Clin Cancer Res* **15**(2): 425–430 (2009).
10. Anand, P., A.B. Kunnumakkara, C. Sundaram, K.B. Harikumar, S.T. Tharakan, O.S. Lai, B. Sung, and B.B. Aggarwal, Cancer is a preventable disease that requires major lifestyle changes, *Pharm Res* **25**(9): 2097–2116 (2008).
11. Parkin, D.M., The global health burden of infection-associated cancers in the year 2002, *Int J Cancer* **118**(2): 3030–3044 (2006).
12. Belpomme, D., P. Irigaray, L. Hardell, R. Clapp, L. Montagnier, S. Epstein, and A.J. Sasco, The multitude and diversity of environmental carcinogens, *Environ Res* **105**(3): 414–429 (2007).
13. Ziegler, R.G., R.N. Hoover, M.C. Pike, A. Hildesheim, A.M. Nomura, D.W. West, A.H. Wu-Williams, L.N. Kolonel, P.L. Horn-Ross, J.F. Rosenthal, and M.B. Hyer, Migration patterns and breast cancer risk in Asian-American women, *J Natl Cancer Inst* **85**(22): 1819–1827 (1993).
14. Haenszel, W. and M. Kurihara, Studies of Japanese migrants. I. Mortality from cancer and other diseases among Japanese in the United States, *J Natl Cancer Inst* **40**(1): 43–68 (1968).
15. Shanmugam, M.K., R. Kannaiyan, and G. Sethi, Targeting cell signaling and apoptotic pathways by dietary agents: Role in the prevention and treatment of cancer, *Nutr Cancer* **63**(2): 161–173 (2011).
16. Li, Y., M.S. Wicha, S.J. Schwartz, and D. Sun, Implications of cancer stem cell theory for cancer chemoprevention by natural dietary compounds, *J Nutr Biochem* **22**(9): 799–806 (2011).
17. Manson, M.M., P.B. Farmer, A. Gescher, and W.P. Steward, Innovative agents in cancer prevention, *Recent Results Cancer Res* **166**: 257–275 (2005).
18. Deorukhkar, A., S. Krishnan, G. Sethi, and B.B. Aggarwal, Back to basics: How natural products can provide the basis for new therapeutics, *Expert Opin Investig Drugs* **16**(11): 1753–1773 (2007).

19. Dorai, T. and B.B. Aggarwal, Role of chemopreventive agents in cancer therapy, *Cancer Lett* **215**(2): 129–140 (2004).
20. Kannaiyan, R., R. Surana, E.M. Shin, L. Ramachandran, G. Sethi, and A.P. Kumar, Targeted inhibition of multiple proinflammatory signaling pathways for the prevention and treatment of multiple myeloma, Gupta, A. (Ed.), in *Multiple Myeloma — An Overview*, InTech, pp. 93–128 (2011).
21. Mitsiades, C.S., N. Mitsiades, V. Poulaki, R. Schlossman, M. Akiyama, D. Chauhan, T. Hideshima, S.P. Treon, N.C. Munshi, P.G. Richardson, and K.C. Anderson, Activation of NF-kappaB and upregulation of intracellular anti-apoptotic proteins via the IGF-1/Akt signaling in human multiple myeloma cells: Therapeutic implications, *Oncogene* **21**(37): 5673–5683 (2002).
22. Fallone, F., S. Britton, L. Nieto, B. Salles, and C. Muller, ATR controls cellular adaptation to hypoxia through positive regulation of hypoxia-inducible factor 1 (HIF-1) expression, *Oncogene* **32**(37): 4387–4396 (2012).
23. Monti, E. and M.B. Gariboldi, HIF-1 as a target for cancer chemotherapy, chemosensitization and chemoprevention, *Current Mol Pharmacol* **4**(1): 62–77 (2011).
24. Yee Koh, M., T.R. Spivak-Kroizman, and G. Powis, HIF-1 regulation: Not so easy come, easy go, *Trends Biochem Sci* **33**(11): 526–534 (2008).
25. Brahimi-Horn, M.C. and J. Pouysségur, HIF at a glance, *J Cell Sci* **122**(Pt 8): 1055–1057 (2009).
26. Semenza, G.L., Evaluation of HIF-1 inhibitors as anticancer agents, *Drug Discov Today* **12**(19–20): 853–859 (2007).
27. Zhan, H., H. Liang, X. Liu, J. Deng, B. Wang, and X. Hao, Expression of Rac1, HIF-1α, and VEGF in gastric carcinoma: Correlation with angiogenesis and prognosis, *Onkologie* **36**(3):102–107 (2013).
28. Zhang, Z.G., Q.N. Zhang, X.H. Wang, and J.H. Tian, Hypoxia-inducible factor 1 alpha (HIF-1α) as a prognostic indicator in patients with gastric tumors: A meta-analysis, *Asian Pac J Cancer Prev* **14**(7): 4195–4198 (2013).
29. Brahimi-Horn, M.C. and J. Pouysségur, Harnessing the hypoxia-inducible factor in cancer and ischemic disease, *Biochem Pharmacol* **73**(3): 450–457 (2007).
30. Onnis, B., A. Rapisarda, and G. Melillo, Development of HIF-1 inhibitors for cancer therapy, *J Cell Mol Med* **13**(9A): 2780–2786 (2009).
31. De Luca, A., M.R. Maiello, A. D'Alessio, M. Pergameno, and N. Normanno, The RAS/RAF/MEK/ERK and the PI3K/AKT signalling pathways: Role in cancer pathogenesis and implications for therapeutic approaches, *Expert Opin Ther Targets* **16**(Suppl. 2): S17–S27 (2012).
32. Qu, J.L., X.J. Qu, M.F. Zhao, Y.E. Teng, Y. Zhang, K.Z. Hou, Y.H. Jiang, X.H. Yang, and Y.P. Liu, Gastric cancer exosomes promote tumour cell proliferation

through PI3K/Akt and MAPK/ERK activation, *Dig Liver Dis* **41**(12): 875–880 (2009).
33. Kang, M.H., S.C. Oh, H.J. Lee, H.N. Kang, J.L. Kim, J.S. Kim, and Y.A. Yoo, Metastatic function of BMP-2 in gastric cancer cells: the role of PI3K/AKT, MAPK, the NF-κB pathway, and MMP-9 expression, *Exp Cell Res* **317**(12): 1746–1762 (2011).
34. Courtney, K.D., R.B. Corcoran, and J.A. Engelman, The PI3K pathway as drug target in human cancer, *J Clin Oncol* **28**(6): 1075–1083 (2010).
35. Yuan, T.L. and L.C. Cantley, PI3K pathway alterations in cancer: Variations on a theme, *Oncogene* **27**(41): 5497–5510 (2008).
36. Engelman, J.A., J. Luo, and L.C. Cantley, The evolution of phosphatidylinositol 3-kinases as regulators of growth and metabolism, *Nat Rev Genet* **7**(8): 606–619 (2006).
37. Mayo, L.D. and D.B. Donner, A phosphatidylinositol 3-kinase/Akt pathway promotes translocation of Mdm2 from the cytoplasm to the nucleus, *Proc Natl Acad Sci USA* **98**(20): 11598–11603 (2001).
38. Chong, M.L., M. Loh, B. Thakkar, B. Pang, B. Iacopetta, and R. Soong, Phosphatidylinositol-3-kinase pathway aberrations in gastric and colorectal cancer: Meta-analysis, co-occurrence and ethnic variation, *Int J Cancer* [Epub ahead of print] (2013).
39. Canbay, E., O.T. Kahraman, D. Bugra, B. Caykara, M.F. Seyhan, T. Bulut, S. Yamaner, and O. Ozturk, Increased gastric cancer risk with PTEN IVS4 polymorphism in a Turkish population, *Genet Test Mol Biomarkers* **17**(3): 249–253 (2013).
40. Goswami, S.K. and D.K. Das, Resveratrol and chemoprevention, *Cancer Lett* **284**(1): 1–6 (2009).
41. Atten, M.J., B.M. Attar, T. Milson, and O. Holian, Resveratrol-induced inactivation of human gastric adenocarcinoma cells through a protein kinase C-mediated mechanism, *Biochem Pharmacol* **62**(10): 1423–1432 (2001).
42. Aggarwal, B.B., Signalling pathways of the TNF superfamily: A double-edged sword, *Nat Rev Immunol* **3**(9): 745–756 (2003).
43. Bertelli, A.A., L. Giovannini, R. Stradi, S. Urien, J.P. Tillement, and A. Bertelli, Evaluation of kinetic parameters of natural phytoalexin in resveratrol orally administered in wine to rats, *Drugs Exp Clin Res* **24**(1): 51–55 (1998).
44. Andlauer, W., J. Kolb, K. Siebert, and P. Fürst, Assessment of resveratrol bioavailability in the perfused small intestine of the rat, *Drugs Exp Clin Res* **26**(2): 47–55 (2000).
45. Zaidi, S.F., K. Ahmed, T. Yamamoto, T. Kondo, K. Usmanghani, M. Kadowaki, and T. Sugiyama, Effect of resveratrol on *Helicobacter pylori*-induced interleukin-8 secretion, reactive oxygen species generation and morphological changes in human gastric epithelial cells, *Biol Pharm Bull* **32**(11): 1931–1935 (2009).

46. Wang, Z., W. Li, X. Meng, and B. Jia, Resveratrol induces gastric cancer cell apoptosis via reactive oxygen species, but independent of sirtuin1, *Clin Exp Pharmacol Physiol* **39**(3): 227–232 (2012).
47. Riles, W.L., J. Erickson, S. Nayyar, M.J. Atten, B.M. Attar, and O. Holian, Resveratrol engages selective apoptotic signals in gastric adenocarcinoma cells, *World J Gastroenterol* **12**(35): 5628–5634 (2006).
48. Zhou, H.B., J.J. Chen, W.X. Wang, J.T. Cai, and Q. Du, Anticancer activity of resveratrol on implanted human primary gastric carcinoma cells in nude mice, *World J Gastroenterol* **11**(2): 280–284 (2005).
49. Holian, O., S. Wahid, M.J. Atten, and B.M. Attar, Inhibition of gastric cancer cell proliferation by resveratrol: Role of nitric oxide, *Am J Physiol Gastrointest Liver Physiol* **282**(5): G809–G816 (2002).
50. Arora, S., S. Singh, G.A. Piazza, C.M. Contreras, J. Panyam, and A.P. Singh, Honokiol: A novel natural agent for cancer prevention and therapy, *Curr Mol Med* **12**(10): 1244–1252 (2012).
51. Liu, S.H., C.C. Shen, Y.C. Yi, J.J. Tsai, C.C. Wang, J.T. Chueh, K.L. Lin, T.C. Lee, H.C. Pan, and M.L. Sheu, Honokiol inhibits gastric tumourigenesis by activation of 15-lipoxygenase-1 and consequent inhibition of peroxisome proliferator-activated receptor-gamma and COX-2-dependent signals, *Br J Pharmacol* **160**(8): 1963–1972 (2010).
52. Shureiqi, I., K.J. Wojno, J.A. Poore, R.G. Reddy, M.J. Moussalli, S.A. Spindler, J.K. Greenson, D. Normolle, A.A. Hasan, T.S. Lawrence, and D.E. Brenner, Decreased 13-S-hydroxyoctadecadienoic acid levels and 15-lipoxygenase-1 expression in human colon cancers, *Carcinogenesis* **20**(10): 1985–1995 (1999).
53. Sheu, M.L., S.H. Liu, and K.H. Lan, Honokiol induces calpain-mediated glucose-regulated protein-94 cleavage and apoptosis in human gastric cancer cells and reduces tumor growth, *PloS One* **2**(10): e1096 (2007).
54. Liu, S.H., K.B. Wang, K.H. Lan, W.J. Lee, H.C. Pan, S.M. Wu, Y.C. Peng, Y.C. Chen, C.C. Shen, H.C. Cheng, K.K. Liao, and M.L. Sheu, Calpain/SHP-1 interaction by honokiol dampening peritoneal dissemination of gastric cancer in nu/nu mice, *PloS One* **7**(8): e43711 (2012).
55. Murakami, A., H. Ashida, and J. Terao, Multitargeted cancer prevention by quercetin, *Cancer Lett* **269**(2): 315–325 (2008).
56. Wang, K., R. Liu, J. Li, J. Mao, Y. Lei, J. Wu, J. Zeng, T. Zhang, H. Wu, L. Chen, C. Huang, and Y. Wei, Quercetin induces protective autophagy in gastric cancer cells: Involvement of Akt-mTOR- and hypoxia-induced factor 1 alpha-mediated signaling, *Autophagy* **7**(9): 966–978 (2011).
57. Boots, A.W., G.R. Haenen, and A. Bast, Health effects of quercetin: From antioxidant to nutraceutical, *Eur J Pharmacol* **585**(2–3): 325–337 (2008).

58. Manna, S.K., Double-edged sword effect of biochanin to inhibit nuclear factor kappaB: Suppression of serine/threonine and tyrosine kinases, *Biochem Pharmacol* **83**(10): 1383–1392 (2012).
59. Wang, P., K. Zhang, Q. Zhang, J. Mei, C.J. Chen, Z.Z. Feng, and D.H. Yu, Effects of quercetin on the apoptosis of the human gastric carcinoma cells, *Toxicol In Vitro* **26**(2): 221–228 (2012).
60. Yu, Z.J., L.Y. He, Y. Chen, M.Y. Wu, X.H. Zhao, and Z.Y. Wang, Effects of quercetin on the expression of VEGF-C and VEGFR-3 in human cancer MGC-803 cells, *Xi Bao Yu Fen Zi Mian Yi Xue Za Zhi.* **25**(8): 678–680 (2009).
61. Qin, Y., L.Y. He, Y. Chen, W.Y. Wang, X.H. Zhao, and M.Y. Wu, Quercetin affects leptin and its receptor in human gastric cancer MGC-803 cells and JAK-STAT pathway, *Xi Bao Yu Fen Zi Mian Yi Xue Za Zhi* **28**(1): 12–16 (2012).
62. Borska, S., M. Chmielewska, T. Wysocka, M. Drag-Zalesinska, M. Zabel, and P. Dziegiel, *In vitro* effect of quercetin on human gastric carcinoma: Targeting cancer cells death and MDR, *Food Chem Toxicol* **50**(9): 3375–3383 (2012).
63. Choi, W.Y., C.Y. Jin, M.H. Han, G.Y. Kim, N.D. Kim, W.H. Lee, S.K. Kim, and Y.H. Choi, Sanguinarine sensitizes human gastric adenocarcinoma AGS cells to TRAIL-mediated apoptosis via down-regulation of AKT and activation of caspase-3, *Anticancer Res* **29**(11): 4457–4465 (2009).
64. Chen, P.Y., K.C. Lin, J.P. Lin, N.Y. Tang, J.S. Yang, K.W. Lu, and J.G. Chung, Phenethyl isothiocyanate (PEITC) inhibits the growth of human oral squamous carcinoma HSC-3 cells through G(0)/G(1) phase arrest and mitochondria-mediated apoptotic cell death, *Evid Based Complement Alternat Med*, doi: 10.1155/2012/718320 (2012).
65. Cheung, K.L. and A.N. Kong, Molecular targets of dietary phenethyl isothiocyanate and sulforaphane for cancer chemoprevention, *AAPS J* **12**(1): 87–97 (2010).
66. Yang, M.D., K.C. Lai, T.Y. Lai, S.C. Hsu, C.L. Kuo, C.S. Yu, M.L. Lin, J.S. Yang, H.M. Kuo, S.H. Wu, and J.G. Chung, Phenethyl isothiocyanate inhibits migration and invasion of human gastric cancer AGS cells through suppressing MAPK and NF-kappaB signal pathways, *Anticancer Res* **30**(6): 2135–2143 (2010).
67. Tang, T., X. Song, Y.F. Liu, and W.Y. Wang, PEITC reverse multi-drug resistance of human gastric cancer SGC7901/DDP cell line, *Cell Biol Int* [Epub ahead of print] (2013).
68. Charoenprasert, S. and A. Mitchell, Factors influencing phenolic compounds in table olives (*Olea europaea*), *J Agric Food Chem* **60**(29): 7081–7095 (2012).
69. Kountouri, A.M., A.C. Kaliora, L. Koumbi, and N.K. Andrikopoulos, *In-vitro* gastric cancer prevention by a polyphenol-rich extract from olives through induction of apoptosis, *Eur J Cancer Prev* **18**(1): 33–39 (2009).

70. Jaganathan, S.K. and E. Supriyanto, Antiproliferative and molecular mechanism of eugenol-induced apoptosis in cancer cells, *Molecules* **17**(6): 6290–6304 (2012).
71. Manikandan, P., R.S. Murugan, R.V. Priyadarsini, G. Vinothini, and S. Nagini, Eugenol induces apoptosis and inhibits invasion and angiogenesis in a rat model of gastric carcinogenesis induced by MNNG, *Life Sci* **86**(25-26): 936–941 (2010).
72. Manikandan, P., G. Vinothini, R. Vidya Priyadarsini, D. Prathiba, and S. Nagini, Eugenol inhibits cell proliferation via NF-κB suppression in a rat model of gastric carcinogenesis induced by MNNG, *Invest New Drugs* **29**(1): 110–117 (2011).
73. Meiyanto, E., A. Hermawan, and Anindyajati, Natural products for cancer-targeted therapy: Citrus flavonoids as potent chemopreventive agents, *Asian Pac J Cancer Prev* **13**(2): 427–436 (2012).
74. Lee, Y.C., T.H. Cheng, J.S. Lee, J.H. Chen, Y.C. Liao, Y. Fong, C.H. Wu, and Y.W. Shih, Nobiletin, a citrus flavonoid, suppresses invasion and migration involving FAK/PI3K/Akt and small GTPase signals in human gastric adenocarcinoma AGS cells, *Mol Cell Biochem* **347**(1–2): 103–115 (2011).
75. Minagawa, A., Y. Otani, T. Kubota, N. Wada, T. Furukawa, K. Kumai, K. Kameyama, Y. Okada, M. Fujii, M. Yano, T. Sato, A. Ito, and M. Kitajima, The citrus flavonoid, nobiletin, inhibits peritoneal dissemination of human gastric carcinoma in SCID mice, *Jpn J Cancer Res* **92**(12): 1322–1328 (2001).
76. Jaramillo, S., S. Lopez, L.M. Varela, R. Rodriguez-Arcos, A. Jimenez, R. Abia, R. Guillen, and F.J. Muriana, The flavonol isorhamnetin exhibits cytotoxic effects on human colon cancer cells, *J Agric Food Chem* [Epud ahead of print] (2010).
77. Kim, J.E., D.E. Lee, K.W. Lee, J.E. Son, S.K. Seo, J. Li, S.K. Jung, Y.S. Heo, M. Mottamal, A.M. Bode, Z. Dong, and H.J. Lee, Isorhamnetin suppresses skin cancer through direct inhibition of MEK1 and PI3-K, *Cancer Prev Res (Phila)* **4**(4): 582–591 (2011).
78. Yao, L., F. Liu, L. Sun, H. Wu, C. Guo, S. Liang, L. Liu, N. Liu, Z. Han, H. Zhang, K. Wu, and D. Fan, Upregulation of PPARgamma in tissue with gastric carcinoma, *Hybridoma* **29**(4): 341–343 (2010).
79. Lu, J., K. Imamura, S. Nomura, K. Mafune, A. Nakajima, T. Kadowaki, N. Kubota, Y. Terauchi, G. Ishii, A. Ochiai, H. Esumi, and M. Kaminishi, Chemopreventive effect of peroxisome proliferator-activated receptor gamma on gastric carcinogenesis in mice, *Cancer Res* **65**(11): 4769–4774 (2005).

80. Ramachandran, L., K.A. Manu, M.K. Shanmugam, F. Li, K.S. Siveen, S. Vali, S. Kapoor, T. Abbasi, R. Surana, D.T. Smoot, H. Ashktorab, P. Tan, K.S. Ahn, C.W. Yap, A.P. Kumar, and G. Sethi, Isorhamnetin inhibits proliferation, invasion, and induces apoptosis through the modulation of peroxisome proliferator-activated receptor-gamma activation pathway in gastric cancer, *J Biol Chem* **287**(45): 38028–38040 (2012).
81. Yanaka, A., J.W. Fahey, A. Fukumoto, M. Nakayama, S. Inoue, S. Zhang, M. Tauchi, H. Suzuki, I. Hyodo, and M. Yamamoto, Dietary sulforaphane-rich broccoli sprouts reduce colonization and attenuate gastritis in *Helicobacter pylori*-infected mice and humans, *Cancer Prev Res (Phila)* **2**(4): 353–360 (2009).
82. Velmurugan, B., V. Bhuvaneswari, and S. Nagini, Effect of S-allylcysteine on oxidant-antioxidant status during N-methyl-N′-nitro-N-nitrosoguanidine and saturated sodium chloride-induced gastric carcinogenesis in Wistar rats, *Asia Pac J Clin Nutr* **12**(4): 488–494 (2003).
83. Velmurugan, B., A. Mani, and S. Nagini, Combination of S-allylcysteine and lycopene induces apoptosis by modulating Bcl-2, Bax, Bim and caspases during experimental gastric carcinogenesis, *Eur J Cancer Prev* **14**(4): 387–393 (2005).
84. Park, H.S., G.Y. Kim, I.W. Choi, N.D. Kim, H.J. Hwang, Y.W. Choi, and Y.H. Choi, Inhibition of matrix metalloproteinase activities and tightening of tight junctions by diallyl disulfide in AGS human gastric carcinoma cells, *J Food Sci* **76**(4): T105–T111 (2011).
85. Tang, H., Y. Kong, J. Guo, Y. Tang, X. Xie, L. Yang, Q. Su, and X. Xie, Diallyl disulfide suppresses proliferation and induces apoptosis in human gastric cancer through Wnt-1 signaling pathway by up-regulation of miR-200b and miR-22, *Cancer Lett* **340**(1): 72–81 (2013).
86. Ling, H., L.Y. Zhang, Q. Su, Y. Song, Z.Y. Luo, X.T. Zhou, X. Zeng, J. He, H. Tan, and J.P. Yuan, Erk is involved in the differentiation induced by diallyl disulfide in the human gastric cancer cell line MGC803, *Cell Mol Biol Lett* **11**(3): 408–423 (2006).
87. Xiang, S.L., X.L. Xiao, H. Ling, Q.J. Liao, X.T. Zhou, L. Dong, and Q. Su, Antitumor effect of diallyl disulfide on human gastric cancer MGC803 cells xenograft in nude mice, *Ai Zheng* **24**(8): 940–944 (2005).
88. Yuan, J.P., G.H. Wang, H. Ling, Q. Su, Y.H. Yang, Y. Song, R.J. Tang, Y. Liu, and C. Huang, Diallyl disulfide-induced G2/M arrest of human gastric cancer MGC803 cells involves activation of p38 MAP kinase pathways, *World J Gastroenterol* **10**(18): 2731–2734 (2004).

89. Badary, O.A., O.A. Al-Shabanah, M.N. Nagi, A.C. Al-Rikabi, and M.M. Elmazar, Inhibition of benzo(a)pyrene-induced forestomach carcinogenesis in mice by thymoquinone, *Eur J Cancer Prev* **8**(5): 435–440 (1999).
90. Lei, X., X. Lv, M. Liu, Z. Yang, M. Ji, X. Guo, and W. Dong, Thymoquinone inhibits growth and augments 5-fluorouracil-induced apoptosis in gastric cancer cells both *in vitro* and *in vivo*, *Biochem Biophys Res Commun* **417**(2): 864–868 (2012).
91. Sasazuki, S., A. Tamakoshi, K. Matsuo, H. Ito, K. Wakai, C. Nagata, T. Mizoue, K. Tanaka, I. Tsuji, M. Inoue, S. Tsugane; and Research Group for the Development and Evaluation of Cancer Prevention Strategies in Japan, Green tea consumption and gastric cancer risk: An evaluation based on a systematic review of epidemiologic evidence among the Japanese population, *Jpn J Clin Oncol* **42**(4): 335–346 (2012).
92. Mu, L.N., Q.Y. Lu, S.Z. Yu, Q.W. Jiang, W. Cao, N.C. You, V.W. Setiawan, X.F. Zhou, B.G. Ding, R.H. Wang, J. Zhao, L. Cai, J.Y. Rao, D. Heber, and Z.F. Zhang, Green tea drinking and multigenetic index on the risk of stomach cancer in a Chinese population, *Int J Cancer* **116**(6): 972–983 (2005).
93. Gutierrez-Orozco, F., B.R. Stephens, A.P. Neilson, R. Green, M.G. Ferruzzi, and J.A. Bomser, Green and black tea inhibit cytokine-induced IL-8 production and secretion in AGS gastric cancer cells via inhibition of NF-kappaB activity, *Planta Med* **76**(15): 1659–1665 (2010).
94. Tanaka, T., T. Ishii, D. Mizuno, T. Mori, R. Yamaji, Y. Nakamura, S. Kumazawa, T. Nakayama, and M. Akagawa, (−)-Epigallocatechin-3-gallate suppresses growth of AZ521 human gastric cancer cells by targeting the DEAD-box RNA helicase p68, *Free Radic Biol Med* **50**(10): 1324–1335 (2011).
95. Onoda, C., K. Kuribayashi, S. Nirasawa, N. Tsuji, M. Tanaka, D. Kobayashim, and N. Watanabe, (−)-Epigallocatechin-3-gallate induces apoptosis in gastric cancer cell lines by down-regulating survivin expression, *Int J Oncol* **38**(5): 1403–1408 (2011).
96. Liu, M., L.Q. Lin, B.B. Song, L.F. Wang, C.P. Zhang, J.L. Zhao, and J.R. Liu, Cranberry phytochemical extract inhibits SGC-7901 cell growth and human tumor xenografts in Balb/c nu/nu mice, *J Agric Food Chem* **57**(2): 762–768 (2009).
97. Zhang, L., J. Ma, K. Pan, V.L. Go, J. Chen, and W.C. You, Efficacy of cranberry juice on Helicobacter pylori infection: A double-blind, randomized placebo-controlled trial, *Helicobacter* **10**(2): 139–145 (2005).
98. Sun, W., Q. Wang, B. Chen, J. Liu, H. Liu, and W. Xu, Gamma-tocotrienol-induced apoptosis in human gastric cancer SGC-7901 cells is associated

with a suppression in mitogen-activated protein kinase signalling, *Br J Nutr* **99**(6): 1247–1254 (2008).
99. Sun, W., W. Xu, H. Liu, J. Liu, Q. Wang, J. Zhou, F. Dong, and B. Chen, Gamma-tocotrienol induces mitochondria-mediated apoptosis in human gastric adenocarcinoma SGC-7901 cells, *J Nutr Biochem* **20**(4): 276–284 (2009).
100. Bi, S., J.R. Liu, Y. Li, Q. Wang, H.K. Liu, Y.G. Yan, B.Q. Chen, and W.G. Sun, Gamma-tocotrienol modulates the paracrine secretion of VEGF induced by cobalt(II) chloride via ERK signaling pathway in gastric adenocarcinoma SGC-7901 cell line, *Toxicology* **274**(1–3): 27–33 (2010).
101. Liu, H.K., Q. Wang, Y. Li, W.G. Sun, J.R. Liu, Y.M. Yang, W.L. Xu, X.R. Sun, and B.Q. Chen, Inhibitory effects of gamma-tocotrienol on invasion and metastasis of human gastric adenocarcinoma SGC-7901 cells, *J Nutr Biochem* **21**(3): 206–213 (2010).
102. Sun, W., W. Xu, H. Liu, J. Liu, Q. Wang, J. Zhou, F. Dong, and B. Chen, Gamma-tocotrienol induces mitochondria-mediated apoptosis in human gastric adenocarcinoma SGC-7901 cells, *J Nutr Biochem.* **20**(4): 276–284 (2009).
103. Manu, K.A., M.K. Shanmugam, L. Ramachandran, F. Li, C.W. Fong, A.P. Kumar, P. Tan, and G. Sethi, First evidence that gamma-tocotrienol inhibits the growth of human gastric cancer and chemosensitizes it to capecitabine in a xenograft mouse model through the modulation of NF-kappaB pathway, *Clin Cancer Res* **18**(8): 2220–2229 (2012).

12

Cancer Preventive and Therapeutic Properties of Fruits and Vegetables Against Commonly Occurring Cancers in Humans

*Javadi Monisha, Ganesan Padmavathi, Vaishali Bakliwal, Naman Katre, Jose Padikkala and Ajaikumar B. Kunnumakkara**

INTRODUCTION

In the previous chapters, we have discussed the chemopreventive and therapeutic effects of fruits and vegetables and their active components used against breast cancer, colon cancer, gynecologic malignancies, head and neck cancer, liver cancer, pancreatic cancer, prostate cancer, and stomach cancer. In addition to such cancers, the beneficial effects of fruits and vegetables have also been studied in other widespread disorders such as brain tumors, bladder cancer, esophageal cancer, bone cancer, leukemia, and lymphoma. However, limited scientific information is available on the effects of fruits and vegetables on these cancers. Therefore, in this chapter, we will discuss the influence of fruits and vegetables on these commonly occurring cancers about which are lesser known.

*Corresponding author: Ajaikumar B. Kunnumakkara, Ph.D., Assistant Professor, Department of Biotechnology Indian Institute of Technology Guwahati, Guwahati, Assam-781039, India. Tel: (+91) 361-258-2231, Fax: (+91) 361-258-2249, Email: kunnumakkara@iitg.ernet.in.

BONE CANCER

Bone cancer is the malignancy in bone tissues, which accounts for 0.2% of overall cancer prevalence. It was estimated that 3,010 new cases and 1,440 deaths of bone cancer would occur in the United States in 2013.[1] Bone tumors are classified based on the site of origin — examples include chondrosarcoma, osteosarcoma, and Ewing's sarcoma. Chondrosarcoma is the most frequent bone cancer with an incidence rate of 40% of all bone cancers and it affects the axial skeleton. It damages cartilage at the pelvis, thigh bone, upper arm, shoulder blade, and ribs. This cancer is common in adults who are 40 years of age and above, and the risk increases with advancing age. It is rarely found in children and adolescents. Osteosarcoma accounts for 28% of bone cancers occurring in individuals 10 to 25 years of age, affecting the knees and upper arms of males. Ewing's sarcoma is highly reported in teenagers, and is found in the pelvis, thighs, or shin bones.

The earliest symptoms of bone cancer are pain and swelling in the area of the tumor, and weakening of bones, causing unexplained bone fracture even with slight trauma; weight loss and fever are additional symptoms. There is no clear defined risk factor for bone cancers; however, people with hereditary genetic syndromes like Li–Fraumeni syndrome and hereditary retinoblastoma are at greater risk of developing these cancers. Further, people with a history of Paget's disease and exposure to radiation during the treatment of other cancers are much more susceptible to bone cancer.

Many molecular alterations have been reported in the development of bone cancer. Loss of heterozygosity (LOH) on chromosomal regions 3q26 and 18q22 has been found to lead to bone cancer.[2] Mutations in both the *p53* and *Rb* genes have been shown to be involved in osteosarcoma pathogenesis. These mutations activate PI3 kinase (PI3K) and then PKB/Akt, leading to the inhibition of proapoptotic factor Bad, thus escaping apoptosis.[3] The upregulation of HIF-1α and VEGF results in the release of many other proangiogenic factors like fibroblast growth factor (FGF), platelet-derived growth factor (PDGF), angiopoietin1 (Ang1), and ephrin-B2, which also leads to bone cancer.[3] It has been reported that activation of the MAPK pathway is responsible for the aggressive behavior of osteosarcoma.[4]

Diagnosis of bone cancer includes bone scans, X-ray, computerized tomography (CT), magnetic resonance imaging (MRI), positron emission tomography (PET), biopsies, and blood tests to ascertain the presence of enzymes such as alkaline phosphatase among others. Once the tumor is detected, it is treated by chemotherapy, radiation therapy, or surgery. Sometimes, instead of surgery, cryosurgery is preferred (using liquid nitrogen to freeze and kill cancer cells).

Anticancer Properties of Fruits and Vegetables Potentially Effective Against Bone Cancer

There is limited information available in the literature about the effect of fruits and vegetables on bone cancer. Among studies previously conducted, Zhang *et al.*[5] investigated the effect of neferine, an alkaloid ingredient in lotus seed embryos, on the proliferation of human osteosarcoma cells and neferine's mechanism of action. This compound was shown to inhibit the proliferation of human osteosarcoma cell lines by inducing cell cycle arrest at G1. This was accomplished by promoting p38 MAPK-mediated p21 stabilization.

In another study, Zhu *et al.*[6] showed that β-ionone induced cell death in human osteosarcoma cells by bringing about cell cycle arrest at the G1/S phase. In addition, this study showed that the β-ionone compound upregulated the Bax protein and downregulated the Bcl2 protein, which led to Bax translocation and cytochrome c release, and subsequently, activated caspase 3 that further resulted in apoptosis in U2OS cells.

The effect of sulforaphane, which is found in broccoli, was also examined in bone cancer cells.[7] The results showed that the treatment of cells with sulforaphane generated a concentration- and time-dependent inhibition of cell growth and the G2/M phase arrest of the cell cycle. Moreover, sulforaphane treatment resulted in a decrease in protein expression of cyclin A and B1 and their activating partners, cyclin-dependent kinases (Cdks) 1 and 2, with concomitant upregulation of p21, a Cdk inhibitor. In addition, several other studies have shown that the phytochemicals present in fruits and vegetables have great potential in the prevention and treatment of bone cancer.[7–9]

BLADDER CANCER

Bladder cancer is the sixth most common type of cancer in the world. It was estimated in 2011 that globally, approximately 386,300 new cases and 150,200 deaths will occur annually due to this disease.[10] Bladder cancer is much more prevalent in males than in females with an incidence ratio of 4:1. The reason why more men develop bladder cancer is due to the androgen receptor, which is more active in males. These tumors are mainly classified into two types: superficial and invasive. Superficial tumors occur in the innermost lining of the gallbladder, while invasive tumors reach the muscle layers of the bladder. Based on their development, these cancers are again classified as papillary (with a wart-like appearance and attached to a stalk) and non-papillary (with a flat appearance) tumors. The main risk factors for these cancers are cigarette smoking, exposure to chemicals at work or long-term bladder infections, and sometimes a result of treatments for other cancers (e.g., radiation and chemotherapy). Gallbladder cancers are very difficult to identify but, generally, symptoms include frank hematuria, abdominal pain, painful urination, fatigue, and weight loss. Frank hematuria occurs in most bladder cancer patients, and is observed when red blood cells are seen in urine.

The alterations in molecular pathways controlling cell homeostasis may result in bladder cancer.[11] Alterations in the p53 and retinoblastoma pathways are usually observed in invasive bladder cancers.[11] Mutations in *TP53* result in loss of expression of *TP21* (coding for CdkI),[12,13] and overexpression of MDM2 proteins.[14] In low-grade papillary tumors, mutations in the FGF receptor 3 gene (FGFR3) activates the Ras/MAPK pathway.[15] Other events, such as overexpression of VEGFR2, STAT3, and loss of alleles on chromosome 9, are also associated with bladder cancers.

Treatment for bladder cancer involves surgical and non-surgical methods, including chemotherapy, radiation, and biological therapy. Surgery may involve transurethral resection (TUR) with fulguration (burning the tumor with high-energy electricity), radical cystectomy (removal of the bladder and lymph nodes), segmental cystectomy (removal of a part of the bladder), and urinary diversion (making a new passage to store urine and to urinate). Even though tumors are removed surgically, sometimes chemotherapy is warranted to kill the remaining cancerous cells. Apart from these treatments, photodynamic therapy has also shown some promising effects; however, it is still in clinical trials.

Anticancer Properties of Fruits and Vegetables Potentially Effective Against Bladder Cancer

There is not a lot of information regarding the role of fruits and vegetables in reducing bladder cancer risk. However, there is some, yet scant, evidence showing that the intake of fruits and vegetables containing vitamins A, C, and E, α-carotene, β-carotene, β-cryptoxanthin, and folate may reduce the risk of bladder cancer in women.[16] Antioxidants present in fruits are known to reduce the effect of free radicals in cigarette smoke thereby reducing bladder cancer risk.[17] Additionally, the intake of cruciferous vegetables, mainly cauliflower, cabbage, cress, bok choy, and broccoli, is known to reduce this type of cancer.[18–21] These vegetables contain isothiocyanates, which are potent chemotherapeutic agents against bladder cancer because of their anti-proliferative effects. For example, broccoli is rich in isothiocyanates (sulforaphane and erucin), while cabbage and cauliflower are rich in allylisothiocyanate.[22–24] Sulforaphane and erucin downregulate survivin, as well as the epidermal growth factor receptor (EGFR), human epidermal growth factor receptor 2 (HER2/neu), and G2/M cell cycle accumulation that induces apoptosis in bladder cancer cells.[24] The anticancer properties of garlic have also been reported to be effective against bladder cancer. Garlic has the capacity to detoxify cancer-causing agents by activating the antioxidant and sulfur-binding properties of cytochrome P450 enzymes.[25] Intake of garlic increases immunity and activates macrophages, natural killer (NK) cells, and lymphokine-activated killer cells (LAK cells) that boost the production of IL-2, TNF, and IFNγ, which in turn, are responsible for antitumor activity. Garlic consumption also aids the suppression of cancer cell immunity to chemotherapy and radiotherapy.[26] S-allylmercaptocysteine (SAMC), a water-soluble component of garlic, inactivates Id-1 (inhibitor of DNA binding 1) and inhibits the survival, proliferation, migration, and invasion of bladder cancer cells.[27]

In large doses, the phytochemical resveratrol found in grapes has been shown to induce apoptosis in bladder cancer cells by deregulating mitochondrial function.[28] Similarly, silibinin has also been shown to induce caspase-dependent and -independent apoptosis acting upon the mitochondria, resulting in the release of the cytochrome complex, Omi/HtrA2, and apoptosis-inducing factor (AIF) in human bladder carcinoma cell line 5637 *in vitro*.[29] Quercetin also has been shown to bring about apoptosis by deactivating mutant p53 and survivin proteins.[30] Apigenin, a flavonoid found in many fruits and vegetables, was shown to alter the PI3K/Akt pathway and Bcl-2 family proteins, thus suppressing proliferation, invasion, and migration in the T24 bladder cancer cell line. Liu *et al.*[31] also showed that apigenin inhibited cell migration in human bladder smooth muscle (hBSM) cells by blocking the MAPK pathway. However, additional studies are required to conclusively prove their potential against bladder cancer.

BRAIN CANCER

Brain tumors are the result of the uncontrolled growth of mutated cells in brain tissues. According to an NCI (National Cancer Institute) report in 2013, 23,130 new cases and 14,080 deaths due to this cancer were documented in the United States that year. These tumors can either be benign or malignant. Gliomas (50.4%), meningiomas (20.8%), pituitary adenomas (15%), and nerve sheath tumors (18%) are the most common types of primary brain tumors. The exact causes for most brain tumors are still unknown. Brain cancers may be attributable to exposure to ionizing radiation and immune suppression, and, to some extent, genetic disorders like neurofibromatosis, tuberous sclerosis, Von Hippel–Lindau disease, and Li–Fraumeni syndrome. The risk for brain tumors increases with age; however, a few brain tumors do occur in young adults and children. The symptoms of brain tumors vary with the size, type, and location of the tumor, but some tumors, like pituitary adenomas, cause no symptoms. Patients with brain tumors may experience headaches, weakness, clumsiness, difficulty in walking, and seizures.

Genetic mutations involved in different molecular pathways, like co-alterations in tumor suppressor genes *TP53*, *p16/CDKN2A*, *p14ARF*, and *PTEN* have been frequently found in glioma cells.[32] Mutations of the *NBS1* gene, which is involved in DNA repair, have caused radio resistance to glioblastoma stem cells.[33] Mutations of the *WRN* gene have resulted in a high risk of cancer.[33] Improper activation of the Hh/Gli pathway has also resulted in brain tumorigenesis.[34]

Treatment of brain cancer depends on the size, location, type, and grade of tumor. The age and health of the patient also play a major role in deciding the treatment method. Surgery, radiation therapy, and chemotherapy are the available methods; however, chemotherapy remains a challenge because of the blood–brain barrier and the non-specificity of potentially toxic drugs. Recent advances in nanotechnology provide tumor-specific detection and treatment.

Anticancer Properties of Fruits and Vegetables Potentially Effective Against Brain Cancer

There are not many reports on the intake of fruits and vegetables in reducing the risk of brain cancer. Nevertheless, the intake of fruits and vegetables during pregnancy has been proven to protect against medulloblastoma/primitive neuroectodermal tumors (PNETs) seen among children,[35] while the intake of salted vegetables may increase the risk of brain cancers.[36] However, many reports suggest that antioxidant phytochemicals may modulate gliomas.[37] For example, resveratrol reduces tumor growth by repressing the expression of nestin, a brain cancer stem cell marker, controlling the overexpression of the *YKL-40* gene in GBM (glioblastoma multiforme) and reduces angiogenesis.[38–40] Silibinin (a phenolic compound from the plant *Silybum marianum*) inhibits cell proliferation by increasing intracellular Ca^{2+} and reactive oxygen species (ROS) generation.[41] Quercetin (a flavonoid found in fruits, vegetables, leaves, and grains) inhibits the invasion and proliferation of glioma cells by altering phospholipase D1 (PLD1) expression and also inhibits NF-κB transactivation.[42] Ellagic acid (a phenolic antioxidant) can be used with chitosan to reduce tumor growth by activating apoptosis and reducing angiogenesis.[43]

ESOPHAGEAL CANCER

The esophagus is a muscular tube that helps in the passage of food from the pharynx to the stomach. Tumors of the esophagus are termed esophageal cancer. Esophageal cancer is the seventh most common cancer among men, worldwide. The incidence rate varies at a rate of 16-fold, with a globally estimated 482,300 new esophageal cancer cases and 406,800 deaths in 2008.[10] Esophageal cancer can be classified into two types: squamous cell carcinoma and adenocarcinoma.

Squamous Cell Carcinoma of the Esophagus

This is the most common type of cancer occurring in the squamous cells, lining the esophagus. It includes the upper and middle regions of the esophagus. These types of tumors are less common in Americans.

Adenocarcinoma of the Esophagus

These cancers develop on the gland cells including those in the lower region of the esophagus near the stomach. These types of cancers are most common in Americans.

Risk factors for these cancers include consumption of alcohol, cigarette smoking, chewing tobacco, and exposure to some solvents, lye (i.e., accidentally swallowing lye), and radiation. Diets with deficiencies of iron, riboflavin, vitamin A, fish, fruits and vegetables, as well as dairy and egg products are associated with an increased risk of esophageal cancers. People with certain medical conditions, such as achalasia, gastroesophageal reflux disease (GERD), Plummer–Vinson syndrome, Barrett's esophagus, and tylosis, are at high risk of developing these cancers.

The symptoms of esophageal cancer manifest only after a tumor has developed. These symptoms include chest pain, fatigue, hoarseness or cough, pain in swallowing (dysphagia), persistent heartburn, weight loss, or bleeding. Various molecular alterations have been implicated in the development of esophageal cancer, which include alterations in epidermal growth factor receptor (EGFR), cyclin D1, telomerase, and the *Rb*, *p53*, *p16*, and *3p* genes.[44] In general, the cell cycle proceeds through the G1, S, G2, and M phases, which requires the activation of growth factors. This results in the binding of cyclins D1 to Cdks, phosphorylating the *Rb* gene. Thus, the cell cycle proceeds through G1 and S.[45] The suppression of the Cdks by the *p53* and *p16* genes[45] or overexpression of cyclin D1 results in control over G1,[45] and can lead to esophageal cancers.[46–48] Mutations in the *Rb* and *p16* genes have been shown to contribute to 20–60% of esophageal cancers, resulting in poor prognosis.[49–53]

Various treatment procedures are available such as esophagectomy (when the tumor is in esophagus), photodynamic therapy (using lasers), radiation therapy, chemotherapy, or sometimes combination of some or all, as well as surgery. Apart from these, biological therapy with the drug Trastuzumab is possible but is not often recommended.

Anticancer Properties of Fruits and Vegetables Potentially Effective Against Esophageal Cancer

Fruits have been shown to be more effective against esophageal cancer than vegetables.[54] However, cruciferous vegetables have been widely known to reduce the risk of esophageal cancer.[55] Freedman *et al.*[54] reported that intake of fruits of family Rosaceae (apples, peaches, nectarines, plums, pears, and strawberries) and Rutaceae (citrus fruits) have protective effects against esophageal cancer. Extracts of the *E. elaterium* fruit were known to induce apoptosis in esophageal cancer cell lines. It has been also reported that consumption of vitamins A, C, and E in the form of fruits and vegetables has shown an inverse relation to esophageal cancer.[56,57] Berries contain vitamins A, C, and E, folic acid, calcium, selenium, β-carotene, α-carotene, and lutein as well as polyphenols such as ellagic, ferulic, and p-coumaric acid. They also contain quercetin and several anthocyanins, as well as phytosterols such as β-sitosterol, stigmasterol, and kaempferol, all of which play an important role in chemoprevention.[58] Therefore, Stoner *et al.*[58] studied the mechanism of chemoprevention in rats fed with freeze-dried strawberries, blackberries, and black raspberries. The resulting data indicated that freeze-dried berries inhibit both initiation and post-initiation events in rat esophageal carcinogenesis, as evidenced by decreases in tumor multiplicity, reduction in adduct formation, reduced proliferative indices, inhibition of preneoplastic lesion formation, and downregulation of COX-2 and iNOS.[58] Further, in a study by Kresty *et al.*,[59] it was shown that the dietary administration of lyophilized black raspberries reduced proliferation, tumor incidence, and preneoplastic lesion formation in rodents.

Some phytochemicals derived from plants, like resveratol and ellagic acid, have been proven effective against esophageal cancers. Resveratrol was shown to induce cell cycle arrest at the G1 phase in esophageal cancer cell lines in a dose-dependent manner, resulting in apoptosis.[60] It has also been shown that resveratrol induced apoptosis in esophageal cancer cell lines by downregulating the *Bcl-2* gene and upregulating the *Bax* gene.[61]

As mentioned earlier, ellagic acid is a natural antioxidant found in blackberries, cranberries, pecans, pomegranates, raspberries, strawberries, walnuts, wolfberries, and grapes. Many studies have reported that the ellagic acid present in berries have lessened esophageal tumorigenesis in rodents given *N*-nitrosobenzylmethylamine or methylbenzylnitrosamine.[62–64] Epigallocatechin-3-gallate also suppressed the growth of esophageal squamous cell carcinoma KYSE 150 cells and epidermoid squamous cell carcinoma A431 cells by suppressing the phosphorylation of EGFR.[65] Therefore, it can be concluded that dietary intake of fruits and vegetables have great potential in the prevention of esophageal cancer.

LEUKEMIA

In a healthy human being, the bone marrow produces three types of cells: red blood cells, white blood cells, and platelets. But because of certain mutations, the bone marrow can produce increased amounts of abnormal white blood cells leading to a type of cancer, leukemia. These white blood cells do not function as normal cells; instead, they grow rapidly, uncontrolled and interfere with normal blood cells, masking their regular functions. Leukemia can spread to the lymph nodes and other parts of the body. According to the Leukemia Research Foundation, an estimated 47,150 new cases were recorded in 2012. Among these, nearly half (23,540) lost the fight against leukemia. Every day, 129 new cases of leukemia are treated, out of which 60 result in failure. There are several different kinds of leukemia and they are classified based on growth of the cells and the type of white blood cell affected. The main types of leukemia are categorized as follows.

Acute Lymphocytic Leukemia (ALL) and Chronic Lymphocytic Leukemia (CLL)

In these types of cancers, the body produces many abnormal lymphocytes (a type of white blood cells). Symptoms include weakness, fever, bleeding under the skin, weight loss, and pain in bones or stomach; or painless swelling of the lymph nodes in the neck, painless lumps in the neck, underarm, stomach, or groin, and a feeling of fullness below the ribs. ALL usually occurs in children two to five years old and in most cases, it can be successfully treated. CLL usually affects adults, mostly males, at the age of 60. Eighty-five percent of ALL patients are children. Almost 70% of T-ALL cases have a gain-of-function mutation in the *NOTCH* gene; on the other hand, B-ALL cases involve a loss-of-function in the genes *PAX5*, *E2A*, and *EBF*,[66,67] or a translocation of chromosomes 12 and 21 for the genes *TEL* and *AML1*.[66] All these aberrations affect the differentiation and maturation of the lymphoid precursors leading to ALL. Treatment for ALL is divided into four phases: induction chemotherapy, consolidation therapy, intensification therapy (to eliminate the remaining leukemia cells), and CNS prophylaxis (to stop metastasis). There are also maintenance treatments with chemotherapeutic drugs (to prevent reoccurrence). In CLL, chromosomal translocations are not observed. CLL is mainly characterized by deletions of the chromosomal regions of 13q14.3, 11q, 17p, and trisomy 12q.[66] The deletions in the regions of chromosome 13 indicate that microRNAs (miR15a and miR-16-1) could be two possible tumor suppressor genes.[68]

Acute Myeloid Leukemia (AML) and Chronic Myeloid Leukemia (CML)

Usually observed in adults, in such cancers, the body produces many abnormal myelocytes (a type of white blood cells). Men are more prone to CML as compared to women. Typically, the symptoms are fatigue, weight loss, night sweats, fever, pain, or a feeling of fullness below the ribs on the left side, weakness, bleeding under the skin, and loss of appetite. Chromosomal aberrations involving transcription factors result in AML. For instance, inversions occurring in chromosome 16 and translocation t(8;21), interfere with the two genes, *CBF1*α and *CBF1*β, which are required for normal hematopoiesis.[69] This creates a chimeric gene that encodes the fusion protein CBF1α/CBF1β, blocking the maturation of myeloid cells. Similar kinds of translocations involving chromosomes t(8;21), t(15;17), and t(9;11) affect the transcription factors. The reciprocal translocation chromosomes in 9 and 22, known as the Philadelphia chromosome (Ph) t(9;22)(q34;q11), contributes 95% to CML.[70] The result of this rearrangement is a 210-kDa fusion protein p210BCR/ABL. The autophosphorylation of p210BCR/ABL activates the RAS/MAPK, PI-3 kinase, c-CBL, CRKL pathways, JAK-STAT, and the Src pathways responsible for transformation and proliferation.[71–75]

Other types of leukemia, such as hairy cell leukemia (HCL), T cell prolymphocytic leukemia (T-PLL) (affecting mature T cells), large granular lymphocytic leukemia (affecting either T cells or NK cells), and adult T cell leukemia (caused by infection with human T lymphotropic virus, HTLV), also occur in adults.

The risk factors for leukemia are exposure to radiation (radiation therapy, bomb blasts, some X-rays), smoking, exposure to chemicals such as benzene as well as during chemotherapy, and infection with the HTLV type I virus (HTLV-I). Leukemia can also be developed as a result of some disorders like Down syndrome, myelodysplastic syndrome, certain other blood disorders, and inherited diseases.

Treatments for leukemia are mainly based on three factors: the type of leukemia, age of the patient, and whether these abnormal cells are found in the brain. Thus, the prescribed treatment may be chemotherapy, radiation therapy, biological therapy, or bone marrow transplantation.

Anticancer Properties of Fruits and Vegetables Potentially Effective Against Leukemia

Fruits and vegetables are rich sources of flavonoids such as anthocyanins and carotenoids, and also of polyphenols and phytochemicals. These help in detoxifying carcinogens, inhibiting carcinogens interacting with target sites, and may trigger tumor progression.[76] One such flavonoid, quercetin, widely found in fruits, vegetables, leaves, and grains, has been proven to enhance apoptosis in human leukemia HL-60 cells by activating caspase 8, extracellular signal-regulated kinase (ERK), and Jun N-terminal kinase (JNK) signaling pathways.[77] Quercetin also has been proven to sensitize leukemia cell lines and B cells to chemotherapeutic drugs.[78] In a similar fashion, resveratrol, found in fruits and vegetables, has also been demonstrated to sensitize AML cells to doxorubicin.[79] Additionally, *Aronia melanocarpa* juice (AMJ) has also been proven to induce apoptosis and inhibit cell proliferation in human leukemia cells by generating cell cycle arrest at the G2/M phase.[80] Furthermore, carrots, which are rich in β-carotene, polyacetylenes, antioxidants, and minerals, are also effective in inducing apoptosis in human leukemia cells.[81] Carotenoids, found in orange-colored fruits and vegetables, including, but not limited, to sweet potatoes, carrots, and tomatoes, have been reported to inhibit the proliferation of leukemia cells. Zhang *et al.*[82] showed that these carotenoids activated peroxisome proliferator-activated receptor gamma (PPARγ), which inhibited the growth of K562 leukemia cells. In addition to carotenoids, astaxanthin, capsanthin, and bixin also exhibited the same properties.

One of the main targets of cancer chemotherapy is the proteosome. Extracts of apple, grape, and onion are known to inhibit proteosome activity in human leukemia cells.[83] Studies have demonstrated that anthocyanins from *Hibiscus sabdariffa Linn.* (Malvaceae), a native plant of Africa, have also induced apoptosis in human leukemia cells by inhibiting the JNK signaling pathway.[84]

Another important phytochemical present in fruits that has been proven to inhibit proliferation and induce apoptosis in human leukemia cells is resveratrol. Resveratrol alters the JAK1/STAT pathway and significantly reduces the phosphorylation of tyrosine residues.[85] It induced apoptosis in the 232B4 human CLL cells in a dose-dependent manner, regulating caspase 3 activity and causing cells cycle arrest at G0/G1.[86] Resveratrol has also been shown to induce apoptosis in the AML HL-60 cell line by increasing intracellular levels of ceramides.[87] It also sensitizes AML cells to histone deacetylase inhibitors, through inhibiting the activity of NF-κB, thus activating the class III histone deacetylase Sirt.[88] In addition, it has also been proven to sensitize doxorubicin-resistant AML cells via downregulation of MRP1 expression.[79] Moreover, in K562/IMA-3 cell lines resistant to imatinib, resveratrol induced apoptosis by activating caspase 3.[89]

In addition to the above-mentioned compounds, many other phytochemicals present in fruits and vegetables have been shown to exhibit anti-leukemic properties. For example, diosgenin, isolated from the tubers of *Dioscorea*, has been demonstrated to inhibit K562 cell proliferation via cell cycle G2/M arrest and induce apoptosis, with disruption of Ca^{2+} homeostasis and mitochondrial dysfunction.[90] Eugenol isolated from

Eugenia caryophyllata (Myrtaceae) induced apoptosis in HL-60 cells, reducing the anti-apoptotic protein Bcl-2 level, and inducing cytochrome c release to the cytosol.[91] Similarly, capsaicin has been observed to bring about apoptosis in HL-60 cells as a result of the activation of caspase 3 and the intracellular Ca^{2+} release pathway.[92] Additionally, Ito *et al.*[93] studied the effects of capsaicin on leukemic cells *in vitro* and *in vivo*. Capsaicin suppressed the growth of leukemic cells through G0/G1 phase cell cycle arrest and induced apoptosis through an increase in production of intracellular ROS *in vitro* and in NOD/SCID mice *in vivo*. These studies suggest that fruits and vegetables and their active components have great potential in the prevention and treatment of leukemia.

LYMPHOMA

Lymphoma is a type of cancer due to the abnormal growth of B and T lymphocytes. Lymphoma can grow in any part of the body including, but not limited to, the lymph nodes, bone marrow, spleen, and blood. B cells induce humoral immunity while the T cells induce cell-mediated immunity, thus protecting against infection and disease. Any alterations in these cells and their subtypes make their behavior abnormal leading to lymphoma.

Lymphoma is broadly categorized as two types: Hodgkin's and non-Hodgkin's lymphoma. It has been estimated that 662,789 individuals in the United States are affected with lymphoma, with 159,846 people living with Hodgkin's lymphoma (active disease or in remission) and 502,943 people living with non-Hodgkin's. Lymphomas occur in high incidence in males; it ranks as the seventh type of cancer in men, and the fifth affecting children. Hodgkin's lymphoma is developed with abnormalities in the B cell lineage, with five subtypes. Non-Hodgkin's lymphoma exists either with abnormalities in the B or T cells, and 30 subtypes have been identified. Both Hodgkin's and non-Hodgkin's lymphomas are similar, but the difference lies at the microscopic level with the presence of Reed–Sternberg (RS) cells in the case of Hodgkin's lymphoma.

The exact causes of lymphoma are not yet clearly known. Risk factors include infections (HIV, Epstein–Barr virus, *Helicobacter pylori*, and hepatitis C and hepatitis B viruses), medical conditions such as autoimmune diseases, the results of immunosuppressive therapy, inherited immunodeficiency diseases, and exposure to chemicals such as benzene, pesticides, and herbicides. In some individuals, a family history of lymphoma also plays a major role in contracting the disease. In 2012, researchers from the Department of Medicine at Stanford University identified factors such as older maternal age, low birth order, and high fetal growth as contributing causes of non-Hodgkin's lymphoma.

Initial symptoms of lymphoma manifest in the swelling of the neck, underarm, and groin. In severe cases, the spleen enlarges. Non-specific symptoms include fever, chills, unexplained weight loss, night sweats, lack of energy, and itching. These non-specific symptoms are not to be confused with the symptoms of normal flu or other viral infections as these symptoms persist for longer time in lymphoma.

Hodgkin's lymphoma is subdivided into classical Hodgkin's lymphoma, involving Hodgkin's and RS (HRS) cells, and nodular lymphocyte-predominant HL (NLPHL) cells. HRS cells are B cells that have acquired immunoglobulin V gene mutations, accounting for 90% of the cells in damaged tissues. Multiple transcription factors including OCT2, BOB1, PU.1, STAT5A, and STAT5B are downregulated in HRS cells.[94–96] The negative regulators of B cells, Notch1, and NK cell factor ID2 are instead highly expressed.[97–99] The genetic lesions in these cells upregulate the NF-κB and JAK/STAT pathways[100] and deregulate the PI3K/AKT and MAPK/ERK pathways.[101,102] NLPHL cells are lymphocyte-predominant and contribute to 0.1–10% of the cells in affected tissues. Most cases of non-Hodgkin's lymphoma involve the activation of proto-oncogenes and disruption of tumor suppressor genes.[103] The translocation in the chromosomes is the key factor for the activation of proto-oncogenes. However, there are two exceptions: translocation of t(2;5) and t(11;18), resulting in genes coding for chimeric proteins.[104,105] The available treatments for lymphoma include chemotherapy, radiotherapy, antibody therapy, and, in some severe conditions, bone marrow transplantation.

Anticancer Properties of Fruits and Vegetables Potentially Effective Against Lymphomas

Fruits and vegetables are known to contain many antioxidants that help in the detoxification of carcinogens.[106] Some reports suggest that a high intake of green leafy and cruciferous vegetables reduce the risk of non-Hodgkin's lymphoma.[107,108] However, the effect of different fruits and vegetables on non-Hodgkin's lymphoma subtypes has been shown to have differing results. Citrus fruits were proven to improve the health of non-Hodgkin's lymphoma patients.[106] In a study conducted by Choi *et al.*,[109] it was reported that tomato extracts reduced the growth of lymphoma U937 cells. Similarly, trypsin inhibitors extracted from *Peltophorum dubium* seeds, as well as from soy beans, also were shown to induce apoptosis in rat lymphoma cells and also in human leukemia Jurkat cells.[110]

It has been demonstrated that resveratrol induced apoptosis in Hodgkin's lymphoma-derived L-428 cells in a dose-dependent manner. At lower concentrations, resveratrol caused cell cycle arrest in the S phase, while at higher concentrations, it induced apoptosis activating caspase 3.[111] It also induced apoptosis in diffuse large B cell lymphoma (DLBCL) by suppressing the AKT/PKB pathway.[112] Cecconi *et al.*[113] used Jeko-1 cells and showed that resveratrol induced apoptosis by altering cyclin D1 (CCND1), p53 (TP53), p21 (CDKN1A), Bcl-2, Bax, Bcl-x_L (BCL2L1), caspase 9 (CASP9), and p27 (CDKN1B). All of these reports demonstrate that resveratrol is an effective phytochemical against lymphoma.

Ellagic acid, found mostly in berries, has also been shown to decrease cell proliferation, cell viability, and ascites fluid accumulation in Dalton's lymphoma mice by the suppression of PKC signaling.[114]

MULTIPLE MYELOMA

Multiple myeloma (MM) is the uncontrolled growth of plasma cells (white blood cells) in the bone marrow, leading to bone damage. It is also known as plasma cell myeloma or Kahler's disease. It is the second most common type of hematological malignancy in the Western world.[115] According to an NCI report, 22,350 new cases and 10,710 deaths are estimated to occur in 2013 in the United States due to this disease.

There are three different forms of MM, classified based on the developmental stage. Monoclonal gammopathy of undetermined significance (MGUS) is a pre-cancerous condition where the cells do not form a tumor. Smoldering (indolent) myeloma patients have a higher amount of myeloma cells than those with MGUS. However, smoldering myeloma does not cause any damage to the body. Symptomatic (active) myeloma causes bone damage, anemia, hypercalcemia (increase of calcium levels in the blood), and kidney problems.

The exact cause for myeloma is unknown, but it is most commonly associated with older people. For unidentified reasons, MM is more prevalent in males than in females. Race and family history can also be factors. Mutations of oncogenes like *c-myc* can cause MM as well. The most common symptoms of MM are hypercalcemia, renal or kidney damage, anemia, weight loss, and bone damage.

The phosphatidylinositol 3-kinase (PI3K) and the Ras/mitogen-activated protein kinase (MAPK) cascades are the main signaling pathways involved in MM development.[116] Overexpression of the B cell transcription factor *Oct-2*, due to IgH (immunoglobulin heavy chain) gene translocations, and containment of the transcription factor PU.1 are associated with this cancer.[117,118] In MM cells, the *MUM1* (multiple myeloma oncogene 1)/*IRF4* (interferon regulatory factor 4) are activated. Some of the genes that are found to be mutated in MM cells are the FK506-binding protein 3 (FKBP3), the monokine induced by IFNγ (MIG), Fas apoptotic inhibitory molecule (Faim), and zinc finger protein 94.[119] Tumor necrosis factor-alpha (TNF-α) and macrophage inflammatory protein-1α support the survival and growth of these cancer cell.[120] Additionally, mutations in MM cells activate the NF-κB pathway.[121] Upregulation of the AKT pathway was also observed in bone marrow monocytes (BMMs) from MM patients.[122]

A complete cure for this cancer is yet to be discovered. However, possible treatments to reduce the severity of symptoms are chemotherapy, radiation therapy, stem cell transplantation, autologous stem cell transplantation (ASCT), and immunosuppression.

Anticancer Properties of Fruits and Vegetables Effective Against MM

Dietary intake of fruits and vegetables, especially the intake of cruciferous and green vegetables, has been demonstrated a reduction in the risk of MM.[123] Consumption of shallots, garlic, and soy has also been found beneficial in lowering the risk of MM.[124] Moreover, phytochemicals present in fruits and vegetables have been shown to inhibit proliferation and induce apoptosis in MM cells. Sulforaphane and phenylethylisothiocyanates of cruciferous vegetables have the potential to induce apoptosis in MM cells.[125] Apignin, a flavonoid found in fruits and vegetables, reduces the proliferation of MM cells by inhibiting the activation of the *STAT3*, *ERK*, *AKT*, and *NF-κB* genes.[126] Further, resveratrol suppresses MM growth with its antiangiogenic effect by controlling matrix metalloproteinase (MMP)-2 and MMP-9 activity.[127] Fisetin, a flavonol obtained from strawberries, induces the formation of ROS in U266 cells. Fisetin provokes apoptosis of these cells by activating caspase 3, regulating Bcl-2, Mcl-1(L), Bax, Bim, and Bad expression.[126] (−)EGCG, a polyphenol from green tea, reduces the amount of peroxiredoxin V (PrdxV) and causes apoptosis in IM9 cells.[129] Nordihydroguaiaretic acid (NDGA), an antioxidant found in *Larrea tridentata* (a medicinal herb), decreases MAPK activation and stimulates apoptosis in MM cells.[130] Honokiol from the *Magnolia* plant, causes apoptosis of MM cells in both caspase-dependent and -independent pathways.[131] Ursolic acid, present in basil, apples, prunes, and cranberries, has been found to inhibit the activation of STAT3, which in turns suppresses the expression of cyclin D1, Bcl-2, Bcl-x_L, survivin, and Mcl-1, thus resulting in the inhibition of proliferation and activation of apoptosis in MM cells.[132] Arabinoxylan rice bran (MGN-3/Biobran) and curcumin (turmeric) synergistically cause cell death in U266 cells by regulating Bax and Bcl-2 molecules.[133] These results therefore provide exciting opportunities in lowering the risk of MM through the intake of fruits and vegetables.

CONCLUSION

In this chapter, we discussed the beneficial effects of fruits and vegetables in reducing the risk of commonly occurring cancers such as of the brain, bladder, bone, and esophagus, as well as leukemia, lymphoma and MM. However, the available literature about the therapeutic effects of fruits and vegetables and their active ingredients against these cancers is still very much limited. Thus, further studies are required to serve as conclusive evidence of their potential effectiveness against these cancers.

REFERENCES

1. Siegel, R., D. Naishadham, and A. Jemal, Cancer statistics, 2013. *CA-Cancer J Clin* **63**(1): 11–30 (2013).
2. Capodanno, A.-M., Bone: Osteosarco. *Atlas Genet Cytogenet Oncol Haematol* (2002). From http://AtlasGeneticsOncology.org/Tumors/OsteosarcID5043.html.
3. Broadhead, M.L., J.C.M. Clark, D.E. Myers, C.R. Dass, and P.F.M. Choong, The molecular pathogenesis of osteosarcoma: A review, *Sarcoma* doi: dx.doi.org/10.1155/2011/959248 (2011).
4. Na, K.Y., Y.W. Kim, and Y.K. Park, Mitogen-activated protein kinase pathway in osteosarcoma, *Pathology* **44**(6): 540–546 (2012).
5. Zhang, X., Z. Liu, B. Xu, Z. Sun, Y. Gong, and C. Shao, Neferine, an alkaloid ingredient in lotus seed embryo, inhibits proliferation of human osteosarcoma cells by promoting p38 MAPK-mediated p21 stabilization, *Eur J Pharmacol* **677**(1–3): 47–54 (2012).
6. Zhu, J., L. Zhang, X. Jin, X. Han, C. Sun, and J. Yan, Beta-ionone-induced apoptosis in human osteosarcoma (U2OS) cells occurs via a p53-dependent signaling pathway, *Mol Biol Rep* **37**(6): 2653–2663 (2010).
7. Wu, S.B., J.J. Su, L.H. Sun, W.X .Wang, Y. Zhao, H. Li, S.P. Zhang, G.H. Dai, C.G. Wang, and J.F. Hu, Triterpenoids and steroids from the fruits of *Melia toosendan* and their cytotoxic effects on two human cancer cell lines, *J Nat Prod* **73**(11): 1898–1906 (2010).
8. Möller, F., O. Zierau, A. Jandausch, R. Rettenberger, M. Kaszkin-Bettag, and G. Vollmer, Subtype-specific activation of estrogen receptors by a special extract of *Rheum rhaponticum* (ERr 731), its aglycones and structurally related compounds in U2OS human osteosarcoma cells, *Phytomedicine* **14**(11): 716–726 (2007).
9. Saleem, A., M. Husheem, P. Härkönen, and K. Pihlaja, Inhibition of cancer cell growth by crude extract and the phenolics of *Terminalia chebula* retz. fruit, *J Ethnopharmacol* **81**(3): 327–336 (2002).
10. Jemal, A., F. Bray, M.M. Center, J. Ferlay, E. Ward, and D. Forman, Global cancer statistics, *CA-Cancer J Clin* **61**(2): 69–90 (2011).
11. Mitra, A.P. and R.J. Cote, Molecular pathogenesis and diagnostics of bladder cancer, *Annu Rev Pathol* **4**: 251–285 (2009).
12. Mitra, A.P., H. Lin, R.J. Cote, and R.H. Datar, Biomarker profiling for cancer diagnosis, prognosis and therapeutic management, *Natl Med J India* **18**(6): 304–312 (2005).
13. Stein, J.P., D.A. Ginsberg, G.D. Grossfeld, S.J. Chatterjee, D. Esrig, M.G. Dickinson, S. Groshen, C.R. Taylor, P.A. Jones, D.G. Skinner, and R.J. Cote, Effect

of p21WAF1/CIP1 expression on tumor progression in bladder cancer, *J Natl Cancer Inst* **90**(14): 1072–1079 (1998).

14. Simon, R., K. Struckmann, P. Schraml, U. Wagner, T. Forster, H. Moch, A. Fijan, J. Bruderer, K. Wilber, M.J. Mihatsch, T. Gasser, and G. Sauter, Amplification pattern of 12q13–q15 genes (*MDM2*, *CDK4*, *GLI*) in urinary bladder cancer, *Oncogene* **21**(16): 2476–2483 (2002).
15. Pasin, E., D.Y. Josephson, A.P. Mitra, R.J. Cote, and J.P. Stein, Superficial bladder cancer: An update on etiology, molecular development, classification, and natural history, *Rev Urol* **10**(1): 31–43 (2008).
16. Park, S.Y., N.J. Ollberding, C.G. Woolcott, L.R. Wilkens, B.E. Henderson, and L.N. Kolonel, Fruit and vegetable intakes are associated with lower risk of bladder cancer among women in the multiethnic cohort study, *J Nutr* **143**(8): 1283–1292 (2013).
17. Kellen, E., M. Zeegers, A. Paulussen, M. Van Dongen, and F. Buntinx, Fruit consumption reduces the effect of smoking on bladder cancer risk. The Belgian case control study on bladder cancer, *Int J Cancer* **118**(10): 2572–2578 (2006).
18. Michaud, D.S., D. Spiegelman, S.K. Clinton, E.B. Rimm, W.C. Willett, and E.L. Giovannucci, Fruit and vegetable intake and incidence of bladder cancer in a male prospective cohort, *J Natl Cancer Inst* **91**(7): 605–613 (1999).
19. Tang, L., G.R. Zirpoli, K. Guru, K.B. Moysich, Y. Zhang, C.B. Ambrosone, and S.E. McCann, Consumption of raw cruciferous vegetables is inversely associated with bladder cancer risk, *Cancer Epidemiol Biomarkers Prev* **17**(4): 938–944 (2008).
20. Munday, R., P. Mhawech-Fauceglia, C.M. Munday, J.D. Paonessa, L. Tang, J.S. Munday, C. Lister, P. Wilson, J.W. Fahey, W. Davis, and Y. Zhang, Inhibition of urinary bladder carcinogenesis by broccoli sprouts, *Cancer Res* **68**(5): 1593–1600 (2008).
21. Tang, L., G.R. Zirpoli, K. Guru, K.B. Moysich, Y. Zhang, C.B. Ambrosone, and S.E. McCann, Intake of cruciferous vegetables modifies bladder cancer survival, *Cancer Epidemiol Biomarkers Prev* **19**(7): 1806–1811 (2010).
22. Tang, L. and Y. Zhang, Mitochondria are the primary target in isothiocyanate-induced apoptosis in human bladder cancer cells, *Mol Cancer Ther* **4**(8): 1250–1259 (2005).
23. Tang, L. and Y. Zhang, Dietary isothiocyanates inhibit the growth of human bladder carcinoma cells, *J Nutr* **134**(8): 2004–2010 (2004).
24. Abbaoui, B., K.M. Riedl, R.A. Ralston, J.M. Thomas-Ahner, S.J. Schwartz, S.K. Clinton, and A. Mortazavi, Inhibition of bladder cancer by broccoli isothiocyanates sulforaphane and erucin: Characterization, metabolism, and interconversion, *Mol Nutr Food Res* **56**(11): 1675–1687 (2012).

25. Lamm, D.L. and D.R. Riggs, Enhanced immunocompetence by garlic: Role in bladder cancer and other malignancies, *J Nutr* **131**(3s): 1067S–1070S (2001).
26. Lamm, D. L, and D.R. Riggs, The potential application of *Allium sativum* (garlic) for the treatment of bladder cancer, *Urol Clin North Am* **27**(1): 157–162 (2000).
27. Hu, H., X.P. Zhang, Y.L. Wang, C.W. Chua, S.U. Luk, Y.C. Wong, M.T. Ling, X.F. Wang, and K.X. Xu, Identification of a novel function of Id-1 in mediating the anticancer responses of SAMC, a water-soluble garlic derivative, in human bladder cancer cells, *Mol Med Rep* **4**(1): 9–16 (2011).
28. Lin, X., G. Wu, W.Q. Huo, Y. Zhang, and F.S. Jin, Resveratrol induces apoptosis associated with mitochondrial dysfunction in bladder carcinoma cells, *Int J Urol* **19**(8): 757–764 (2012).
29. Zeng, J., Y. Sun, K. Wu, L. Li, G. Zhang, Z. Yang, Z. Wang, D. Zhang, Y. Xue, Y. Chen, G. Zhu, X. Wang, and D. He, Chemopreventive and chemotherapeutic effects of intravesical silibinin against bladder cancer by acting on mitochondria, *Mol Cancer Ther* **10**(1): 104–116 (2011).
30. Ma, L., J.M. Feugang, P. Konarski, J. Wang, J. Lu, S. Fu, B. Ma, B. Tian, C. Zou, and Z. Wang, Growth inhibitory effects of quercetin on bladder cancer cell, *Front Biosci* **11**: 2275–2285 (2006).
31. Liu, Q., X Chen, G Yang, X Min, and M. Deng, Apigenin inhibits cell migration through MAPK pathways in human bladder smooth muscle cells, *Biocell* **35**(3): 71–79 (2011).
32. Ishii, N., D. Maier, A. Merlo, M. Tada, Y. Sawamura, A.C. Diserens, and E.G. Van Meir, Frequent co-alterations of *TP53*, *p16/CDKN2A*, *p14ARF*, *PTEN* tumor suppressor genes in human glioma cell lines, *Brain Pathol* **9**(3): 469–479 (1999).
33. Cheng, L., Q. Wu, Z. Huang, O.A. Guryanova, Q. Huang, W. Shou, J.N. Rich, and S. Bao, L1CAM regulates DNA damage checkpoint response of glioblastoma stem cells through NBS1, *EMBO J* **30**(5): 800–813 (2011).
34. Ruiz i Altaba, A., B. Stecca, and P. Sánchez, Hedgehog–Gli signaling in brain tumors: Stem cells and paradevelopmental programs in cancer, *Cancer Lett* **204**(2): 145–157 (2004).
35. Bunin, G.R., L.H. Kushi, P.R. Gallagher, L.B. Rorke-Adams, M.L. McBride, and A. Cnaan, Maternal diet during pregnancy and its association with medulloblastoma in children: A children's oncology group study (United States), *Cancer Causes Control* **16**(7): 877–891 (2005).
36. Hu, J., C. La Vecchia, E. Negri, L. Chatenoud, C. Bosetti, X. Jia, R. Liu, G. Huang, D. Bi, and C. Wang, Diet and brain cancer in adults: A case-control study in northeast China, *Int J Cancer* **81**(1): 20–23 (1999).

37. Pouliquen, D., C. Olivier, E. Hervouet, F. Pedelaborde, E. Debien, M.T. Le Cabellec, C. Gratas, T. Homma, K. Meflah, F.M. Vallette, and J. Menanteau, Dietary prevention of malignant glioma aggressiveness, implications in oxidant stress and apoptosis, *Int J Cancer* **123**(2): 288–295 (2008).
38. Castino, R., A. Pucer, R. Veneroni, F. Morani, C. Peracchio, T.T. Lah, and C. Isidoro, Resveratrol reduces the invasive growth and promotes the acquisition of a long-lasting differentiated phenotype in human glioblastoma cells, *J Agric Food Chem* **59**(8): 4264–4272 (2011).
39. Zhang, W., K. Murao, X. Zhang, K. Matsumoto, S. Diah, M. Okada, K. Miyake, N. Kawai, Z. Fei, and T. Tamiya, Resveratrol represses YKL-40 expression in human glioma U87 cells, *BMC Cancer* **10**: 593 (2010).
40. Chen, J.C., Y. Chen, J.H. Lin, J.M. Wu, and S.H. Tseng, Resveratrol suppresses angiogenesis in gliomas: Evaluation by color Doppler ultrasound, *Anticancer Res* **26**(2A): 1237–1245 (2006).
41. Kim, K.W., C.H. Choi, T.H. Kim, C.H. Kwon, J.S. Woo, and Y.K. Kim, Silibinin inhibits glioma cell proliferation via Ca^{2+}/ROS/MAPK-dependent mechanism *in vitro* and glioma tumor growth *in vivo*, *Neurochem Res* **34**(8): 1479–1490 (2009).
42. Park, M.H. and S. Min Do, Quercetin-induced downregulation of phospholipase D1 inhibits proliferation and invasion in U87 glioma cells, *Biochem Biophys Res Commun* **412**(4): 710–715 (2011).
43. Kim, S., M.W. Gaber, J.A. Zawaski, F. Zhang, M. Richardson, X.A. Zhang, and Y. Yang, The inhibition of glioma growth *in vitro* and *in vivo* by a chitosan/ellagic acid composite biomaterial, *Biomaterials* **30**(27): 4743–4751 (2009).
44. Alidina, A., T. Siddiqui, I. Burney, W. Jafri, F. Hussain, M. Ahmed, Esophageal cancer — a review, *J Pak Med Assoc* **54**(3): 136–141 (2004).
45. Cohen, E.W. and C.M. Rudin, Molecular biology of esophageal cancer, Posner, M.C., E.E. Vokes, and R.R. Weichselbaum (Eds.), in *Cancer of the Upper Gastrointestinal Tract*, London: BC Decker (2002).
46. Itakura, Y., H. Sasano, C. Shiga, Y. Furukawa, K. Shiga, S. Mori, and H. Nagura, Epidermal growth factor receptor overexpression in esophageal carcinoma. An immunohistochemical study correlated with clinicopathologic findings and DNA amplification, *Cancer* **74**(3): 795–804 (1994).
47. Kitagawa, Y., M. Ueda, N. Ando, S. Ozawa, N. Shimizu, and M. Kitajima, Further evidence for prognostic significance of epidermal growth factor receptor gene amplification in patients with esophageal squamous cell carcinoma, *Clin Cancer Res* **2**(5): 909–914 (1996).
48. Shimada, Y., M. Imamura, G. Watanabe, S. Uchida, H. Harada, T. Makino, and M. Kano, Prognostic factors of oesophageal squamous cell carcinoma from the perspective of molecular biology, *Br J Cancer* **80**(8): 1281–1288 (1999).

49. Adelaide, J., G. Monges, C. Derderian, J.F. Seitz, and D. Birnbaum, Oesophageal cancer and amplification of the human cyclin D gene *CCND1/PRAD1*, *Br J Cancer* **71**(1): 64–68 (1995).
50. Takeuchi, H., S. Ozawa, N. Ando, C.H. Shih, K. Koyanagi, M. Ueda, and M. Kitajima, Altered *p16/MTSI/CDKN2* and *cyclin D1/PRAD-1* gene expression is associated with the prognosis of squamous cell carcinoma of the esophagus, *Clin Cancer Res* **3**(12 Pt. 1): 2229–2236 (1997).
51. Xing, E.P., G.Y. Yang, L.D. Wang, S.T. Shi, and C.S. Yang, Loss of heterozygosity of *Rb* gene correlates with PRb protein expression and associates with p53 alteration in human esophageal cancer, *Clin Cancer Res* **5**(5): 1231–1240 (1999).
52. Hashimoto, N., M. Tachibana, D.K. Dhar, H. Yoshimura, and N. Nagasue, Expression of p53 and RB proteins in squamous cell carcinoma of the esophagus: Their relationship with clinicopathologic characteristics, *Ann Surg Oncol* **6**(5): 489–494 (1999).
53. Grana, X. and E.P. Reddy, Cell cycle control in mammalian cells: Role of cyclins, cyclin dependent kinases (CDKs), growth suppressor genes and cyclin-dependent kinase inhibitors (CKIs), *Oncogene* **11**(2): 211–219 (1995).
54. Freedman, N.D., Y. Park, A.F. Subar, A.R. Hollenbeck, M.F. Leitzmann, A. Schatzkin, and C.C. Abnet, Fruit and vegetable intake and esophageal cancer in a large prospective cohort study, *Int J Cancer* **121**(12): 2753–2760 (2007).
55. Yamaji, T., M. Inoue, S. Sasazuki, M. Iwasaki, N. Kurahashi, T. Shimazu, S. Tsugane; and Japan Public Health Center-based Prospective Study Group, Fruit and vegetable consumption and squamous cell carcinoma of the esophagus in Japan: The JPHC study, *Int J Cancer* **123**(8): 1935–1940 (2008).
56. Lukić, M., A. Šegec, I. Šegec, L. Pinotić, K. Pinotić, B. Atalić, K. Šolić, and A. Včev, The impact of the vitamins A, C and E in the prevention of gastroesophageal reflux disease, Barrett's oesophagus and oesophageal adenocarcinoma, *Coll Antropol* **36**(3): 867–872 (2012).
57. Tzonou, A., L. Lipworth, A. Garidou, L.B. Signorello, P. Lagiou, C. Hsieh, and D. Trichopoulos, Diet and risk of esophageal cancer by histologic type in a low-risk population, *Int J Cancer* **68**(3): 300–304 (1996).
58. Stoner, G.D., T. Chen, L.A. Kresty, R.M. Aziz, T. Reinemann, and R. Nines, Protection against esophageal cancer in rodents with lyophilized berries: Potential mechanisms, *Nutr Cancer* **54**(1): 33–46 (2006).
59. Kresty, L.A., M.A. Morse, C. Morgan, P.S. Carlton, J. Lu, A. Gupta, M. Blackwood, and G.D. Stoner, Chemoprevention of esophageal tumorigenesis by dietary administration of lyophilized black raspberries, *Cancer Res* **61**(16): 6112–6119 (2001).

60. Tang, Q., G. Li, X. Wei, J. Zhang, J.F. Chiu, D. Hasenmayer, D. Zhang, and H. Zhang, Resveratrol-induced apoptosis is enhanced by inhibition of autophagy in esophageal squamous cell carcinoma, *Cancer Lett* **336**(2): 325–337 (2013).
61. Zhou, H.B., Y. Yan, Y.N. Sun, and J.R. Zhu, Resveratrol induces apoptosis in human esophageal carcinoma cells, *World J Gastroenterol* **9**(3): 408–411 (2003).
62. Barch, D.H. and C.C. Fox, Dietary ellagic acid reduces the esophageal microsomal metabolism of methylbenzylnitrosamine, *Cancer Lett* **44**(1): 39–44 (1989).
63. Mandal, S. and G.D. Stoner, Inhibition of *N*-nitrosobenzylmethylamine-induced esophageal tumorigenesis in rats by ellagic acid, *Carcinogenesis* **11**(1): 55–61 (1990).
64. Barch, D.H. and C.C. Fox, Selective inhibition of methylbenzylnitrosamine-induced formation of esophageal O6-methylguanine by dietary ellagic acid in rats, *Cancer Res* **48**(24 Pt. 1): 7088–7092 (1988).
65. Hou, Z., S. Sang, H. You, M.J. Lee, J. Hong, K.V. Chin, and C.S. Yang, Mechanism of action of (−)-epigallocatechin-3-gallate: Auto-oxidation-dependent inactivation of epidermal growth factor receptor and direct effects on growth inhibition in human esophageal cancer KYSE 150 cells, *Cancer Res* **65**(17): 8049–8056 (2005).
66. Kumar, V., A.K. Abbas, N. Fausto, and J. Aster, *Robbins & Cotran Pathologic Basis of Disease* (8th Edn.), Elsevier (2010).
67. Mullighan, C.G., S. Goorha, I. Radtke, C.B. Miller, E. Coustan-Smith, J.D. Dalton, K. Girtman, S. Mathew, J. Ma, S.B. Pounds, X. Su, C.H. Pui, M.V. Relling, W.E. Evans, S.A. Shurtleff, and J.R. Downing, Genome-wide analysis of genetic alterations in acute lymphoblastic leukemia, *Nature* **446**(7137): 758–764 (2007).
68. Calin, G.A. and C.M. Croce, Genomics of chronic lymphocytic leukemia microRNAs a new player with clinical significance, *Semin Oncol* **33**(2): 167–173 (2006).
69. De Bruijn, M.F. and N.A. Speck, Core-binding factors in hematopoiesis and immune function, *Oncogene* **23**(24): 4238–4248 (2004).
70. Nowell, P. and D. Hungerford, A minute chromosome in human chronic granulocytic leukemia, *Science* **132**: 1497 (1960).
71. Raitano, A.B., J.R. Halpern, T.M. Hambuch, and C.L. Sawyers, The *Bcr-Abl* leukemia oncogene activates Jun kinase and requires Jun for transformation, *Proc Natl Acad Sci USA* **92**(25): 11746–11750 (1995).
72. Sawyers, C.L., J. McLaughlin, and O.N. Witte, Genetic requirement for Ras in the transformation of fibroblasts and hematopoietic cells by the *Bcr-Abl* oncogene, *J Exp Med* **181**(1): 303–313 (1995).

73. Skorski. T, P. Kanakaraj, M. Nieborowska-Skorska, M.Z. Ratajczak, S.C. Wen, G. Zon, A.M. Gewirtz, B. Perussia, and B. Calabretta, Phosphatidylinositol-3 kinase activity is regulated by BCR/ABL and is required for the growth of Philadelphia chromosome-positive cells, *Blood* **86**(2): 726–736 (1995).
74. Skorski, T., A. Bellacosa, M. Nieborowska-Skorska, R. Martinez, J.K. Choi, R. Trotta, P. Wlodarski, D. Perrotti, T. O. Chan, M.A. Wasik, P.N. Tsichlis, and B. Calabretta, Transformation of hematopoietic cells by BCR/ABL requires activation of a P1-3k/Akt-dependent pathway, *EMBO J* **16**(20): 6151–6161 (1997a).
75. Salesse, S. and C.M. Verfaillie, BCR/ABL: From molecular mechanisms of leukemia induction to treatment of chronic myelogenous leukemia, *Oncogene* **21**(56): 8547–8559 (2002).
76. Tatman, D. and H. Mo, Volatile isoprenoid constituents of fruits, vegetables and herbs cumulatively suppress the proliferation of murine B16 melanoma and human HL-60 leukemia cells, *Cancer Lett* **175**(2): 129–139 (2002).
77. Lee, W.J., Y.R. Chen, and T.H. Tseng, Quercetin induces FasL-related apoptosis, in part, through promotion of histone H3 acetylation in human leukemia HL-60 cells, *Oncol Rep* **25**(2): 583–591 (2011).
78. Spagnuolo, C., M. Russo, S. Bilotto, I. Tedesco, B. Laratta, and G.L. Russo, Dietary polyphenols in cancer prevention: The example of the flavonoid quercetin in leukemia, *Ann NY Acad Sci* **1259**: 95–103 (2012).
79. Kweon, S.H., J.H. Song, and T.S. Kim, Resveratrol-mediated reversal of doxorubicin resistance in acute myeloid leukemia cells via downregulation of MRP1 expression, *Biochem Biophys Res Commun* **395**(1): 104–110 (2010).
80. Sharif, T., M. Alhosin, C. Auger, C. Minker, J.H. Kim, N. Etienne-Selloum, P. Bories, H. Gronemeyer, A. Lobstein, C. Bronner, G. Fuhrmann, and V.B. Schini-Kerth, *Aronia melanocarpa* juice induces a redox-sensitive p73-related caspase 3-dependent apoptosis in human leukemia cells, *PLoS One* **7**(3): e32526 (2012).
81. Zaini, R., M.R. Clench, and C.L. Le Maitre, Bioactive chemicals from carrot (*Daucus carota*) juice extracts for the treatment of leukemia, *J Med Food* **14**(11): 1303–1312 (2011).
82. Zhang, X., W.E. Zhao, L. Hu, L. Zhao, and J. Huang, Carotenoids inhibit proliferation and regulate expression of peroxisome proliferators-activated receptor gamma (PPARγ) in K562 cancer cells, *Arch Biochem Biophys* **512**(1): 96–106 (2011).
83. Chen, D., K.G. Daniel, M.S. Chen, D.J. Kuhn, K.R. Landis-Piwowar, and Q.P. Dou, Dietary flavonoids as proteasome inhibitors and apoptosis inducers in human leukemia cells, *Biochem Pharmacol* **69**(10): 1421–1432 (2005).

84. Hou, D.X., T. Ose, S. Lin, K. Harazoro, I. Imamura, M. Kubo, T. Uto, N. Terahara, M. Yoshimoto, and M. Fujii, Anthocyanidins induce apoptosis in human promyelocytic leukemia cells: Structure–activity relationship and mechanisms involved, *Int J Oncol* **23**(3): 705–712 (2003).
85. Li, T., W. Wang, and T. Li, Regulatory effect of resveratrol on JAK1/STAT3 signal transduction pathway in leukemia, *Zhongguo Shi Yan Xue Ye Xue Za Zhi* **16**(4): 772–776 (2008).
86. Gokbulut, A.A., E. Apohan, and Y. Baran, Resveratrol and quercetin-induced apoptosis of human 232B4 chronic lymphocytic leukemia cells by activation of caspase-3 and cell cycle arrest, *Hematology* **18**(3): 144–150 (2013).
87. Cakir, Z., G. Saydam, F. Sahin, and Y. Baran, The roles of bioactive sphingolipids in resveratrol-induced apoptosis in HL60: Acute myeloid leukemia cells, *J Cancer Res Clin Oncol* **137**(2): 279–286 (2011).
88. Yaseen, A., S. Chen, S. Hock, R. Rosato, P. Dent, Y. Dai, and S. Grant, Resveratrol sensitizes acute myelogenous leukemia cells to histone deacetylase inhibitors through reactive oxygen species-mediated activation of the extrinsic apoptotic pathway, *Mol Pharmacol* **82**(6): 1030–1041 (2012).
89. Can, G., Z. Cakir, M. Kartal, U. Gunduz, and Y. Baran, Apoptotic effects of resveratrol, a grape polyphenol, on imatinib-sensitive and resistant K562 chronic myeloid leukemia cells, *Anticancer Res* **32**(7): 2673–2678 (2012).
90. Liu, M.J., Z. Wang, Y. Ju, R.N. Wong, and Q.Y. Wu, Diosgenin induces cell cycle arrest and apoptosis in human leukemia K562 cells with the disruption of Ca^{2+} homeostasis, *Cancer Chemother Pharmacol* **55**(1): 79–90 (2005).
91. Yoo, C.B., K.T. Han, K.S. Cho, J. Ha, H.J. Park, J.H. Nam, U.H. Kil, and K.T. Lee, Eugenol isolated from the essential oil of *Eugenia caryophyllata* induces a reactive oxygen species-mediated apoptosis in HL-60 human promyelocytic leukemia cells, *Cancer Lett* **225**(1): 41–52 (2005).
92. Tsou, M.F., H.F. Lu, S.C. Chen, L.T. Wu, Y.S. Chen, H.M. Kuo, S.S. Lin, and J.G. Chung, Involvement of Bax, Bcl-2, Ca^{2+} and caspase-3 in capsaicin-induced apoptosis of human leukemia HL-60 cells, *Anticancer Res* **26**(3A): 1965–1971 (2006).
93. Ito, K., T. Nakazato, K. Yamato, Y. Miyakawa, T. Yamada, N. Hozumi, K. Segawa, Y. Ikeda, and M. Kizaki, Induction of apoptosis in leukemic cells by homovanillic acid derivative, capsaicin, through oxidative stress: Implication of phosphorylation of p53 at Ser-15 residue by reactive oxygen species, *Cancer Res* **64**(3): 1071–1078 (2004).
94. Stein, H., T. Marafioti, H.D. Foss, H. Laumen, M. Hummel, I. Anagnostopoulos, T. Wirth, G. Demel, and B. Falini, Down-regulation of BOB.1/OBF.1 and Oct2 in classical Hodgkin disease but not in lymphocyte predominant

Hodgkin disease correlates with immunoglobulin transcription, *Blood* **97**(2): 496–501 (2001).

95. Torlakovic, E., A. Tierens, H.D. Dang, and J. Delabie, The transcription factor PU.1, necessary for B-cell development is expressed in lymphocyte predominance, but not classical Hodgkin's disease, *Am J Pathol* **159**(5): 1807–1814 (2001).
96. Scheeren, F.A., S.A. Diehl, L.A. Smit, T. Beaumont, M. Naspetti, R.J. Bende, B. Blom, K. Karube, K. Ohshima, C.J. van Noesel, and H. Spits, IL-21 is expressed in Hodgkin lymphoma and activates STAT5; evidence that activated STAT5 is required for Hodgkin lymphomagenesis, *Blood* **111**(9): 4706–4715 (2008).
97. Jundt, F., O. Acikgöz, S.H. Kwon, R. Schwarzer, I. Anagnostopoulos, B. Wiesner, S. Mathas, M. Hummel, H. Stein, H.M. Reichardt, and B. Dörken, Aberrant expression of Notch1 interferes with the B-lymphoid phenotype of neoplastic B cells in classical Hodgkin lymphoma, *Leukemia* **22**(8): 1587–1594 (2008).
98. Mathas, S., M. Janz, F. Hummel, M. Hummel, B. Wollert-Wulf, S. Lusatis, I. Anagnostopoulos, A. Lietz, M. Sigvardsson, F. Jundt, K. Jöhrens, K. Bommert, H. Stein, and B. Dörken, Intrinsic inhibition of transcription factor E2A by HLH proteins ABF-1 and Id2 mediates reprogramming of neoplastic B cells in Hodgkin lymphoma, *Nat Immunol* **7**(2): 207–215 (2006).
99. Renné, C., J.I. Martin-Subero, M. Eickernjäger, M.L. Hansmann, R. Küppers, R. Siebert, and A. Bräuninger, Aberrant expression of ID2, a suppressor of B-cell-specific gene expression, in Hodgkin's lymphoma, *Am J Pathol* **169**(2): 655–664 (2006).
100. Schmitz, R., J. Stanelle, M.L. Hansmann, and R. Küppers, Pathogenesis of classical and lymphocyte-predominant Hodgkin lymphoma, *Annu Rev Pathol* **4**: 151–174 (2009).
101. Zheng, B., P. Fiumara, Y.V. Li, G. Georgakis, V. Snell, M. Younes, J.N. Vauthey, A. Carbone, and A. Younes, MEK/ERK pathway is aberrantly active in Hodgkin disease: A signaling pathway shared by CD30, CD40, and RANK that regulates cell proliferation and survival, *Blood* **102**(3): 1019–1027 (2003).
102. Renné, C., K. Willenbrock, R. Küppers, M.L. Hansmann, and A. Bräuninger, Autocrine and paracrine activated receptor tyrosine kinases in classical Hodgkin lymphoma, *Blood* **105**(10): 4051–4059 (2005).
103. Dalla-Favera, R. and G. Gaidano, Molecular biology of lymphomas, DeVita, V.T. Jr, S. Hellman, and S.A. Rosenberg (Eds.), in *Cancer: Principles and Practice of Oncology*, Philadelphia: Lippincott Williams, and Wilkins (2001), pp. 2215–2235.
104. Morris, S.W., M.N. Kirstein, M.B. Valentine, K.G. Dittmer, D.N. Shapiro, D.L. Saltman, and AT. Look, Fusion of a kinase gene, ALK, to a nucleolar protein gene, NPM, in NHL, *Science* **267**(5196): 316–317 (1995).

105. Dierlamm, J., M. Baens, I. Wlodarska, M. Stefanova-Ouzounova, J.M. Hernandez, D.K. Hossfeld, C. De Wolf-Peeters, A. Hagemeijer, H. Van den Berghe, and P. Marynen, The apoptosis inhibitor gene *AP12* and a novel 18q gene, *MLT*, are recurrently rearranged in the t(11;18)(q21;21) associated with MALT lymphomas, *Blood* **93**(11): 3601–3609 (1999).
106. Han, X., T. Zheng, F. Foss, T.R. Holford, S. Ma, P. Zhao, M. Dai, C. Kim, Y. Zhang, Y. Bai, and Y. Zhang, Vegetable and fruit intake and non-Hodgkin lymphoma survival in Connecticut women, *Leuk Lymphoma* **51**(6): 1047–1054 (2010).
107. Chiu, B.C., S. Kwon, A.M. Evens, T. Surawicz, S.M. Smith, and D.D. Weisenburger, Dietary intake of fruit and vegetables and risk of non-Hodgkin lymphoma, *Cancer Causes Control* **22**(8): 1183–1195 (2011).
108. Zhang, S.M., D.J. Hunter, B.A. Rosner, E.L. Giovannucci, G.A. Colditz, F.E. Speizer, and W.C. Willett, Intakes of fruits, vegetables, and related nutrients and the risk of non-Hodgkin's lymphoma among women. *Cancer Epidemiol Biomarkers Prev* **9**(5): 477–485 (2000).
109. Choi, S.H., H.R. Kim, H.J. Kim, I.S. Lee, N. Kozukue, C.E. Levin, and M. Friedman, Free amino acid and phenolic contents and antioxidative and cancer cell-inhibiting activities of extracts of 11 greenhouse-grown tomato varieties and 13 tomato-based foods, *J Agric Food Chem* **59**(24): 12801–12814 (2011).
110. Troncoso, M.F., V.A. Biron, S.A. Longhi, L.A. Retegui, and C. Wolfenstein-Todel, *Peltophorum dubium* and soybean Kunitz-type trypsin inhibitors induce human Jurkat cell apoptosis, *Int Immunopharmacol* **7**(5): 625–636 (2007).
111. Frazzi, R., R. Valli, I. Tamagnini, B. Casali, N. Latruffe, and F. Merli, Resveratrol-mediated apoptosis of Hodgkin lymphoma cells involves SIRT1 inhibition and FOXO3a hyperacetylation, *Int J Cancer* **132**(5): 1013–1021 (2013).
112. Hussain, A.R., S. Uddin, R. Bu, O.S. Khan, S.O. Ahmed, M. Ahmed, and K.S. Al-Kuraya, Resveratrol suppresses constitutive activation of AKT via generation of ROS and induces apoptosis in diffuse large B cell lymphoma cell lines, *PLoS One* **6**(9): e24703 (2011).
113. Cecconi, D., A. Zamò, A. Parisi, E. Bianchi, C. Parolini, A.M. Timperio, L. Zolla, and M. Chilosi, Induction of apoptosis in Jeko-1 mantle cell lymphoma cell line by resveratrol: A proteomic analysis, *J Proteome Res* **7**(7): 2670–2680 (2008).
114. Mishra, S. and M. Vinayak, Ellagic acid checks lymphoma promotion via regulation of PKC signaling pathway, *Mol Biol Rep* **40**(2): 1417–1428 (2013).
115. Collins, C.D., Problems monitoring response in multiple myeloma, *Cancer Imaging* **5**(Spec. No. A): S119–S126 (2005).

116. Misso, G., S. Zappavigna, M. Castellano, G. De Rosa, M.T. Di Martino, P. Tagliaferri, P. Tassone, and M. Caraglia, Emerging pathways as individualized therapeutic target of multiple myeloma, *Expert Opin Biol Ther* (Suppl. 1): S95–S109 (2013).
117. Toman, I., J. Loree, A.C. Klimowicz, N. Bahlis, R. Lai, A. Belch, L. Pilarski, and T. Reiman, Expression and prognostic significance of Oct2 and Bob1 in multiple myeloma: Implications for targeted therapeutics, *Leuk Lymphoma* **52**(4): 659–667 (2011).
118. Tatetsu, H., S. Ueno, H. Hata, Y. Yamada, M. Takeya, H. Mitsuya, D.G. Tenen, and Y. Okuno, Down-regulation of PU.1 by methylation of distal regulatory elements and the promoter is required for myeloma cell growth, *Cancer Res* **67**(11): 5328–5336 (2007).
119. Uranishi, M., S. Iida, T. Sanda, T. Ishida, E. Tajima, M. Ito, H. Komatsu, H. Inagaki, and R. Ueda, Multiple myeloma oncogene 1 (*MUM1*)/interferon regulatory factor 4 (*IRF4*) upregulates monokine induced by interferon-gamma (MIG) gene expression in B-cell malignancy, *Leukemia* **19**(8): 1471–1478 (2005).
120. Tsubaki, M., M. Komai, T. Itoh, M. Imano, K. Sakamoto, H. Shimaoka, N. Ogawa, K .Mashimo, D. Fujiwara, T. Takeda, J. Mukai, K. Sakaguchi, T. Satou, and S. Nishida, Inhibition of the tumour necrosis factor-alpha autocrine loop enhances the sensitivity of multiple myeloma cells to anticancer drugs, *Eur J Cancer* **49**(17): 3708–3717 (2013).
121. Fuchs, O., Targeting of NF-kappaB signaling pathway, other signaling pathways and epigenetics in therapy of multiple myeloma, *Cardiovasc Hematol Disord Drug Targets* **13**(1): 16–34 (2013).
122. Cao, H., K. Zhu, L. Qiu, S. Li, H. Niu, M. Hao, S. Yang, Z. Zhao, Y. Lai, J.L. Anderson, J. Fan, H.J. Im, D. Chen, G.D. Roodman, and G. Xiao, Critical role of AKT in myeloma-induced osteoclast formation and osteolysis, *J Biol Chem* **288**(42): 30399–30410 (2013).
123. Hosgood, H.D., D. Baris, S.H. Zahm, T. Zheng, and A.J. Cross, Diet and risk of multiple myeloma in Connecticut women, *Cancer Causes Control* **18**(10): 1065–1076 (2007).
124. Wang, Q., Y. Wang, Z. Ji, X. Chen, Y. Pan, G. Gao, H. Gu, Y. Yang, B.C. Choi, and Y.Yan, Risk factors for multiple myeloma: A hospital-based case-control study in northwest China. *Cancer Epidemiol* **36**(5): 439–444 (2012).
125. Jakubikova, J., D. Cervi, M. Ooi, K. Kim, S. Nahar, S. Klippel, D. Cholujova, M. Leiba, J.F. Daley, J. Delmore, J. Negri, S. Blotta, D.W. McMillin, T. Hideshima, P.G. Richardson, J. Sedlak, K.C. Anderson, and C.S. Mitsiades, Anti-tumor activity and signaling events triggered by the isothiocyanates,

sulforaphane and phenethyl isothiocyanate, in multiple myeloma, *Haematologica* **96**(8): 1170–1179 (2011).
126. Zhao, M., J. Ma, H.Y. Zhu, X.H. Zhang, Z.Y. Du, Y.J. Xu, and X.D. Yu, Apigenin inhibits proliferation and induces apoptosis in human multiple myeloma cells through targeting the trinity of CK2, Cdc37 and Hsp90, *Mol Cancer* **10**: 104 (2011).
127. Hu, Y., C.Y. Sun, J. Huang, L. Hong, L. Zhang, and Z.B. Chu, Antimyeloma effects of resveratrol through inhibition of angiogenesis, *Chin Med J (Engl)* **120**(19): 1672–1677 (2007).
128. Jang, K.Y., S.J. Jeong, S.H. Kim, J.H. Jung, J.H. Kim, W. Koh, C.Y. Chen, and S.H. Kim Activation of reactive oxygen species/AMP activated protein kinase signaling mediates fisetin-induced apoptosis in multiple myeloma U266 cells, *Cancer Lett* **319**(2): 197–202 (2012).
129. Ren, L., H.Y. Yang, H.I. Choi, K.J. Chung, U. Yang, I.K. Lee, H.J. Kim, D.S. Lee, B.J. Park, and T.H. Lee, The role of peroxiredoxin V in (−)-epigallocatechin 3-gallate-induced multiple myeloma cell death, *Oncol Res* **19**(8–9): 391–398 (2011).
130. Meyer, A.N., C.W. McAndrew, and D.J. Donoghue, Nordihydroguaiaretic acid inhibits an activated fibroblast growth factor receptor 3 mutant and blocks downstream signaling in multiple myeloma cells, *Cancer Res* **68**(18): 7362–7370 (2008).
131. Ishitsuka, K., T. Hideshima, M. Hamasaki, N. Raje, S. Kumar, H. Hideshima, N. Shiraishi, H. Yasui, A.M. Roccaro, P. Richardson, K. Podar, S. Le Gouill, D. Chauhan, K. Tamura, J. Arbiser, and K.C. Anderson, Honokiol overcomes conventional drug resistance in human multiple myeloma by induction of caspase-dependent and -independent apoptosis, *Blood* **106**(5): 1794–1800 (2005).
132. Pathak, A.K., M. Bhutani, A.S. Nair, K.S. Ahn, A. Chakraborty, H. Kadara, S. Guha, G. Sethi, and B.B. Aggarwal, Ursolic acid inhibits STAT3 activation pathway leading to suppression of proliferation and chemosensitization of human multiple myeloma cells, *Mol Cancer Res* **5**(9): 943–955 (2007).
133. Ghoneum, M. and S. Gollapudi, Synergistic apoptotic effect of arabinoxylan rice bran (MGN-3/Biobran) and curcumin (turmeric) on human multiple myeloma cell line U266 *in vitro*, *Neoplasma* **58**(2): 118–123 (2011).

Index